CANCER ETIOLOGY, DIAGNOSIS AND TREATMENTS

AN INTRODUCTION TO CANCER THERAPY

Cancer Etiology, Diagnosis and Treatments

Additional books and e-books in this series can be found on Nova's website under the Series tab.

CANCER ETIOLOGY, DIAGNOSIS AND TREATMENTS

AN INTRODUCTION TO CANCER THERAPY

NEVILLE CHARRON

EDITOR

nova
Medicine & Health
New York

NOTICE TO THE READER

Library of Congress Cataloging-in-Publication Data

Names: Charron, Neville, author.
Title: An introduction to cancer therapy / Neville Charron.
Description: New York : Nova Science Publishers, [2020] | Series: Cancer etiology, diagnosis and treatments | Includes bibliographical references and index.
Identifiers: LCCN 2020038879 (print) | LCCN 2020038880 (ebook) | ISBN 9781536184501 (hardcover) | ISBN 9781536185874 (adobe pdf)
Subjects: LCSH: Cancer--Treatment. | Cancer--Immunotherapy.
Classification: LCC RC270.8 .C44 2020 (print) | LCC RC270.8 (ebook) | DDC 616.99/406--dc23
LC record available at https://lccn.loc.gov/2020038879
LC ebook record available at https://lccn.loc.gov/2020038880

Published by Nova Science Publishers, Inc. † New York

CONTENTS

PREFACE

This compilation attempts to provide readers with brief and concise information on different types of cancer, their origins, and available treatment options. Protein kinase inhibitors, currently in clinical practice and under research for potential clinical usefulness, are also reviewed. Currently employed gene therapy strategies, obstacles, and challenges in cancer gene therapy are presented, focusing on the latest nanotechnological advancements in this field including gene transfer methods, vectors, and their current successful applications in cancer gene therapy. Lastly, sulfamethoxazole is examined for its history of combating several microbial infections by affecting folic acid biosynthesis inhibiting dihydropteroate synthetase.

Chapter 1 - The curse of cancer has been bane of multi-cellular organisms since the beginning of time. With rapid improvements made in medicine made by pioneers starting from 15th century, our understanding of our own physiology has increased to unprecedented levels. Foremost cause of death in multi-cellular organisms is cancer and this curse can originate in any part of our body with blood cells, bones, tissues, lymph nodes or in simple words everything that makes us alive can be a source of cancerous growth. Modern medical science has been chipping away at the question on why, how, where cancer originates and our understanding in the twenty first century though not by any means anywhere near complete with much of what causes cancer still needs to be understood, at least provides us with broad contours of how different cancers originate, what are some of the genetic mutations that trigger cancer, what are the treatment options available. This chapter attempt to provide readers with brief and concise information of different types of cancer, their origins, and the available treatment options. Cancer rates are shooting up across the world with rate of increased close to 50% growth year on year. After reading this chapter the reader should have broad understanding on the above topics.

Chapter 2 - Cancer is a major human health problem, worldwide. Significant progress has been achieved over the past 35 years in understanding the molecular basis of cancer, contributing to the development of new targeted therapies. Kinases - receptor tyrosine kinases (RTK) and non-receptor tyrosine kinases (NRTKs), play a fundamental role in cell proliferation, survival, and migration. They are constitutively overexpressed and/or activated in several solid and hematological malignant disorders, associated with cancer development, progression and metastasis constituting, therefore, a potential treatment target. Therapies against deregulated RTKs comprise the targeting of the intracellular tyrosine kinase domain by reversible or irreversible tyrosine kinase inhibitors (TKIs) as well as, binding to extracellular domains. A considerable number of small molecule inhibitors have been developed, and many are already on clinical practice such as, TKIs inhibitors (*Gefitinib, Lapatinib*), and several monoclonal antibodies that bind to extracellular regions, including antibodies against EGFR (*Cetuximab and Panitumumab*), HER2 (*Trastuzumab and Panitumumab*), VEGFR1/R2 (*Bevacizumab, Ramucirumab*) and PDGFRα (*Olaratumab*). Non-receptor tyrosine kinases (NRTKs) are cytoplasmic proteins or proteins anchored to cell membrane that trigger intracellular signals derived primarily from RTK and from other growth factor receptors. Several specific kinase inhibitors have also been developed to target mutated kinases and inhibit their activity playing a central role on the control of carcinogenesis. In general, TKIs exhibit excellent clinical results as they are efficacious and well tolerated. Imatinib (IMA), a BCR-ABL inhibitor, was the first TKI approved, initially indicated for chronic myeloid leukemia (CML), and later for acute lymphoblastic leukemia (ALL), Philadelphia positive. It is also a useful therapeutic agent for gastrointestinal stromal tumors (GIST), due to the well-recognized oncogenic mutations seen in the RTK, KIT. Although IMA remains one of the gold standards for first-line CML treatment, the emergence of IMA resistance led to the development and use, in this setting, of second and third-generation TKIs, *Nilotinib, Dasatinib, Bosutinib* and *Ponatinib*, respectively. *Ibrutinib* is the first approved Bruton's tyrosine kinase (BTK) inhibitor that has shown clinical activity against B-cell malignancies. *Ruxolitinib* is the first JAK inhibitor approved for the treatment of intermediate and high-risk myelofibrosis. Other TKIs that target tyrosine kinase receptors including, *Midostaurin* (FLT3 F691), *Erlotinib and Gefitinib* (EGFR T790) and *Sunitinib*, were approved for treatment of newly diagnosed FLT3-mutated AML, advanced systemic mastocytosis, non-small-cell lung cancer (NSCLC) and renal cell carcinoma (RCC), respectively. *Vemurafenib* and *Dabrafenib* are BRAF inhibitors which approved for melanoma treatment, in cases exhibiting the specific BRAF/V600E mutation. Although, 75% of patients with this BRAF mutation respond to *Vemurafenib*, resistance to this drug occurs, leading to de development of novel BRAF inhibitors such as, *Regorafenib* and *Encorafenib,* to overcome this condition. *Vandetanib* has been approved for the treatment of medullar thyroid cancer exhibiting RET kinase activity and, *Crizotinib* is currently used to treat patients with ALK-positive non-small cell lung cancer. *Sorafenib*, a multi-kinase inhibitor is indicated in the treatment of hepatocellular carcinoma, renal cell carcinoma, and thyroid carcinoma. This drug inhibits several tyrosine kinases, and the serine/threonine kinases RAF, MEK1/2 and ERK1/2 kinases. Activation of the phosphoinositide 3-kinase (PI3K) signaling pathway is frequently observed in breast cancer and in some hematological cancers. The delta PI3K inhibitors, *Idelalisib* and *Duvelisib*, have been approved for the treatment of indolent B cell neoplasias. *Copanlisib* extends existing treatment options for indolent non-Hodgkin lymphoma (NHL) and shows promising response rates in aggressive NHL, especially in DLBCL of the activated B-cell type. Other kinases, as Aurora A kinase (AAK), Cyclin-Dependent Kinases (CDK) and Polo-like kinases (PLK), play a pivotal role in cancer cells mitosis and activates EMT during the metastatic process

(Figure 2). The development of AAK inhibitors including *Alisertinib, Danusertib, Barasertib, Tozasertib, Hesperidin* and *Radotinib,* has been promoted. Several CDK inhibitors entered clinical trials such as, *Roscovitine (Seliciclib)* and the natural product derivative flavopiridol (*Alvocidib*). The clinical response evaluation to the CDK inhibitor *Alvocidib* in hematological tumors was limited and was associated with non-acceptable toxicities. *Palbociclib, Abemaciclib and Ribociclib*, which are CDK4/6-selective inhibitors have been already approved for the treatment of metastatic breast cancer (HR+, HER2-) in combination with endocrine therapy. Clinical trials with PLK1 inhibitors, *Rigosertib, Volasertib* and *Poloxin*, are ongoing to evaluating their potential clinical benefit in sensitizing tumors to chemotherapy. Twenty-eight kinase inhibitors deserved FDA approval since the initial development of Imatinib; *Brigatinib* and *Osimertinib*, were the latest and they are indicated to treat metastatic NSCLC ALK-positive. Despite a such considerable number of already approved kinase inhibitors, more than three thousand of new kinase inhibitors are still under ongoing phase I-III clinical trials. Yet and so far, one may consider that only a small fraction of the *kinome* is currently being targeted. Protein kinase inhibitors, currently in clinical practice and under research for potential clinical usefulness, will be reviewed in this chapter.

Chapter 3 - Cancer ranks second among the causes of death in developed countries. It is stated that 9.6 million people died in 2018 due to cancer. The clinical failure of conventional cancer treatments like chemotherapy, radiotherapy, and surgery necessitates novel therapeutic strategies that minimize the side effects and enhance long-term patient survival. In the past two decades, there have been dramatic scientific and technological advances in cancer genomic research, and consequently, gene therapy has emerged as a promising approach for cancer treatment. Since gene therapy is developed, 60% of research is focused on cancer. In its most general definition, gene therapy can be described the correction of a genetic deficiency by inserting a wild type version of a defective or missing gene into the somatic cells, by silencing the gene that causes a disease, or by inserting new genes to overcome a disease thereby treating a disorder or disease. There are several prospective strategies for gene therapy of cancer. These are suicide gene therapy, anti-angiogenic gene therapy, immunomodulatory gene therapy, chemoprotection approach, RNA interference therapy, and pro-apoptotic gene therapy. In this chapter, the currently employed gene therapy strategies, obstacles, and challenges in cancer gene therapy were presented. The theme was focused on the latest nanotechnological advancements in this field including gene transfer methods, vectors, and their current successful applications in cancer gene therapy.

Chapter 4 - Drug development in the field of oncology is facing an acute 'productivity crisis,' where the success rate for new drugs from Phase I trial to US Food and Drug Administration (FDA) approval in the period 2003 to 2011 was around 6.7%. A figure that is about half the rate for non-oncological drugs. This apparent slow pace of new oncology drug production is occurring against two challenges, one of increased cancer incidence across the globe, and the other of existing significant therapeutic resistance in many types of malignant disease. To overcome these hurdles, the Repurposing Drugs in Oncology (ReDO) project is focused to find existing and widely-used non-cancer drugs with hidden attributes of anticancer potential. In contrast to the de novo development of new molecules, drug repurposing begins with known pharmaceutical agents with a prehistory of clinical use. In this regard, Sulfamethoxazole (SMX) has long been known for combating several microbial infections. It affects folic acid biosynthesis inhibiting dihydropteroate synthetase. Although some toxic effects of SMX and its derivatives have been reported in patients, specific target of SMX or its derivatives in eukaryotic system has not been identified precisely. Earlier some sulfonamide group of compounds like E-7010 and many others were found to selectively inhibit microtubule assembly by binding to tubulin at the colchicine site. A wealth of information exists regarding inhibitory activity of sulfonamides against a panel of human cancer cell lines. Because the sulfonamide moiety (O=S=O) is common to many anticancer sulphur group drugs, it is tempting to explore SMX for its anticancer potential. Binding interaction of SMX with microtubule and lactate dehydrogenase is indicative of additional mode of action of SMX along with the cytotoxicity exhibited by the drug against Hela cancer cell lines.

In: An Introduction to Cancer Therapy
Editor: Neville Charron
ISBN: 978-1-53618-450-1

Chapter 1

UNDERSTANDING CANCER: TYPES AND THERAPEUTICS

***Deepti Malik*[1]*, Gitika Batra*[2]*, Saniya Mahendiratta*[1]*, Ajay Prakash*[1] *and Bikash Medhi*[1,*]**

[1]Department of Pharmacology, Post Graduate Institute of Medical Education and Research, Chandigarh, India

[2]Department of Neurology, Post Graduate Institute of Medical Education and Research, Chandigarh, India

ABSTRACT

The curse of cancer has been bane of multi-cellular organisms since the beginning of time. With rapid improvements made in medicine made by pioneers starting from 15th century, our understanding of our own physiology has increased to unprecedented levels. Foremost cause of death in multi-cellular organisms is cancer and this curse can originate in any part of our body with blood cells, bones, tissues, lymph nodes or in simple words everything that makes us alive can be a source of cancerous growth. Modern medical science has been chipping away at the question on why, how, where cancer originates and our understanding in the twenty first century though not by any means anywhere near complete with much of what causes cancer still needs to be understood, at least provides us with

* Corresponding Author's E-mail: drbikashmedhi@gmail.com.

broad contours of how different cancers originate, what are some of the genetic mutations that trigger cancer, what are the treatment options available. This chapter attempt to provide readers with brief and concise information of different types of cancer, their origins, and the available treatment options. Cancer rates are shooting up across the world with rate of increased close to 50% growth year on year. After reading this chapter the reader should have broad understanding on the above topics.

INTRODUCTION

What molecular events trigger cancer progression? What causes a normal cell phenotype to change into a transformed phenotype? How a balance that keeps the proper cell surface to volume ratio in normal cells gets disrupted in a transformed cell? How is the fine balance maintained by homeostatic control mechanisms in cells disrupted resulting in tumour, or neoplasm?

Answer to these questions is what we call the morphing of healthy cells to carcinogenic cells.

Normal body cells maintain a proper cell surface to volume ratio by regulating different processes like cell growth, division and apoptosis in a synchronized manner. The cells in the human body have a constant life span under normal circumstances. They grow, divide and replace worn-out or dying cells, maintaining a constant cell number (Hanahan and Weinberg 2011). When cells outgrows abnormally in number without following the cells apoptotic signals, a tumour forms, which is characterized by destabilization of the homeostatic balance maintaining cell growth and division. Acquisition of six essential characteristics in normal cells lead to the expression of the transformed phenotype: Self-sustaining proliferation, ability to block the signals that stop proliferation, ability to escape apoptosis, unbridled replication ability, sustained excessive formation of blood vessels and malignant invasion of tissue and metastasis (Hanahan and Weinberg 2000). Defining feature of cancereous cells structure are large nuclei, asymmetrical size and shape prominent nucleoli, scarce and intensely coloured cytoplasm, poorly developed Golgi apparatus with the manifestation of abnormal mitotic divisions and acquisition of macrophage like properties (Baba and Câtoi 2007).

TYPES OF CANCER BASED ON SITE OF FORMATION

There are broadly two classifications for tumours -Benign and Malignant. Benign tumours are the ones which are contained and never invade the surrounding tissue whilst malignant tumours are virulent, exhibit metastasis, with cancerous cells breaking free from tumour and invading blood or lymphatic vessels, leading to formation of new tumours in different parts of body (Waldum et al. 2008).

The tissue from which the tumour originated is primary way of classification:

- Carcinomas: Cancers can form in endodermal or ectodermal germ layer during normal embryogenesis or epithelial lining of organs and glands (Hassanpour and Dehghani 2017). Typical examples of carcinomas are cases of lung, Colon, Breast and Prostate.
- Leukemias and Lymphomas: To understand leukaemias and lymphomas we first need to understand how haematopoietic stem cells maintain their population. Haematopoietic stem cells are present in bone marrow of all humans. Haematopoietic stem cells renew themselves automatically and they sustain their population by cell division and have ability to give rise to all the blood cells from the myeloid or lymphoid lineage (Kondo 2010), (Bryder, Rossi, and Weissman 2006). The self-renewal concept means that when it happens correctly results in 50% daughter cells which are characterized by cell lineage differentiating into lymphoid and myeloid precursors of blood cells and rest 50% of the cells do not show any kind of differentiation resulting in equilibrium in the number of stem cells. This phenomenon is known as asymmetric cell division (Gordon, 2005) whereas in symmetric division stem cells divide into 100% similar stem cells (Seita and Weissman 2010). Myeloid lineage produces dendritic cells, eosinophils monocytes, basophils, neutrophils, erythrocytes, platelets, whereas lymphoid lineage results in T-cells, B-cells and NK cells (Seita and Weissman 2010).

- Leukemias: Leukemias are kind of cancer of blood/bone marrow directly caused by uncontrolled division of white blood cells (Terwilliger and Abdul-Hay 2017). Blood cells are produced by bone marrow and released into the bloodstream where these cells have a defined life span with a certain percentage dying and certain percentage of blood cells been released(Terwilliger and Abdul-Hay 2017). Somatic mutations can affect lymphoid and myeloid progenitor cells resulting into production of cancerous blood cells which do not die easily, slowly accumulating and over numbering the normal cells leading to cancer (Yamashita et al. 2020).

TYPES OF LEUKEMIA

Acute

Leukemias can be classified as acute, a rapidly progressing disease characterized by massive increase of immature blood cells (le Viseur et al. 2008). These immature blood cells tend to accumulate in bone marrow of humans, making it impossible for bone marrow to produce normal blood cells prompting immediate treatment as the spill over of immature blood cells from bone marrow to the bloodstream can lead to spread of cancer to the whole body. This is a more prevalent form of leukemia (le Viseur et al. 2008).

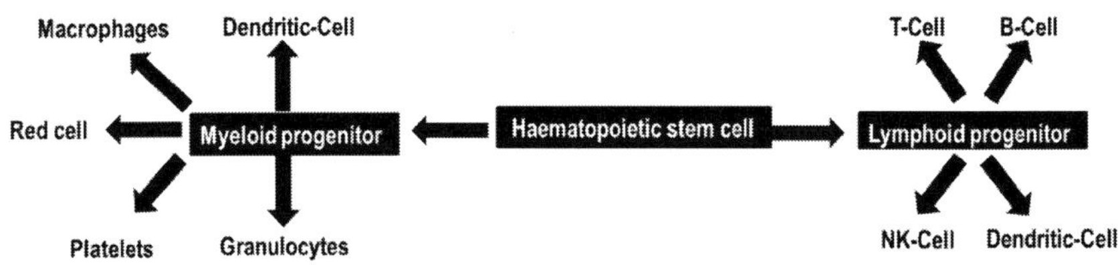

Figure 1. **Haematopoietic stem cells (HSCs) differentiation pathways**: HSCs can differentiate to different blood cells ranging from myeloid to lymphoid lineage. Myeloid lineage produces dendritic cells, eosinophils monocytes, basophils, neutrophils, erythrocytes, platelets, whereas lymphoid lineage results in NK cells, B-cells and T-cells. (Seita and Weissman 2010).

Chronic

Leukemias where the cancerous cell production is slower allowing more mature cells to be formed thus leading to the slow spread of the disease. This cancer is typically found in adults above the age of 50 (Hallek 2019).

Lymphocytic and Myelogenous

Leukemias can originate in lymphoid or myeloid lineages.

Lymphoblastic leukemia is malignant disorder resulting from the somatic mutation that arises at any stage of the development in the lymphoid progenitor cell that is destined to produce lymphocytes (Figure 1); (le Viseur et al. 2008). Myeloid leukemias originate from the mutation arising in the myeloid progenitor cells. Myeloid progenitor cells lead tp origination of platelets, white cells and red blood cells (Weiskopf et al. 2016)

Clubbing the above-mentioned classifications helps us define different type of leukemia

- Acute lymphoblastic leukemia (ALL) young children are typically impacted by ALL (Terwilliger and Abdul-Hay 2017). ALL can be classified as
    - precursor T-cell ALL
    - precursor B-cell ALL
    - acute biphenotypic
    - Burkitt's leukaemia.
- Chronic lymphocytic leukemia (CLL) Older humans are typically impacted. Children are rarely diagnosed with CLL (Hallek 2019). CLL can be classified as
    - Hairy cell leukemia
    - T-cell prolymphocytic leukemia
    - B-cell prolymphocytic leukaemia
- Acute myelogenous leukemia (AML) Adult males are generally diagnosed with AML. AML is classified based on the stage at which

the cancer developed and which kind of cell was involved in development of cancer (Saultz and Garzon 2016). Typical classifications range from M0 to M7. M0-5 has their origin in white blood cells while M6 typically originates in RBC's and M7 has its origin in blood platelets(Saultz and Garzon 2016) Typical examples of AML are

  - Acute myelomonocytic
  - Acute monocytic
  - Acute promyelocytic (APL)
  - Acute myelomonocytic with eosinophilia

- Chronic myelogenous leukemia (CML) can be diagnosed in adults and infrequently in children (Cortes, Talpaz, and Kantarjian 1996). Typical examples of CML are
  - Chronic granulocytic leukaemia
  - Juvenile CML
  - Chronic neutrophilic leukaemia (CNL)
  - Atypical CML (aCML)

LYMPHOMAS

Lymphoma is a cancer that originates in bodies lymph nodes/glands, spleen, thymus gland or bone marrow. It typically occurs when lymphocytes division gets out of control and the cells do not die as programmed and accumulate either in armpits, neck or groin leading to the development of tumors and spreading to other parts of the body (Matasar and Zelenetz 2008).

Types of Lymphoma

- Hodgkin's lymphoma also Hodgkin's disease): originates in upper body mostly in the neck, chest of armpit, is very easy to detect and has the most positive probability of having good prognosis. Hodgkin's lymphoma is characterized by Reed-Sternberg cells (Shanbhag and Ambinder 2018).

- Non-Hodgkin's lymphoma (NHL) originates in lymph nodes and is more common type of lymphoma. Typical patients are above 55. It is not easy to detect and by the time diagnosis is done the disease has reached an advanced stage. The cells called Reed-Sternberg cells are not present. NHL can be classified by the rate of growth of cancer, either "indolent" or "aggressive" (Connors 2013).
  - Indolent NHL is characterized by slow growth not requiring immediate treatment with treatment starting only when symptoms show up.
  - Aggressive NHL is characterized by rapid growth requiring immediate treatment. Treatment requires intensive chemotherapy for stage I or II. Aggressive NHL can lead to unbridled cancerous cell growth leading to large sites of disease in the body. Aggressive NHL is more common in children.

Indolent and aggressive NHL typically results in fatigue, weight loss, fever and enlarged lymph nodes (Connors 2013).

Types of Hodgkin Lymphoma

Hodgkin lymphoma can be characterized as

- Classical Hodgkin lymphoma (cHL): Majority of the cases of Hodgkin lymphoma are cHL. Reed-Sternberg cells are the characteristic abnormal lymphocytes defining cHL. Four subtypes of cHL are based on lymph node structure and cells (Shanbhag and Ambinder 2018). Subtypes of Classical Hodgkin lymphoma are:
  - Nodular sclerosis Hodgkin lymphoma,
  - Lymphocyte-rich classical Hodgkin lymphoma,
  - Mixed cellularity Hodgkin lymphoma
  - Lymphocyte-depleted Hodgkin lymphoma
- Nodular sclerosis: Most prevalent sub-type of classical Hodgkin lymphoma. Children and young adults specifically women are

diagnosed by Nodular sclerosis impacting chest and/or neck causing fibrous marks in the lymph nodes(Mani and Jaffe 2009).

- Mixed cellularity: About quarter of cHL cases are of the type Mixed cellularity and mostly diagnosed in older adults affecting abdomen (Ansell 2018).
- Lymphocyte-rich: mostly diagnosed in men with nodular lymphocyte-predominant and often develops into non-Hodgkin lymphoma called diffuse large B-cell lymphoma (Ansell 2018).
- Lymphocyte-depleted: extremely rare and impacts geriatric humans or those afflicted with HIV (Ansell 2018).

Types of Non-Hodgkin's Lymphoma (NHL)

- B-cell lymphoma. Most prevalent non-Hodgkin's lymphoma accounting for more than quarter of cases worldwide. It's a fast-growing NHL and impacts B-lymphocytes. B-cell lymphoma (BCL) can be diagnosed in anywhere in the body and impact one or multiple sites in the human body. Typically, is diagnosed in adults over 60 and has a high probability of being cured (Jiang, Bennani, and Feldman 2017). Subtypes of BCL are :
    - Primary cutaneous DLBCL, leg type
    - Epstein-Barr virus (EBV)-positive DLBCL
    - T-cell/histiocyte-rich B-cell lymphoma
- T-cell lymphoma. Much rarer as compared to B-cell Lympoma, mostly prevalent in Asian countries (Marginean et al. 2018).
- Natural Killer (NK) cell lymphoma. Extremely rare with rate of occurrence of less than one percent (Marginean et al. 2018).

SARCOMAS

Tumors originating in connective tissues of the body. The word 'Sarcoma' originates form Greek word which literally means fleshy growth (Hoang et al. 2018)

Types of Sarcomas

Soft Tissue Sarcomas

Sarcomas originating in soft tissues are a typically rare kind of cancer. Tumours caused by soft tissue sarcoma can become quite big in size before their presence is discovered. They generally originate as a soft painless lump. With tumour growth pain/soreness is felt at nerves near the tissue where the tumour is growing get pressed. Soft tissue sarcomas have the ability to metastasize leading to the formation of secondary tumours (Hoang et al. 2018).

Types of Soft Tissue Sarcomas

- Alveolar Soft-Parts Sarcoma,
- Angiosarcoma- (impacts blood cells and/or lymph vessels),
- Dermatofibrosarcoma Protuberans- a skin lesion,
- Epithelioid Sarcomas – typically impacts younger humans hands/feet.
- Extraosseoustumors: They are giant cell tumors, there are three types of Extraosseoustumors
    - osteosarcomas,
    - Ewing's sarcoma- kind of bone sarcoma impacting soft tissues.
    - Fibrosarcoma- affecting fibroblasts
- Gastrointestinal Stromal Tumor (GIST)-impacting neuromuscular cells of the gut
- Kaposi Sarcoma (affects the skin)
- Leiomyosarcoma (smooth muscle tumor)
- Uterine Sarcoma
- Liposarcoma (sarcoma of fat tissue)
- Malignant Fibrous Histiocytoma (MFH)
- Malignant Neurilemomas
- Mesenchymomas, Myxoma
- Rhabdomyosarcomas- children are typically diagnosed and are found in muscles.

- Synovial Cell Sarcoma – impacts arm/leg joints and Vascular Sarcomas

Bone Sarcomas

Bone Sarcomas can be both type malignant or benign. Benign bone sarcomas can be easily treated and are rarely malignant (Franchi 2012). Typically these cancers will grow within the bone and are known as primary bone cancers. If the bone sarcoma spreads from bone to rest of the body it is known as Secondary Sarcoma (Franchi 2012).

Types of Bone Sarcoma

- Chondrosarcoma**:** originates in cartilage cells and affectsadults older than 40.
- Osteosarcoma: affects teenagers and young adults and typically originates in knees, shinbone or upper arm.
- Chordoma: typically affects older adults in the age of 40-50 affecting sacrum or the skull.

Risk Factors

An individual's probability of been impacted by any kind of cancer depends upon broadly on two kind of factors. The first kind of factors is genetic in nature and second sort is based on the kind of lifestyle the individual leads (Hanahan and Weinberg 2011). The various risk factors at play are cigarette-smoking, obesity, age, chronic inflammation, lack of physical activity, radiation exposure, poor diet, virus infections, infectious agents, immuno-suppression, alcohol intake and hereditary factors (Hanahan and Weinberg 2000)

Recently research has shown that altered expression of microRNAs (miRNAs) play crucial role in triggering cancer development (Ha 2011). miRNAs have a crucial impact on most biological processes and there has been a surge of recent research to understand their roles in preventing or curing multiple multifactorial diseases (Hwang & Mendell 2006). microRNAs are characterized by RNA sequences (19-23 nucleotides) which are short and single stranded and have the ability to bind to 3'-UTR sequences of specific genes leading to degradation of mRNA leading to reduced gene levels (Malik & Kaul 2015).Thus, mutations in such miRNAs could lead to the overexpression of an oncogene or the reduction of a tumour suppressor gene (Wahida et al. 2010, Sharma et al. 2015). miR-21, miR-155, miR-23, miR-191, miR-196b are overexpressed in breast cancer (Yan et al. 2008, Kaul and Malik 2012), miR-191,199a and miR155 (Ramamurthy et al. 2016) are overexpressed in AML. miR-2909 potentially plays role in immunomodulation (Kaul et al. 2019), energy metabolism (Malik & Kaul 2018, Kaushik et al. 2019) and its altered expression leading to many diseases including rheumatoid arthritis (Malik et al. 2015) and pediatric acute lymphoblastic leukaemia (Malik et al. 2014).

CANCER THERAPEUTICS

Cancer treatment has made giant stripes in recent years with chemotherapy playing a central role in increasing the efficacy of treatment and becoming the first line of defence for most primary tumours along with surgery. This approach paid rich dividends and was preferred way of cancer therapy for keeping in check and treating localized tumours well into 1960's. One of the major challenges with this approach is that most cancers microscopically metastasize throughout subjects body which leads to reoccurrence of disease even after initial remission leading to the need of regular chemotherapy with objective of controlling metastases. With advances been made the use of cytotoxic drugs with chemotherapy has stopped with increasing use of cancer specific agents leading to the age of "targeted therapy", sometimes also called "molecularly targeted drugs," "molecularly targeted therapies," "precision medicines etc. In the following sections we will be talking in detail about different kinds of therapies available for treatment of cancer.

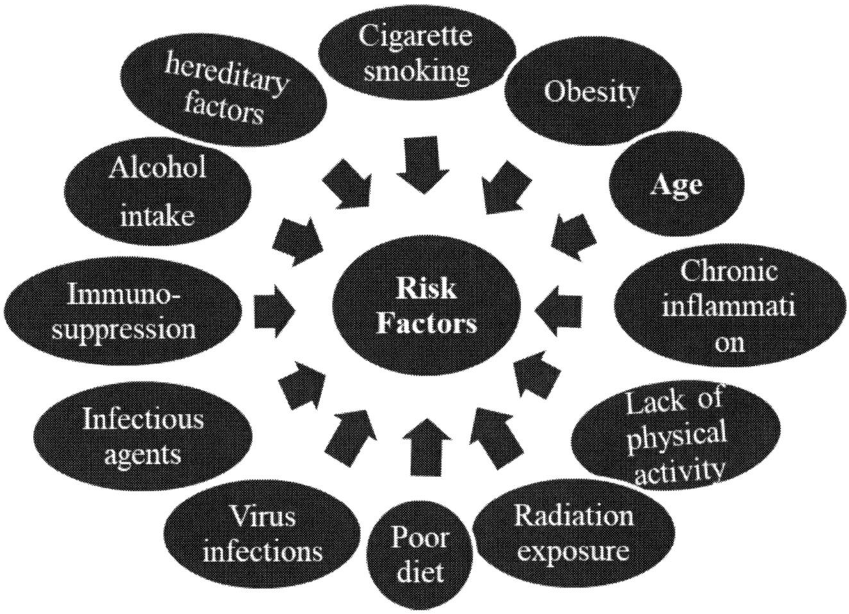

Figure 2. Cancer Risk Factors.

RADIOTHERAPY

It was Röntgen who discovered the X-rays in 1895, and Marie Curie was awarded the 2nd Nobel Prize for her pioneering research in radium hence, marking the year 2011 as the "Year of Radiation Therapy" to celebrate century of advances. It was first clinically used in 1896 and further technological advancements has fully transformed the clinical Radiation Therapy (RT) leading to precise delivery of radiations for improved clinical outcomes (Grubbe 1933; Bernier, Hall, and Giaccia 2004).

With the refinement in the understanding of radiobiology the focus and criteria has shifted to personalize the cancer treatment with the combination of biological precision with physical targeting. At present, RT is being chiefly used as treatment modality covering 50% of all cancer victims, being used either in a standalone fashion or in conjuction with surgery and chemotherapy (Delaney et al. 2005). Ionizing radiations forming ions are used for the cancer cell destruction through which it pass by depositing energy leading to cancer cell death (Ringborg et al. 2003).

Radiations can be delivered to site of cancer via two methods: External beam radiation which is commonly used in clinical setting and can be given from outside the body through the use of high-energy rays. Another method is brachytherapy which are the internal radiations routinely used for the treatment of gynecological and prostrate malignancies. Brachytherapy uses radiations from certain radioactive sources inside the body capped in catheters or placed directly into tumors therefore providing its utility in conditions where retreatment is required (Baskar et al. 2012).

It is known that RT can only be effective if it maximally eradicates the tumor cells sparing the normal cells. Technology has created such instrumentation enabling its delivery precisely targeting tumor cells with a considerable reduction of injury to normal tissues (Chen and Kuo 2017). The use of RT in western countries has been providing an important means of treatment modality in uncomplicated locoregional tumors. Considering the advances in technology in 3D conformal radiation treatments, the use of stereotactic (body) radiotherapy (SBRT), intensity-modulated radiation therapy (IMRT) and improved imaging systems (i.e., image-guided radiation therapy, IGRT), has improved. This has led to precise delivery of matching radiation towards the cancer cells while minimally invading the normal tissues (Baumann et al. 2016).

TECHNIQUES USED IN RADIOTHERAPY

The use of RT in clinical setting utilizes high precision RT techniques with the motive of specifically targeting the tissues surrounded by cancerous cells. Following techniques have been used:

3D Conformal Radiotherapy (3D CRT)

3D radiation therapy has replaced 2D radiation therapy which was using X-ray imaging based rectangular fields. The new 3D CRT is based on CT imaging to allow for accurate localization of tumor which aims to deliver the radiations to the gross tumor volume (GTV), clinical target volume (CTV), and planning target volume (PTV) (Morgan-Fletcher 2001).

Intensity Modulated Therapy (IMRT)

The advanced form of 3DCRT is Intensity modulated RT (IMRT) which was introduced in the early 1990's (Veldeman et al. 2008) and was made available for use in breast cancer. Many studies have documented its use for those patients who require complex breast treatments (McCormick and Hunt 2011) and also making it suitable for left-sided breast cancers for lessening the cardiac dose, re-irradiation, contra-lateral breast irradiation and bed irradiation for deep tumors. IMRT uses computer-controlled multi-leaf collimators (MLC's) and certain advanced treatment designs capable of creating variations in the desired dose in radiation field in contrast to standard methods using try and error approach for dose distribution (Vicini et al. 2002).

IMRT allows for delivery of different doses to various parts of the tumor such as a hypoxic area is determined through functional imaging which can receive a boost dose. Similar approaches are under investigation as an alternative to conventional RT such as use of simultaneous integrated boost (SIB) and the delivery of dose-escalated conventionally fractionated or hypo-fractionated RT using IMRT techniques for different anatomical sites such as breast, (Hamilton et al. 2016) head and neck (Feng et al. 2007) and prostrate (Timon et al. 2016).

Certain studies have been conducted to see the clinical outcomes of IMRT which was mainly retrospective studies except in 3 prospective randomized studies done (Pignol et al. 2008; Mukesh et al. 2013) with the pivotal aim of investigating treatment induced toxicity and quality of life (QOL) in breast cancer patients. The study reported increased dose homogeneity and a decrease in toxicity in its initial stages.

Above all the use of IMRT poses some after effects as a larger dimension of normal tissue also receives some amount of radiations leading to secondary malignancies and an increased theoretical risk from 1% to 1.75% as demonstrated by Hall and Wuu (Hall and Wuu 2003) Examples of IMRT solutions include TomoTherapy Hi-Art (Accuray, Inc., Sunnyvale, CA, USA), (Mackie et al. 1993) (Mackie et al. 1993) and volumetric-modulated arc therapy (RapidArc, Varian Medical Systems, Inc., Paolo Alto, CA, USA and VMAT, Elekta, AB, Stockholm, Sweden) (Otto 2008).

Particle Beam Therapy

Particle Beam Therapy uses proton rather than photons used in IMRT which has the advantage of reduced radiations towards the normal tissue. Although these advantages are theoretical still independent clinical evaluation needs to be done for its strengths and weakness (Mohan and Grosshans 2017). The use of this therapy is for the cancer of the eye, base of skull and spine specifically for pediatric patients (Matloob, Nasir, and Choi 2016) with lower frequency of vision and hearing impairment and neuro-degeneration compared to other modes of RT (Leroy et al. 2016).

Stereotactic Body Therapy (SBRT)

A highly technology-driven treatment method among the hypofractionated radiation treatment was introduced following IMRT known as Stereotactic body RT (SBRT) (Potters et al. 2010). This technique is safe and efficacious for treating across a range of anatomic locations along with its capability of producing a steep gradient outside the target (Lo et al. 2010). Studies also reported its effectiveness in laryngeal cancer with only 5 treatment fractions (NCT01984502, ClinicalTrials.gov). Accurate target delineation and implementing inter- and intra-fraction tumor motion compensation strategies (especially in lung and upper abdomen tumors) are prerequisites for SBRT (Tipton et al. 2011). Many systems are available for SBRT and some of which are based on traditional LINAC gantry, for instance Versa HD (Elekta, AB, Stockholm, Sweden) (Narayanasamy et al.

2016) in contrast to greater non-coplanar beam arrangements CyberKnife® (Accuray, Inc., Sunnyvale, CA, USA) (Adler Jr et al. 1997). SBRT can challenge the surgery which is the gold standard with its local ablative capabilities and itself can become a standard treatment for patients with operable early stage lung cancer but are at higher risk of mortality (Abbas, Danish, and Krasna 2016).

Image-Guided Radiotherapy (IGRT)

With further advancements in treatment options it becomes essential to avoid any errors during the treatment as there is a probability of missing the tumor (Langen and Jones 2001). To evade these errors IGRT plays an important role through its detection efficiency for errors acquired via pre-radiotherapy imaging allowing for corrections. It can be understood citing an example of daily cone-beam CT scans prior each treatment (Jaffray et al. 2002). IGRT is advantageous over IMRT due to its improved accuracy in making dose escalation feasible and allowing for refinement of therapeutic ratio for various tumor sites (Gill et al. 2011).

Stereotactic Radio-Surgery (Gamma Knife)

Gamma Knife works on the principle of stereotactic radio-surgery converging multiple beams in three dimensions targeting the tumor with intense dose of radiations sparing the surrounding tissues. It has wide variety of applications which includes malignant tumors arising in the brain, blood vessel defects (arterio-venous malformations) and functional problems (trigeminal neuralgia) (Combs et al. 2005) but its use is limited owing to high cost, limited access, inability to treat extracranial lesions and not suitable for targeting tumors larger than 2.5 cm in size.

Another form of stereotactic radio-surgery is X-Knife and Cyber Knife or Robotic radio-surgery where the former uses linear accelerator for treatment delivery but with less precision than Gamma Knife (Ahn et al.

2000) while the latter uses real time image guidance technology and computer-controlled robotics for delivering high doses of radiations. It has the advantage of completing the treatment in a week but high cost limits its use (Dieterich and Pawlicki 2008).

There are certain limitations to RT caused due to intrinsic radio-resistance of tumor cells leading to increased recurrence therefore there emerged a need to identify new molecules for improving the radio-sensitivity (Lambin et al. 2017). One of the methods to overcome this problem is to combine the RT with chemotherapy or targeted agents. Another strategy is the use of "omics" by means of expression of genes, proteins and metabolites (Chung et al. 2007) where response towards treatment is predicted through screening of genetic polymorphisms or gene expression analysis and post-translational polymorphism (Scott et al. 2017).

CHEMOTHERAPY

Chemotherapy works by using drugs that have the ability yo either kill or destroy tumor cells. Multiple drugs are simuletaneously used to kill the tumor or to inhibit the growth as well as the further spread of the tumor cells and also for symptomatic relief to the patient. Chemotherapy is used along with radiation therapy or surgery. Studies show the more efficacy of combination chemotherapy as compared to the single drug chemotherapy (Devita VT et al. 1975). Neoadjuvant chemotherapy is given before the surgery or radiation therapy so as to decrease the size of the tumor for localized radiation therapy or surgery whereas adjuvant chemotherapy is used after the surgery or radiation therapy so as to kill the remaining cancer cells (Springfeld C et al. 2020). But chemotherapy has one major drawback as it also affects the normal healthy cells of the body along with the cancer cells which sometimes alters the major cells of the body (Mead GM et al. 1982).

Cytotoxic Drugs

Cytotoxic drugs are also known as cytostatics as it involves the use of various agents the causes cytotoxicity mainly in the cancer cells and destroy the tumor cells. Most of the cytotoxic drugs alter the replication and cell division to kill the tumor cells (Ismael, et al. 2008). There are various types of cytotoxic drugs that alter the cell division of the cancerous cells such as:

- Alkylating agents: These drugs alter the DNA structure by cross linking or fragmenting the DNA which ultimately alters the function of the DNA of the cancerous cells. These drugs are also known as DNA damaging agents. Some of the alkylating agents are temozolamide, lomustine, melphalan, cyclophosphamide, and, etc (Ralhan R et al. 2007). High dose of these alkylating agents show cytotoxicity (causes leukemia) as it affects the normal cell as well (Tucker MA et al. 1987). Therefore, platinum based alkylating agents are extensively used instead of above mentioned ones such as cisplatin that does not destroys bone marrow and does not causes leukemia (Dilruba S et al. 2016).
- Antimetabolite drugs: Antimetabolites alter the normal metabolism of the tumor cells which ultimately stops the tumor cells growth. These drugs inhibit purine or pyrimidine biosynthesis. Examples of antimetabolite drugs are methotrexate, 5-fluorouracil, gemcitabine, 6-mercaptopurine and, etc. (Luengo A et al. 2017).
- Mitotic inhibitors: Mitotic inhibitors are also known as microtubule inhibitors. Microtubule polymerization and de-polymerization is an important process during the cell division. Some drugs inhibit these processes via working on tubulin protein and block the spindle assembly or disassembly, chromosome segregation and, cell division or the formation of new daughter cells (for example, Colchicine) (Gascoigne, K. E., and Taylor, S. S. 2009). Some drugs stabilize microtubule assembly such as paclitaxel. Other inhibitors include vincristine and vinblastine which destabilizes the microtubule that causes mitotic arrest and finally cell death of the cancer cells (Mukhtar E et al. 2014).

- Topoisomerase inhibitors: Topoisomerase releases the tension in the DNA during the replication process. It unlinks the DNA via forming a nick or a break in the DNA strand. Therefore, inhibition of the topoisomerase increases the tension or coiling in the DNA, no closing of DNA strand and that leads to DNA breakage, cell cycle arrest and ultimately leading to apoptosis (Hande KR. 2008). Some drugs inhibits topoisomerase I and other topoisomerase II such as camptothecin (Pommier Y. 2006) or topotecan and etoposide (Hande K. 1998) respectively.
- Anti-cancer antibiotics: Certain antibiotics (anthracyclins) shows anticancer activity via acting on various processes such as intercalating agent such as actinomycin-D which inhibits elongation of RNA chain during transcription and inhibits RNA synthesis. Some antibiotics generate free radicals such as superoxide and hydroxyl radicals which cause DNA strand breakage and also inhibit topoisomerase II. For example, doxorubicin (Hande KR. 2008) and bleomycin. Bleomycin can also intercalate between DNA strands to inhibit RNA synthesis. Low doses of these antibiotics are more favorable due to low toxicity (Booser DJ., and Hortobagyi GN. 1994).

Steroids and Hormone Antagonists

Steroids are given during or after chemotherapy session to give a feeling of euphoria to the patient. Steroids also regulate the body weight nausea allergic response and, haemoglobin levels of the patient receiving cancer chemotherapy. Studies show the anti-inflammatory action of various hormones such as glucocorticosteroid (Prednisone and Dexamethasone). Aromatase inhibitors, 5-α-reductase inhibitors anti-androgen, and GnRH analogues are some of the hormone and its antagonists available in the market (Dreicer R et al. 1992). In breast cancer, estrogen binds to its receptors present on mammary cells and causes the growth of these cells and ultimately the formation of tumor. Selective Estrogen Receptor

Downregulators (ERDs) namely Fulvestrant steroid drugs removes estrogen receptor and inhibits its dimerization. Therefore, causing estrogen receptor down-regulation and decreases the growth of tumor. Some non-steroidal Selective Estrogen Receptor Modulators (Tamoxifen) competes with the estrogen for receptor binding and shows antagonistic action on breast cells and blood vessels to inhibit the tumor growth (Flötotto, T et al. 2001).

TARGETED THERAPY: SMALL MOLECULES AND MONOCLONAL ANTIBODIES

Targeted cancer therapy involves the small molecules or drugs that specifically block the cancer progression and metastasis by interfering with molecular targets that are associated with cancer cell without damaging the normal cells (Wahl DR., and Lawrence TS. 2017). These molecular targets regulate the cancer proliferation, progression and cancer spread (Lee YT et al. 2018). There are various FDA approved small molecules for the treatment of different types of cancer (Table 1). Some of the molecular targets involved in targeted cancer therapy are mentioned below:

Table 1. FDA-Approved molecular targeted drugs for the treatment of cancer**

Drug/Antibody	Molecular Target	Cancer treatment/Therapeutic Indication
Kinase Inhibitors: 1. Imatinib 2. Gefitinib, Erlotinib 3. Sorafenib, Vandetanib 4. Ribociclib 5. Alectinib 6. Ibrutinib 7. Cobimetinib 8. Everolimus 9. Regorafenib	1. BCR-Abl, PDGFR 2. EGFR 3. VEGFR, RAF 4. CDK4/6 5. ALK 6. BTK 7. MEK1/2 8. FKBP12/mTOR 9. RET, FLT, FGFR, MAPK, PDGFR	1. CML or ALL, gastrointestinal stromal tumor 2. NSCLC, pancreatic cancer 3. RCC, HCC, medullary thyroid cancer 4. Metastatic breast cancer (combination therapy) 5. ALK positive NSCLC 6. CLL, marginal zone and mantle cell lymphoma 7. *BRAF* positive melanomas (combination therapy) 8. Breast cancer (HER2 negative), RCC, pancreatic neuroendocrine cancer 9. Colorectal cancer, stomach cancer
Proteosome Inhibitors: 1. Carfilzomib 2. Bortezomib	1. PSMB(1,2,5,8,9,10) 2. PSMB (1,2,5), PSMD (1,2)	1. Multiple myeloma 2. Multiple myeloma, lymphoma
PARP Inhibitors: 1. Olaparib 2. Niraparib	1. PARP (1,2,3) 2. PARP (1,2)	1. Advanced ovarian cancer (gBRCA-mutated) 2. Epithelial ovarian cancer, peritoneal cancer

Drug/Antibody	Molecular Target	Cancer treatment/Therapeutic Indication
Epigenetic Modulators: 1. Varinostat, Balinostat 2. Romidepsin	1. HDAC (1,2,3,6) 2. HDAC (1,2,3,6)	1. Lymphoma 2. Lymphoma
Monoclonal antibodies: 1. Bevacizumab 2. Cetuzimab 3. Trastuzumab emtansin, Pertuzumab 4. Ibritumomab tiuxetan, Tositumomab, Rituximab 5. Gemtuzumab ozogamicin, Ofatumumab 6. Alemtuzumab 7. Brentuximab vedotin 8. Ramucirumab 9. Pambrolizumab 10. Nivolumab 11. Ipilimumab	1. VEGFA 2. EGFR 3. ERBB2or HER2+ (ADC) 4. MS4A1 or CD20 (RIC) 5. CD33 (ADC) 6. CD52 7. CD30 or TNFRSF8 8. KDR 9. PD-L1 or PDCD1 10. PD-L1 or PDCD1 11. CTLA4	1. Colorectal cancer, RCC, NSCLC, Glioblastoma 2. Colorectal cancer, head & neck cancer 3. HER2+ metastatic breast cancer and stomach cancer 4. Non-Hodgkin's Lymphoma 5. Leukemia (AML) 6. Leukemia (CLL) 7. Hodgkin's Lymphoma 8. Stomach cancer 9. Melanoma 10. Melanoma, HCC, RCC, NSCLC 11. Melanoma

** Data taken from Ref. Roskoski R, (2019); Sun J et al. (2017); and Lee YT et al. (2018)

* PDGF, platelet-derived growth factor; ALL, acute lymphoblastic lymphoma; CML, chronic myeloid leukemia; EGFR, epidermal growth factor receptor; NSCLC, non-small-cell lung carcinoma; VEGFR, vascular endothelial growth factor receptor; RAF, rapidly Accelerated Fibrosarcoma; RCC, renal cell carcinoma; HCC, hepatocellular carcinoma; CDK, cyclin-dependent kinase; ALK, anaplastic lymphoma receptor tyrosine kinase; BTK, Bruton's tyrosine kinase; MAPK/MEK, mitogen-activated protein kinase; FKBP12, FK506-binding protein 12; mTOR, mechanistic target of rapamycin; RET, rearranged during transfection; FGFR, Fibroblast growth factor receptor; PSMB, Proteasome β subunits; HDAC, Histone deacetylases; PARP, poly-ADP-ribose polymerase; BRCA, breast cancer gene; ADC, antibody-drug conjugate; CD, cluster of differentiation; TNFR, Tumor necrosis factorreceptor; KDR, Kinase Insert Domain Receptor; PD-L1, programmed death-ligand 1; CTLA4, cytotoxic T-lymphocyte-associated protein 4.

Growth Factor Kinase and Cyclin-Dependent Kinase (CDK) Inhibitors

These inhibitors work by blocking the kinase activity of the growth factor receptor and their downstream signal transduction (Shawver LK et al. 2002). Growth factor kinase (tyrosine kinase) inhibition is one of the most used agents for the cancer therapy as it directly stops the cancer growth (Arora A. 2005). Next, CDKs are involved cell cycle progression, inhibition of CDKs lead to cell cycle arrest and finally, apoptosis of cancer cells (Whittaker SR et al. 2017).

Apoptosis Inducers

These molecules or drugs act by inducing cell death, (apoptosis) of the cancer cells. Cancer cells have various mechanisms to evade the apoptosis

LaCasse E et al. 1998). Other than modulation of pre-apoptotic molecules and anti-apoptotic molecules, MDM2 inhibition also increases p53-induced apoptosis of cancer cells (Vassilev LT. 2007).

Angiogenesis Inhibitors

Various anti-angiogenic agents inhibit the blood vessel formation, so it deprives the cancer cells of nutrients which are required for their growth (Yang Y. 2013). Therefore, angiogenesis inhibitors restrict the growth and metastasis of cancer cells. Vascular endothelial growth factor (VEGF), certain cytokines like IL-8, MMPs are involved in angiogenesis. They are the pro-inducers of angiogenesis along with Hypoxia Inducible Factor-1 (HIF-1). Inhibition of these pro-inducers decreases the angiogenesis as well as metastasis of tumor cells (El-Kenawi AE., and El-Remessy AB. 2013).

Proteosome Inhibitors

Ubiquitin-Proteosome complex is involved in the breakdown of various cellular protein like misfiled or damaged or unfolded proteins. This complex contains many subunits such as 19S cap and 20S subunit which together makes the 26S proteasome. Inhibition of 26S proteasome causes the accumulation of damaged proteins (Deepti VD et al. 2016).

Poly ADP-Ribose Polymerase Inhibitors (PARP Inhibitors)

These molecules block the activity of PARP (a set of enzymes), which is involved in DNA repair. Inhibiting the PARP activity lead to the accumulation of damaged DNA in the cancer cells and ultimately causes cell death (Slade D et al. 2020). Inhibition of PARP-1 decreases significant cancer growth followed by PARP-2 and PARP-3. PARP inhibition ultimately cause selective killing of cells bearing BRCA1/2 mutations via disrupting DNA replication, repair and transcription pathways (Lin KY., and Kraus WL. 2017).

Cell Cycle Checkpoint Inhibitors

Cell cycle checkpoint inhibitors generally include molecular targets such as Chk1 and Wee, which regulate the cell cycle arrest. In a normal cell, whenever some DNA damage occur the repair mechanism by the help of cell cycle checkpoint. These inhibitors ultimately stop the cell cycle of cancer cells (Visconti R et al. 2016). Haynes Bet al. 2018 showed that Chk1 inhibition can also overcome the resistance induced due to PARP inhibitors in case of cancers with Homologous Recombination (HR) defects.

Epigenetic Modulators/Modifiers/Mediators

These agents regulate the expression of deregulated genes without altering the DNA sequences. Epigenetic reprogramming is associated with the inactivation of various tumor-suppressor genes and activation of oncogenes (Brown G et al. 2010). HDAC is a major molecular epigenetic target that regulates various processes such as apoptosis, cell proliferation, growth and metastasis. Studies have also shows the inhibition of HDAC decreases cancer progression and increases cell death of tumor cells (Khan, O., and La Thangue N. B. 2011). Studies show that BET inhibitors or Bromodomain inhibitors regulate the immune response pathway and control the cancer growth (Ramadoss M., and Mahadevan V. 2018).

Telomerase Inhibitor

Cancer cells sustain their telomere length by the help of telomerase enzyme. Telomerase is highly expressed in various cancers but not in normal cells. Telomerase inhibition causes the shortening of telomere and leads to replicative senescence and apoptosis. Telomerase inhibitors also cause rapid apoptosis without the telomere shortening through some alternative pathway. (Cunningham AP et al. 2006). Targeting human Telomerase reverse transcriptase (hTERT) leads to alter enzyme activity and no further maintenance of telomere length to kill cancer cells is under use for various types of cancers (Jafri MA et al. 2016).

Cancer Stem Cells

Cancer stem cells are the cells present in the tumor that leads to the tumor initiation, metastasis and resistance towards various chemotherapeutics options (Sandoval et al. 2014.). These cells have the ability to self-renew but their expansion and differentiation is highly dis-regulated. Thus, these cancer stem cell or tumor initiating cells contributes to one of the reason for recurrence of cancer in the patients already treated with radiotherapy along with chemotherapy (Kuşoğlu et al. 2019). Identification of cancer stem cells within a tumor is very import to target these cells and their identification is done by using fluorescence-activated cell sorting method for various cancer stem cell markers (surface or intracellular markers such as CD133, CD44 and CD24) (Dawood et al. 2014). Studies showing the inhibition of various cancer stem cells pathway have shown the decrease expression of cancer stem cell markers, resistance toward the chemotherapeutic agents and the complete removal of tumor cells (Ginestier et al. 2010; Chao et al. 2011).

Photodynamic Therapy (PDT)

Photodynamic therapy (PDT) is one of the powerful drug-device for the targeted therapy of cancer. Various studies highlight the high selectivity and specificity of PDT towards the malignant tumor cells. It does not cause any harm to the normal cells in the body (Dolmans et al. 2003). Generally, PDT consists of three parts: a light sensitive photo-sensitizer (PS), light radiating source and an oxygen source (Agostinis et al. 2011). During the PD therapy session, first, photosensitizer is administered followed by irradiation of the tumor with an appropriate wavelength which corresponds to the absorbance band of the light sensitive photo-sensitizer. Then, the light excites the photosensitizer which leads to the generation of various reactive oxygen species (singlet oxygen form) and these ROS generates local inflammatory response (Korbelik et al. 2006). PDT works by various mechanisms to eradicate the tumor cells such as induction of cell death pathways leading to apoptosis (Mroz et al. 2011), damaging microvasculature (Chen et al. 2002) and generation of inflammatory response along with immune response against the cancer cells (systematic antitumor immunity) (Korbelik et al. 2006). Therefore, PDT therapy imparts specific killing of tumor cells with low toxicity and relapse in the patients undergoing PDT therapy (Agostinis et al. 2011). Combination of PDT along with chemotherapy and radiotherapy shows successful reduction in tumor growth and significant killing of tumor cells (Lee et al. 2018).

Immunotherapy

Immune system has the inherent property of differentiating between self from non-self due to T-cell receptor binding to peptide complexes with major histocompatibility complex (MHC) class I molecule presented on the surface of all cells, including tumor cells. Still, for T-cell activation this complex is not sufficient as it needs a co-stimulatory or co-inhibitory signal and this property is exploited by tumor cells to escape the destruction (Schreiber, Old, and Smyth 2011). Several studies have demonstrated the intricate relationship between cancer and immune system making it practical and feasible for significant developments in tumor immunotherapy. There have been advances and promising clinical benefit from the modulators of the immune system recently approved by FDA for malignancies such as melanoma, renal cell carcinoma and non-small cell lung cancer (Kalyan et al. 2018). In 2013 Science voted Cancer immunotherapy as "breakthrough of the year" owing to observable success in clinical trials (Yang 2015) but the responses were variable within the same cohort and with same malignancy (Ventola 2017). Identification of specific biomarkers, immune checkpoint inhibitors and certain predictive tools can be helpful in improving the response rates as well as ease the identification of patients who can respond to immunotherapy (Pardoll 2015). At present the most studied form of cancer therapy is immunotherapy which works via acting on immune system along with chemotherapy.

Studies have shown the involvement of both innate and adaptive immunity in anti-cancer treatment where the former functions by releasing signals required for the stimulation of B-cells and T-cells. (Dranoff 2004; Woo, Corrales, and Gajewski 2015; Binder 2014). Adaptive immune system primarily comprises of B cells, CD8+ cytotoxic T cells as well as CD4+ helper T cells (Liu and Zeng 2012). Certain molecules such as antigen presenting cells (APC) recognize antigens and present them to naïve T-cells thus linking the innate and the adaptive immune system (Liu and Zeng 2012). Studies have shown the contribution of both the types of immunity for completely conquering cancer (Kakimi et al. 2017) where CD8+ cytotoxic T lymphocytes (CTLs) are chief warriors fighting against cancer. (Lesterhuis, Haanen, and Punt 2011). For an antitumor response tumor antigen should be recognized (Borghaei, Smith, and Campbell 2009).

NK cells also have ability to kill cancer cells via mechanisms: secretion of TNF-α, perforin, cytoplasmic granules and granzymes, expression of death receptor-mediated apoptosis, and expression of CD16 leading to antibody dependent cellular cytotoxicity (ADCC) (Brehm et al. 2014). Even macrophages hep in clearing the apoptotic cancer cells and are characterized as (Brehm et al. 2014; Becker et al. 2016) pro-inflammatory M1 or anti-inflammatory M2 macrophages.

Current Therapeutic Strategies

Currently, various treatment strategies such as immune check-point inhibitors, engineered T cell therapy, novel tumor antigens via next-generation sequencing have been developed for a new beginning of cancer immunotherapy (Becker et al. 2016; Dustin 2016). Cancer immunotherapy can be administered into two forms: active and passive, where former includes mAbs, lymphocytes or cytokines enhancing the already existing anti-tumor response (Dustin 2016); and the latter functions by stimulating the immune system to destroy the cancer cells via vaccination, non-specific immunomodulation, or targeting specific antigen receptors (Dustin 2016). Promising therapies have been described:

Monoclonal Antibodies

The function of monoclonal antibodies (mAbs) is to target the deregulated signal transduction pathways in cancer which have also been used in the treatment of solid as well as hematological malignancies (Dustin 2016; Maleki et al. 2013). The type of mAbs which are in use includes naked, conjugated and bispecific mAbs (Gül and van Egmond 2015) with naked mAbs being the most common which acts to boost the immune system and marks the cancer cells to get destroyed by the immune system.

An example of naked mAb is Alemtuzumab used for the treatment of chronic lymphocytic leukemia by its binding to CD52 antigen on lymphocytes (Neumann et al. 2016). Similarly others also function through their attachment to the antigens on the cancer cells ceasing their growth as in the case of traztuzumabuseful for breast and stomach cancer acting against HER2 (Pivot et al. 2015). The role of conjugated mAb's is to direct the entrance of chemotherapeutic agents or radioactive substances by joining to them (Teillaud 2012). Certain chemolabeled antibodies are also there with chemotherapeutic agents attached to them. For instance brentuximabvedotintargeting CD30 antigen present on the lymphocytes and useful for treating Hodgkin lymphoma and anaplastic large cell lymphoma (Chen and Chen 2015; Chen et al. 2015). Blinatumomab is a bispecific mAb approved for the treatment of acute lymphocytic leukemia (ALL) is made of 2 parts; one binds to CD3 and the other to CD19 and is used to treat acute lymphocytic leukemia (ALL) (Oak and Bartlett 2015). Possible side effects includes fever, chills, headache, weakness, nausea, diarrhea, rashes and hypotension (Thill 2015).

Cancer Vaccines

They work with the stimulation of the immune system and restoring its activity to fight against cancer (Ye et al. 2018). They can be further of two types' i.e., preventive vaccines and therapeutic vaccines (Speiser and Flatz 2014). They make the cancer cells easily recognizable by the immune system and help in preventing it to develop. Two vaccines have been approved by FDA i.e., hepatitis B virus (HBV) vaccines and human papilloma virus (HPV) vaccines (Hurley et al. 2016). They work via the activation of immune system aided by targeted T cells for the destruction of cancer cells. For example in case of prostate cancer treatment the activation process is carried out by isolating the patient's peripheral blood mononuclear cells and activating it *ex-vivo* in combination with recombinant fusion protein containing a prostate antigen prostatic acid phosphatase (PAP) conjugated to granulocyte-macrophage colony-stimulating factor (GM-CSF) and then administered back to the patient for activating PAP-specific T-cells. Inflammation is the most common side-effect known to occur with cancer vaccines (Sathyanarayanan and Neelapu 2015).

Adoptive T Cell Therapies and T Cell Engineering

Adoptive cell transfer is specifically used for hematologic malignancies as well as solid tumors (Restifo, Dudley, and Rosenberg 2012) and they have also showed promising results in clinical studies by using tumor-infiltrating lymphocytes (TIL's) in metastatic melanoma patients (Schmitt et al. 2015). Use of this therapy is limited due to expanding the viable TIL's but CAR- and T-cell engineered cells overcome this problem (Stone et al. 2012). Despite achieving encouraging results use of TCR technology is still in its infancy and is less attractive because of its MHC restricted nature limiting its development (Park, Rosenberg, and Morgan 2011).

CARs have antibody like structure compared to TCR's which gave them the ability to recognize MHC non restricted structures on target cell surfaces. In order to further improve the function of CAR certain components can be changed such as epitope-recognition part (Jackson and Brentjens 2015). Through modification these CAR T cells are expanded and administered back to the lymphodepleted cancer patients for the eradication of cancer

(Yang 2015). CD19 expressed on normal B-cells is the most investigated CAR target and studies have demonstrated 90% complete remission in refractory or relapsed ALL with anti-CD19 CAR T cells (Kusabuka et al. 2016). There are certain difficulties of this therapy in targeting of solid tumors as no suitable antigen could be found to be targeted (Klebanoff, Rosenberg, and Restifo 2016) in addition to its optimization for alleviating the toxicity (Liu et al. 2018).

Immune Checkpoint Blockade Therapy

Various checkpoint pathways are present in the immune system involved in T-cell activation and modulation of anti-tumor immunity (Thomas, Teicher, and Hassan 2016). This class of drugs facilitates the immune response, and molecules which are chiefly involved includes T-cell surface molecules CTLA-4, PD-1, T-cell immunoglobulin and mucin domain containing protein 3 (Tim-3) and lymphocyte activation gene-3 (LAG-3) (Makkouk and Weiner 2015). Ipilimumab was approved by FDA in 2011 as anti-CTLA4 for treating metastatic melanoma which led to a new era of cancer immunotherapy and similarly pembrolizumab and nivolumab were also approved in 2014 as anti-PD1 for the same disease (Barbee et al. 2015). Another anti-PD-L1 inhibitor atezolizumab (Kates et al. 2016) was approved for the treatment of bladder cancer and nivolumab for Hodgkin lymphoma. Checkpoint inhibitors also possess certain side-effects such as gastrointestinal, dermatologic, endocrine, hepatic and some inflammatory events (Ciccarese et al. 2016). Cancer immunotherapy is challenged by various factors creating problems for its translation into clinical setting which can be sorted with the use of Next-generation sequencing (NGS) (Charoentong et al. 2012). NGS aids in providing a novel insight into molecular machinery of the cancer cells. Another approach is biomarker-driven clinical trials which provide the advantage of recognizing the somatic mutations leading to potential targeted inhibition. (Mouw et al. 2017) Lastly, combination therapy can provide suitable dosing options with promising efficacy (Ishihara et al. 2017). To summarize, cancer immunotherapy made it possible to cure cancer patients with the development of cancer vaccines, CAR-T cell and checkpoint inhibitors. Combining immunotherapy with other therapies can prove to be a potential treatment strategy and a key treatment success with the recognition and management of toxicity.

Gene Therapy

During the last two decades there have been advances in human genomics which reveals host genome somatic aberrations as a very common cause of cancer. It was Rogers et al. who demonstrated first proof-of-concept for gene transfer via viral vectors where he observed the utility of virus to transfer foreign genetic material into the cells of interest (Rogers and Pfuderer 1968) which he further tested it in humans. These experiments made Roger the first person for performing the human gene therapy trial. In his study a wild-type Shope papilloma virus was used to introduce the gene for arginase into two subjects suffering from disorder of urea cycle (i.e., hyperargininemias) (Rogers et al. 1973; Terheggen et al. 1975). According to his hypothesis this gene would have naturally encoded the gene for arginase activity but the results were negative showing no change in arginine levels as well as no variations in clinical consequences.

Finally, US FDA approved 1st gene therapy protocol conducted in 1989. This protocol mentioned the use of tumor infiltrating lymphocytes (TIL's) extracted from patients of advanced melanoma conjugated with a marker gene *ex vivo* and further expanded *in vitro*, and final re-infusion into the patients (Rosenberg et al. 1990). Similarly, Cline et al. made another breakthrough in gene therapy by treating thalassaemia patients, by extracting their bone marrow cells followed by tranfection with human globulin gene containing plasmids *ex vivo* and delivering back to the patients (Wirth and Ylä-Herttuala 2014; Beutler 2001). This study was considered a milestone as it was carried out without the consent of the University of California, Los Angeles (UCLA) Institutional Review Board and also demonstrated the technicality and complexity of gene therapy.

Gene Therapy in Clinic

Despite several advances in the field of molecular biology and genetic engineering approach of using gene therapy have not shown much promise. Nonetheless, it can hold a potential of providing success in future owing to its promising results of long-term survival in a couple of studies. Below are some gene therapies being successfully translated clinically:

p53, one of the most important gene getting affected in many cancer types has been a subject for gene therapy. In 2001, a genetically modified Ad gene in E1B region known as ONYX-015 (*dl*1520), with an absence of a 55 kd gene (for restricting viral replication to p53 mutant cells), was tested in non-small cell lung carcinoma patients (Ahrendt et al. 2003). Phase I clinical trials observed well tolerability of the virus and its capability of shrinking the tumor with partial response rate not up-to the expectations as demonstrated in pre-clinical studies (response only in 3 patients out of 15). During a follow up in Phase II trial, intratumoral injections were administered in two cycles giving a response rate of 28% in treatment group in contrast to 12% in controls. When ONYX-50 was given alone or along with a chemotherapeutic agent in Phase III clinical trial, a response rate of 72.7% was seen compared to 40.4% in control group. Apart from this another clinical study was conducted utilizing prostate specific therapeutic adenovirus, CG7870 with viral replication under regulation of prostate cancer-specific promoter. However, the results were disappointing as there were no signs of tumor regression except a reduction of 25-49% in PSA levels in 5 patients (Reid, Warren, and Kirn 2002).

Gendicine was the first commercialized gene therapy for head and neck squamous cell cancer treatment, synthesized from an engineered adenovirus expressing wild type-*p53* regulated by *Rous sarcoma virus* (Raty et al. 2008). The efficacy of this therapy was evaluated in a Phase III clinical trial recruiting 132 patients where complete regression was observed in 64% of patients when used along with radiotherapy. Similarly, Advexin® (INGN 201; originally a product of Introgen Therapeutics, Inc., Austin, TX) was also reviewed for its clinical benefit in several cancers (Gabrilovich 2006).

Additionally clinical trials conducted with other tumor suppressor genes such as tumor necrosis factor alpha, TRAIL, interleukin-2, and *mda*-7/IL-24 genes exhibited promising results. In 2005, several investigators in their study published efficacy and well tolerability of replication incompetent adenovirus expressing *mda-7*/IL-24, Ad.*mda-7* (INGN-241) in patients with advanced cancers (Cunningham et al. 2005; Tong et al. 2005;Lebedeva et al. 2005; Fisher et al. 2007). Induction of apoptosis was observed with multiple intratumoral injections of Ad.*mda-7* owing to MDA-7/IL-24 expression resulting in shrinkage of more than 50% of the lesion with no signs of toxicity in 44% of the patients suggesting it to be safe and efficacious. Interestingly, it was demonstrated that MDA-7/IL-24 administration to patients induced significantly greater apoptosis compared to the ones who received Ad.p53 in non-small-cell lung cancer. A 64-year old patient of metastatic melanoma showed a considerable response compared to a patient with squamous cell carcinoma of the penis that showed a less dramatic response (Fisher 2005; Su et al. 2005; Gao et al. 2008; Sauane et al. 2008).

Modes of Transmission of the Genes

There has been development of several methods aiding in the transfer of genetic material into the target cells with the use of vectors. Two major categories are there which help in the transfer process which includes: viral (or bacterial) and non-viral vectors. Viral vectors usually function through its binding to the target cells and introducing the genetic material into it as part of their replication process. After their entrance into the target cells, transgenes can also be transferred which are being carried by the virus. Non-viral vectors make use of different approaches such as physical, chemical, as well as other modes of genetic transfer. Transfection is a process of transferring genetic material directly into cells while transduction is a process of moving them into cells with the help of a viral or bacterial vector. The safety and easy modifiability of non-viral vectors makes it advantageous over the viral vectors but is limited by lower transfection efficiency (Shirley, Heller, and Heller 2014).

Safety of Gene Therapy

In spite of tragic death of Jesse Gelsinger with the use of gene therapy via adenoviral vectors still satisfactory data of several gene therapies on safety has been collected. It should be noted that using viral vectors as a part of gene therapy can act as human pathogens leading to unwanted immune response due to the presence of antibodies against it. For instance, immune response can be generated in the form of cytokines if an adenovirus is injected into a human body, difference being this response will be serotype dependent. This was observed in a study by Thoma et al, where administration of adenovirus of the serotype 11 (Ad11) or 5 (Ad5) produced different responses with no/mild responses with Ad11 and moderate/severe toxicity with Ad5 (Thoma et al. 2013).

Several approaches have been developed to improve the safety profile of gene therapy such as targeting strategies for enhancing the delivery of gene transfer vectors hence improving the gene expression. This strategy will lead to better safety outcomes by improving the specificity as well as the transduction efficiency which are the major short-comings of gene therapy. This has been achieved by re-engineering the viral vectors using epitope insertion, chemical modification, and molecular evolution (Wang, Faust, and Rabinowitz 2011). Kim et al, in their Phase I trial have modified the RGD fiber knob on adenoviruses, for improvement of viral infectivity of cancer cells (Kim et al. 2011).

Further to improve the specificity and transduction efficiency modifications can be done on the viral surface proteins. For example, pseudotyping has been performed on lentiviral vectors by infusing cell type specific ligand or antibody to the viral envelope (Barnett, Crews, and Douglas 2002). This has certain limitations of compromising the vector entry into the cell resulting in low vector titers (Mátrai, Chuah, and Vanden Driessche 2010). In addition to this tissue-specific or conditional promoters can also be used such as use of hypoxia-specific regulatory systems whose function will be restricted to ischemic tissues (Kim, Mahato, and Lee 2009). Gene therapy has evolved to be a fascinating and a promising approach for treating various diseases including cancer. Current protocol focus on gene transfer vectors and *ex vivo* approaches of gene transfer with a limitation of low transduction efficiency posing as the biggest challenge of gene therapy along with involvement of high cost in vector manufacturing. Additionally gene therapy in combination with other modalities can offer benefit compared to using it alone. Genomic analysis of the patient and its tumour along with host immunity assessment can lead to determination of a suitable gene therapy. Further advances in biological research will make cheaper gene vectors which can be availed commercially thus transforming the future of gene therapy.

Stem Cell Transplant/Therapy

Stem cell transplant is generally used for haematological malignancies, leukemia and lymphoma. Nowadays various other cancers also involve the stem cell transplant based treatment modalities such as multiple myeloma and neuroblastoma. Even for other cancers such as pancreatic cancer colorectal cancer, stem cells may show potential therapeutic option (Chopra N et al. 2019). The preferred stem cells for the transplant or therapy is embryonic stem cells (ESC) and adult stem cells (ASC). Due to ethical issues, it is difficult to use ESC (Sagar J et al. 2007). ASC are taken from the bone marrow or peripheral blood. Generally, during the treatment, healthy blood-forming stem cells (multipotent stem cells) are injected into the patients whose cells have been destroyed due to the chemotherapy or radiation therapy or chemotherapy. Stem cell transplant can be autologous (stem cells of the patient itself), synergic (stem cells from the identical twin) and, allogenic (stem cells from an immunologically compatible donor such as relatives). Stem cells work directly as well as indirectly to decrease the tumor volume. In case of direct action, a Graft-versus-tumor reaction is generated in which the graft cells (donor stem cells) targets the tumor cells whereas when working indirectly stem cells increase the production of patient's own stem cells and also increases their efficiency to fight against cancer cells. Allogenic stem cells transplant (allo-SCT) also causes relapse in some cases; various immunotherapies are used along with allo-SCT or during the relapse shows improvement in case of acute myeloid leukemia (Sterling Cand Webster J., 2020).

Hormone Therapy

Hormone therapy is a type of a treatment that inhibits the growth of those cells which uses hormones for their growth and proliferation such as breast cancer, ovarian cancer and prostate cancer. Hormone therapy includes the use of small molecules or drugs that either inhibits the production of hormones or the action of hormones. In some cases, it also involves the removal of hormone producing gland. Hormone therapy generally involves breast cancer, prostate cancer, and ovarian cancer (Capper CP et al. 2016). Some other cancers also use hormone therapy such as parathyroid cancer (Grani G et al. 2019). Tamoxifen (FDA approved), and toremifene are the drugs that act on estrogen receptor and inhibit the estrogen action or estrogen mediated signaling pathway, ultimately prevent the cancer growth. These drugs mainly target the estrogen or progesterone receptors positive breast cancer. Fulvestrant (FDA approved) removes the estrogen receptor instead of blocking it, therefore abolishes the estrogen action. These drugs are effective in case of pre-menopausal breast cancer but, not in high risk post-menopausal breast cancer (Flötotto, T et al. 2001). For post-menopausal breast cancer, Raloxifene is the drug of choice which is approved by FDA (Provinciali N et al. 2016). Above mentioned drugs inhibit the hormone activity not the production of the hormones. Certain FDA approved drugs inhibit the production of estrogen such as anastrozole, exemestane, and letrozole. These drugs come under the class of aromatase inhibitors. These drugs are mainly used to treat the advanced stage post-menopausal breast cancer but studies have reported that these inhibitors cause cardiotoxicity in breast cancer patients (Foglietta J et al. 2017). Prostate cancer occurs due to the altered activity of male hormone i.e., testosterone. Therefore, in prostate cancer various drugs are used to block the receptor or testosterone activity or the production of testosterone. Studies show hormone therapy also increases the risk of other cancers and IBDs (Axelrad JE et al. 2020).

Conclusion

Cancer is a disease which has the ability to strike any part of the body. The scourge has been the part of multi cellular organisms from the beginning of time. After reading this chapter the users should be able to identify the different types of cancer, their site of formation, which cells/body parts do the various cancers impact, mechanism of formation, what gives the cancer the ability to spread across the human bodies. The student would have also understood the factors that influence whether the caner is benign or malignant, risk factors involved. We then describe the various treatment options available and the therapies which are still under investigation/research. The student should get a fair idea of existing treatments available, there advantages, disadvantages, probability of treatment, possible side effects. The fight against cancer is going to be a long one but there are few behavior patterns that all of us can inculcate for minimizing the chances of cancer. These are:

- By quitting smoking if you smoke
- Maintain a healthy lifestyle and body mass index
- Be physically active and exercise regularly.
- Do not eat processed foods.
- Moderate Alcohol consumption
- Avoid Excessive exposure to Sun.

Also in the end today one third of the cancers are potentially treatable but with progress being made in different approaches of treatment this number is going to keep in increasing with time.

References

Abbas, G., Danish, A. & Krasna, M. J. (2016). Stereotactic body radiotherapy and ablative therapies for lung cancer. *Surgical Oncology Clinics*, *25*(3), 553-566.

Adler, Jr. J. R., Chang, S. D., Murphy, M. J., Doty, J., Geis, P. & Hancock, S. L. (1997). The Cyberknife: a frameless robotic system for radiosurgery. *Stereotactic and functional neurosurgery*, *69*(1-4), 124-128.

Agostinis, P., Berg, K., Cengel, K. A., Foster, T. H., Girotti, A. W., Gollnick, S. O., Hahn, S. M., Hamblin, M. R., Juzeniene, A., Kessel, D., Korbelik, M., Moan, J., Mroz, P., Nowis, D., Piette, J., Wilson, B. C. & Golab, J. (2011). Photodynamic therapy of cancer: an update. *CA: a Cancer Journal for Clinicians*, *61* (4), 250–281.

Ahn, Y. C., Lee, K. C., Kim, D. Y., Huh, S. J., Yeo, I. H., Lim, D. H., Kim, M. K., Shin, K. H., Park, S. & Chang, S. H. (2000). Fractionated stereotactic radiation therapy for extracranial head and neck tumors. *International Journal of Radiation Oncology* Biology* Physics*, *48*(2), 501-505.

Ahrendt, S. A., Hu, Y., Buta, M., McDermott, M. P., Benoit, N., Yang, S. C., Wu, L. & Sidransky, D. (2003). p53 mutations and survival in stage I non-small-cell lung cancer: results of a prospective study. *Journal of the National Cancer Institute*, *95*(13), 961-970.

Ansell, S. M. (2018). "Hodgkin Lymphoma: 2018 Update on Diagnosis, Risk-Stratification, and Management." *American Journal of Hematology*, *93* (5), 704–15.

Arora, A. (2005). Role of Tyrosine Kinase Inhibitors in Cancer Therapy. *Journal of Pharmacology and Experimental Therapeutics*, *315* (3), 971–979.

Axelrad, J. E., Bazarbashi, A., Zhou, J., Castañeda, D., Gujral, A., Sperling, D., Glass, J., Agrawal, M., Hong, S., Lawlor, G., Hudesman, D., Chang, S., Shah, S., Yajnik, V., Ananthakrishnan, A., Khalili, H., Colombel, J. F., Itzkowitz, S. & New York Crohn's and Colitis Organization. (2020). Hormone Therapy for Cancer Is a Risk Factor for Relapse of Inflammatory Bowel Diseases. *Clinical Gastroenterology and Hepatology : the Official Clinical Practice Journal of the American Gastroenterological Association*, *18* (4), 872–880.e1.

Baba, A. L. & Cornel, C. (2007). *Tumor Cell Morphology*. The Publishing House of the Romanian Academy. https://www.ncbi.nlm.nih.gov/books/NBK9553/.

Barbee, M. S., Ogunniyi, A., Horvat, T. Z. & Dang, T. O. (2015). Current status and future directions of the immune checkpoint inhibitors ipilimumab, pembrolizumab, and nivolumab in oncology. *Annals of Pharmacotherapy*, *49*(8), 907-937.

Barnett, B. G., Crews, C. J. & Douglas, J. T. (2002). Targeted adenoviral vectors. *Biochimica et Biophysica Acta (BBA)-Gene Structure and Expression*, *1575*(1-3), 1-14.

Baskar, R., Lee, K. A., Yeo, R. & Yeoh, K. W. (2012). Cancer and radiation therapy: current advances and future directions. *International journal of medical sciences*, *9*(3), 193.

Baumann, M., Krause, M., Overgaard, J., Debus, J., Bentzen, S. M., Daartz, J., Richter, C., Zips, D. & Bortfeld, T. (2016). Radiation oncology in the era of precision medicine. *Nature Reviews Cancer*, *16*(4), 234.

Becker, P. S., Suck, G., Nowakowska, P., Ullrich, E., Seifried, E., Bader, P., Tonn, T. & Seidl, C. (2016). Selection and expansion of natural killer cells for NK cell-based immunotherapy. *Cancer Immunology, Immunotherapy*, *65*(4), 477-484.

Bernier, J., Hall, E. J. & Giaccia, A. (2004). Radiation oncology: a century of achievements. *Nature Reviews Cancer*, *4*(9), 737-747.

Beutler, E. (2001). The cline affair. *Molecular Therapy*, *4*(5), 396-397.

Binder, R. J. (2014). Functions of heat shock proteins in pathways of the innate and adaptive immune system. *The Journal of Immunology*, *193*(12), 5765-5771.

Borghaei, H., Smith, M. R. & Campbell, K. S. (2009). Immunotherapy of cancer. *European journal of pharmacology*, *625*(1-3), 41-54.

Brehm, C., Huenecke, S., Esser, R., Kloess, S., Quaiser, A., Betz, S., Zimmermann, O., Soerensen, J., Passweg, J. R., Klingebiel, T. & Schwabe, D. (2014). Interleukin-2-stimulated natural killer cells are less susceptible to mycophenolate mofetil than non-activated NK cells: possible consequences for immunotherapy. *Cancer Immunology, Immunotherapy*, *63*(8), 821-833.

Brown, G., Vicente-Dueñas, C. & Sánchez-García, I. (2020). Editorial: Epigenetic Reprogramming and Cancer Development. *Frontiers in Cell and Developmental Biology*, *8*, 12.

Bryder, D., Derrick, J. R. & Irving, L. W. (2006). "Hematopoietic Stem Cells." *The American Journal of Pathology*, *169* (2), 338–46.

Capper, C. P., Rae, J. M. & Auchus, R. J. (2016). The Metabolism, Analysis, and Targeting of Steroid Hormones in Breast and Prostate Cancer. *Hormones and Cancer*, *7* (3), 149–164.

Chao, M. P., Alizadeh, A. A., Tang, C., Jan, M., Weissman-Tsukamoto, R., Zhao, F., Park, C. Y., Weissman, I. L. & Majeti, R. (2011). Therapeutic antibody targeting of CD47 eliminates human acute lymphoblastic leukemia. *Cancer Research*, *71* (4), 1374–1384.

Charoentong, P., Angelova, M., Efremova, M., Gallasch, R., Hackl, H., Galon, J. & Trajanoski, Z. (2012). Bioinformatics for cancer immunology and immunotherapy. *Cancer Immunology, Immunotherapy*, *61*(11), 1885-1903.

Chen, H. H. & Kuo, M. T. (2017). Improving radiotherapy in cancer treatment: promises and challenges. *Oncotarget*, *8*(37), 62742.

Chen, R. & Chen, B. (2015). Brentuximab vedotin for relapsed or refractory Hodgkin's lymphoma. *Drug design, development and therapy*, *9*, 1729.

Chen, R., Hou, J., Newman, E., Kim, Y., Donohue, C., Liu, X., Thomas, S. H., Forman, S. J. & Kane, S. E. (2015). CD30 downregulation, MMAE resistance, and MDR1 upregulation are all associated with resistance to brentuximab vedotin. *Molecular cancer therapeutics*, *14*(6), 1376-1384.

Chen, B., Roskams, T. & de Witte, P. A. (2002). Antivascular tumor eradication by hypericin-mediated photodynamic therapy. *Photochemistry and Photobiology*, *76* (5), 509–513.

Chopra, N., Choudhury, S., Bhargava, S., Wajid, S. & Ganguly, N. K. (2019). Potentials of "stem cell-therapy" in pancreatic cancer: An update. *Pancreatology: official journal of the International Association of Pancreatology (IAP) ... [et al.]*, *19* (8), 1034–1042.

Chung, C. H., Wong, S., Ang, K. K., Hammond, E. H., Dicker, A. P., Harari, P. M. & Le, Q. T. (2007). Strategic plans to promote head and neck cancer translational research within the radiation therapy oncology group: a report from the translational research program. *International Journal of Radiation Oncology* Biology* Physics*, *69*(2), S67-S78.

Ciccarese, C., Alfieri, S., Santoni, M., Santini, D., Brunelli, M., Bergamini, C., Licitra, L., Montironi, R., Tortora, G. & Massari, F. (2016). New toxicity profile for novel immunotherapy agents: focus on immune-checkpoint inhibitors. *Expert opinion on drug metabolism & toxicology*, *12*(1), 57-75.

Combs, S. E., Widmer, V., Thilmann, C., Hof, H., Debus, J. & Schulz-Ertner, D. (2005). Stereotactic radiosurgery (SRS) treatment option for recurrent glioblastoma multiforme (GBM). *Cancer: Interdisciplinary International Journal of the American Cancer Society*, *104*(10), 2168-2173.

Connors, J. M. (2013). "Non-Hodgkin Lymphoma: The Clinician's Perspective—a View from the Receiving End." *Modern Pathology*, *26* (S1), S111–18.

Cortes, J. E., Moshe, T. & Hagop Kantarjian. (1996). "Chronic Myelogenous Leukemia: A Review." *The American Journal of Medicine*, *100* (5), 555–70.

Cunningham, C. C., Chada, S., Merritt, J. A., Tong, A., Senzer, N., Zhang, Y., Mhashilkar, A., Parker, K., Vukelja, S., Richards, D. & Hood, J. (2005). Clinical and local biological effects of an intratumoral injection of mda-7 (IL24; INGN 241) in patients with advanced carcinoma: a phase I study. *Molecular therapy*, *11*(1), 149-159.

Cunningham, A. P., Love, W. K., Zhang, R. W., Andrews, L. G. & Tollefsbol, T. O. (2006). Telomerase inhibition in cancer therapeutics: molecular-based approaches. *Current Medicinal Chemistry*, *13* (24), 2875–2888.

Dawood, S., Austin, L. & Cristofanilli, M. (2014). Cancer stem cells: implications for cancer therapy. *Oncology (Williston Park, N.Y.)*, *28* (12), 1101–1110.

Deepti, V. D., Manohar, H. D., Meena kumari, K. & Patil, N. (2016). Proteosome inhibitors: A targeted therapy. *Research Journal of Pharmaceutical, Biological and Chemical Sciences*, *7* (5), 488-497.

Delaney, G., Jacob, S., Featherstone, C. & Barton, M. (2005). The role of radiotherapy in cancer treatment: estimating optimal utilization from a review of evidence-based clinical guidelines. *Cancer: Interdisciplinary International Journal of the American Cancer Society*, *104*(6), 1129-1137.

Devita, V. T., Young, R. C. & Canellos, G. P. (1975). Combination versus single agent chemotherapy: A review of the basis for selection of drug treatment of cancer. *Cancer*, *35* (1), 98–110.

Dieterich, S. & Pawlicki, T. (2008). Cyberknife image-guided delivery and quality assurance. *International Journal of Radiation Oncology* Biology* Physics*, *71*(1), S126-S130.

Dilruba, S. & Kalayda, G. V. (2016). Platinum-based drugs: past, present and future. *Cancer Chemotherapy and Pharmacology*, *77* (6), 1103–1124.

Dolmans, D. E., Fukumura, D. & Jain, R. K. (2003). Photodynamic therapy for cancer. *Nature Reviews. Cancer*, *3* (5), 380–387.

Dranoff, G. (2004). Cytokines in cancer pathogenesis and cancer therapy. *Nature Reviews Cancer*, *4*(1), 11-22.

Dreicer, R. & Wilding, G. (1992). Steroid Hormone Agonists and Antagonists in the Treatment of Cancer. *Cancer Investigation*, *10* (1), 27–41.

Dustin, M. L. (2016). Cancer immunotherapy: killers on sterols. *Nature*, *531*(7596), 583-584.

El-Kenawi, A. E. & El-Remessy, A. B. (2013). Angiogenesis inhibitors in cancer therapy: mechanistic perspective on classification and treatment rationales. *British Journal of Pharmacology*, *170* (4), 712–729.

Feng, F. Y., Kim, H. M., Lyden, T. H., Haxer, M. J., Feng, M., Worden, F. P., Chepeha, D. B. & Eisbruch, A. (2007). Intensity-modulated radiotherapy of head and neck cancer aiming to reduce dysphagia: early dose–effect relationships for the swallowing structures. *International Journal of Radiation Oncology* Biology* Physics*, *68*(5), 1289-1298.

Fisher, P. B. (2005). Is mda-7/IL-24 a “magic bullet” for cancer?. *Cancer research*, *65*(22), 10128-10138.

Fisher, P. B., Sarkar, D., Lebedeva, I. V., Emdad, L., Gupta, P., Sauane, M., Su, Z. Z., Grant, S., Dent, P., Curiel, D. T. & Senzer, N. (2007). Melanoma differentiation associated gene-7/interleukin-24 (mda-7/IL-24): novel gene therapeutic for metastatic melanoma. *Toxicology and applied pharmacology*, *224*(3), 300-307.

Flötotto, T., Djahansouzi, S., Gläser, M., Hanstein, B., Niederacher, D., Brumm, C. & Beckmann, M. W. (2001). Hormones and Hormone Antagonists: Mechanisms of Action in Carcinogenesis of Endometrial and Breast Cancer. *Hormone and Metabolic Research*, *33* (8), 451–457.

Foglietta, J., Inno, A., de Iuliis, F., Sini, V., Duranti, S., Turazza, M., Tarantini, L. & Gori, S. (2017). Cardiotoxicity of Aromatase Inhibitors in Breast Cancer Patients. *Clinical Breast Cancer*, *17* (1), 11–17.

Franchi, A. (2012). "Epidemiology and Classification of Bone Tumors." *Clinical Cases in Mineral and Bone Metabolism*, *9* (2), 92–95.

Gabrilovich, D. I. (2006). INGN 201 (Advexin®): adenoviral p53 gene therapy for cancer. *Expert opinion on biological therapy*, *6*(8), 823-832.

Gao, P., Sun, X., Chen, X., Wang, Y., Foster, B. A., Subjeck, J., Fisher, P. B. & Wang, X. Y. (2008). Secretable chaperone Grp170 enhances therapeutic activity of a novel tumor suppressor, mda-7/IL-24. *Cancer research*, *68*(10), 3890-3898.

Gascoigne, K. E. & Taylor, S. S. (2009). How do anti-mitotic drugs kill cancer cells? *Journal of Cell Science*, *122* (15), 2579–2585.

Gill, S., Thomas, J., Fox, C., Kron, T., Rolfo, A., Leahy, M., Chander, S., Williams, S., Tai, K. H., Duchesne, G. M. & Foroudi, F. (2011). Acute toxicity in prostate cancer patients treated with and without image-guided radiotherapy. *Radiation Oncology*, *6*(1), 145.

Ginestier, C., Liu, S., Diebel, M. E., Korkaya, H., Luo, M., Brown, M., Wicinski, J., Cabaud, O., Charafe-Jauffret, E., Birnbaum, D., Guan, J. L., Dontu, G. & Wicha, M. S. (2010). CXCR1 blockade selectively targets human breast cancer stem cells *in vitro* and in xenografts. *The Journal of Clinical Investigation*, *120* (2), 485–497.

Grani, G., Ramundo, V., Verrienti, A., Sponziello, M. & Durante, C. (2019). Thyroid hormone therapy in differentiated thyroid cancer. *Endocrine*, *66* (1), 43–50.

Grubbe, E. H. (1933). Priority in the therapeutic use of X-rays. *Radiology*, *21*(2), 156-162.

Gül, N. & van Egmond, M. (2015). Antibody-dependent phagocytosis of tumor cells by macrophages: a potent effector mechanism of monoclonal antibody therapy of cancer. *Cancer research*, *75*(23), 5008-5013.

Ha, T.Y. (2011). MicroRNAs in Human Diseases: From Autoimmune Diseases to Skin, Psychiatric and Neurodegenerative Diseases. Immune Netw, 11(5), 227–244.

Hall, E. J. & Wuu, C. S. (2003). Radiation-induced second cancers: the impact of 3D-CRT and IMRT. *International Journal of Radiation Oncology* Biology* Physics*, *56*(1), 83-88.

Hallek, M. (2019). "Chronic Lymphocytic Leukemia: 2020 Update on Diagnosis, Risk Stratification and Treatment." *American Journal of Hematology*, *94* (11), 1266–87.

Hamilton, D. G., Bale, R., Jones, C., Fitzgerald, E., Khor, R., Knight, K. & Wasiak, J. (2016). Impact of tumour bed boost integration on acute and late toxicity in patients with breast cancer: A systematic review. *The Breast*, *27*, 126-135.

Hanahan, D. & Robert, A. W. (2000). "The Hallmarks of Cancer." *Cell*, *100* (1), 57–70.

Hanahan, D. & Robert, A. W. (2011). "Hallmarks of Cancer: The next Generation." *Cell*, *144* (5), 646–74.

Hande, K. R. (1998). Etoposide: four decades of development of a topoisomerase II inhibitor. *European journal of cancer (Oxford, England: 1990)*, *34* (10), 1514–1521.

Hande, K. R. (2008). Topoisomerase II inhibitors. *Update on Cancer Therapeutics*, *3* (1), 13–26.

Hassan, S. & de Vos, J. (2018). Stem cell Transplantation, *ABC of Clinical Haematology*, Chapter-12, fourth edition.

Hassanpour, S. H. & Mohammadamin, D. (2017). Review of Cancer from Perspective of Molecular." *Journal of Cancer Research and Practice*, *4* (4), 127–29.

Haynes, B., Murai, J. & Lee, J. M. (2018). Restored Replication Fork Stabilization, a Mechanism of PARP Inhibitor Resistance, Can Be Overcome by Cell Cycle Checkpoint Inhibition. *Cancer Treatment Reviews*, *71*, 1–7.

Hoang, N. T., Luis, A. A., Michael, J. M. & Bhairavi, T. (2018). "A Review of Soft-Tissue Sarcomas: Translation of Biological Advances into Treatment Measures." *Cancer Management and Research*, *10*, 1089–1114.

Hurley, L. P., Bridges, C. B., Harpaz, R., Allison, M. A., Leary, S. T. O., Crane, L. A., Brtnikova, M., Stokley, S., Beaty, B. L., Jimenez-Zambrano, A. & Kempe, A. (2016). Physician attitudes toward adult vaccines and other preventive practices, United States, 2012. *Public Health Reports*, *131*(2), 320-330.

Hwang, H.W. & Mendell J.T. (2006). MicroRNAs in cell proliferation, cell death, and tumorigenesis. *Br J Cancer*, 94(6), 776–780.

Ishihara, D., Pop, L., Takeshima, T., Iyengar, P. & Hannan, R. (2017). Rationale and evidence to combine radiation therapy and immunotherapy for cancer treatment. *Cancer Immunology, Immunotherapy*, *66*(3), 281-298.

Ismael, G. F. V., Rosa, D. D., Mano, M. S. & Awada, A. (2008). Novel cytotoxic drugs: Old challenges, new solutions. *Cancer Treatment Reviews*, *34*(1), 81–91.

Jackson, H. J. & Brentjens, R. J. (2015). Overcoming antigen escape with CAR T-cell therapy. *Cancer discovery*, *5*(12), 1238-1240.

Jaffray, D. A., Siewerdsen, J. H., Wong, J. W. & Martinez, A. A. (2002). Flat-panel cone-beam computed tomography for image-guided radiation therapy. *International Journal of Radiation Oncology* Biology* Physics*, *53*(5), 1337-1349.

Jafri, M. A., Ansari, S. A., Alqahtani, M. H. & Shay, J. W. (2016). Roles of telomeres and telomerase in cancer, and advances in telomerase-targeted therapies. *Genome Medicine*, *8* (1), 69.

Jiang, M. N., Nora, B. & Andrew, L. F. (2017). "Lymphoma Classification Update: B-Cell Non-Hodgkin Lymphomas." *Expert Review of Hematology*, *10* (5), 405–15.

Kakimi, K., Karasaki, T., Matsushita, H. & Sugie, T. (2017). Advances in personalized cancer immunotherapy. *Breast Cancer*, *24*(1), 16-24.

Kalyan, A., Kircher, S., Shah, H., Mulcahy, M. & Benson, A. (2018). Updates on immunotherapy for colorectal cancer. *Journal of gastrointestinal oncology*, *9*(1), 160.

Kates, M., Sopko, N. A., Matsui, H., Drake, C. G., Hahn, N. M. & Bivalacqua, T. J. (2016). Immune checkpoint inhibitors: a new frontier in bladder cancer. *World journal of urology*, *34*(1), 49-55.

Kaul, D., Malik, D. (2012). MIR196B (microRNA 196b). *Atlas Genet Cytogenet Oncol Haematol.*;16(5):357-360.

Kaul, D., Malik, D., Wani, S. (2019). Cellular miR-2909 RNomics governs the genes that ensure immune checkpoint regulation. *Molecular and cellular biochemistry*, 451, (1-2), 37-42

Kaushik, H., Malik, D., Parsad, D., Kaul D. (2019). Mitochondrial respiration is restricted by miR-2909 within human melanocytes. *Pigment cell & melanoma research*, 32 (4), 584-587.

Khan, O. & La Thangue, N. B. (2011). HDAC inhibitors in cancer biology: emerging mechanisms and clinical applications. *Immunology and Cell Biology*, *90* (1), 85–94.

Kim, H. A., Mahato, R. I. & Lee, M. (2009). Hypoxia-specific gene expression for ischemic disease gene therapy. *Advanced drug delivery reviews*, *61*(7-8), 614-622.

Kim, K. H., Ryan, M. J., Estep, J. E., Miniard, B. M., Rudge, T. L., Peggins, J. O., Broadt, T. L., Wang, M., Preuss, M. A., Siegal, G. P. & Hemminki, A. (2011). A new generation of serotype chimeric infectivity-enhanced conditionally replicative adenovirals: the safety profile of Ad5/3-Δ24 in advance of a phase I clinical trial in ovarian cancer patients. *Human gene therapy*, *22*(7), 821-828.

Klebanoff, C. A., Rosenberg, S. A. & Restifo, N. P. (2016). Prospects for gene-engineered T cell immunotherapy for solid cancers. *Nature medicine*, *22*(1), 26.

Kusabuka, H., Fujiwara, K., Tokunaga, Y., Hirobe, S., Nakagawa, S. & Okada, N. (2016). Highly efficient gene transfer using a retroviral vector into murine T cells for preclinical chimeric antigen receptor-expressing

T cell therapy. *Biochemical and biophysical research communications*, *473*(1), 73-79.

Kondo, M. (2010). “Lymphoid and Myeloid Lineage Commitment in Multipotent Hematopoietic Progenitors.” *Immunological Reviews*, *238* (1), 37–46.

Korbelik, M. (2006). PDT-associated host response and its role in the therapy outcome. *Lasers in Surgery and Medicine*, *38* (5), 500–508.

Kuşoğlu, A. & Biray Avcı, Ç. (2019). Cancer stem cells: A brief review of the current status. *Gene*, *681*, 80–85.

LaCasse, E. C., Baird, S., Korneluk, R. G. & MacKenzie, A. E. (1998). The inhibitors of apoptosis (IAPs) and their emerging role in cancer. *Oncogene*, *17* (25), 3247–3259.

Lambin, P., Zindler, J., Vanneste, B. G., Van De Voorde, L., Eekers, D., Compter, I., Panth, K. M., Peerlings, J., Larue, R. T., Deist, T. M. & Jochems, A. (2017). Decision support systems for personalized and participative radiation oncology. *Advanced drug delivery reviews*, *109*, 131-153.

Langen, K. M. & Jones, D. T. L. (2001). Organ motion and its management. *International Journal of Radiation Oncology* Biology* Physics*, *50*(1), 265-278.

Lebedeva, I. V., Sauane, M., Gopalkrishnan, R. V., Sarkar, D., Su, Z. Z., Gupta, P., Nemunaitis, J., Cunningham, C., Yacoub, A., Dent, P. & Fisher, P. B. (2005). mda-7/IL-24: exploiting cancer’s Achilles’ heel. *Molecular Therapy*, *11*(1), 4-18.

Lee, H., Han, J., Shin, H., Han, H., Na, K. & Kim, H. (2018). Combination of chemotherapy and photodynamic therapy for cancer treatment with sonoporation effects. *Journal of Controlled Release: Official Journal of the Controlled Release Society*, *283*, 190–199.

Lee, Y. T., Tan, Y. J. & Oon, C. E. (2018). Molecular targeted therapy: Treating cancer with specificity. *European Journal of Pharmacology*, *834*, 188–196.

Lee, Y. T., Tan, Y. J. & Oon, C. E. (2018). Molecular targeted therapy: Treating cancer with specificity. *European Journal of Pharmacology*, *834*, 188–196.

Leroy, R., Benahmed, N., Hulstaert, F., Van Damme, N. & De Ruysscher, D. (2016). Proton therapy in children: a systematic review of clinical effectiveness in 15 pediatric cancers. *International Journal of Radiation Oncology* Biology* Physics*, *95*(1), 267-278.

Lesterhuis, W. J., Haanen, J. B. & Punt, C. J. (2011). Cancer immunotherapy–revisited. *Nature reviews Drug discovery*, *10*(8), 591-600.

Lin, K. Y. & Kraus, W. L. (2017). PARP Inhibitors for Cancer Therapy. *Cell*, *169* (2), 183.

Liu, E., Tong, Y., Dotti, G., Shaim, H., Savoldo, B., Mukherjee, M., Orange, J., Wan, X., Lu, X., Reynolds, A. & Gagea, M. (2018). Cord blood NK cells engineered to express IL-15 and a CD19-targeted CAR show long-term persistence and potent antitumor activity. *Leukemia*, *32*(2), 520-531.

Liu, Y. & Zeng, G. (2012). Cancer and innate immune system interactions: translational potentials for cancer immunotherapy. *Journal of immunotherapy (Hagerstown, Md.: 1997)*, *35*(4), 299.

Lo, S. S., Fakiris, A. J., Chang, E. L., Mayr, N. A., Wang, J. Z., Papiez, L., Teh, B. S., McGarry, R. C., Cardenes, H. R. & Timmerman, R. D. (2010). Stereotactic body radiation therapy: a novel treatment modality. *Nature reviews Clinical oncology*, *7*(1), 44.

Luengo, A., Gui, D. Y. & Vander Heiden, M. G. (2017). Targeting Metabolism for Cancer Therapy. *Cell chemical biology*, *24* (9), 1161–1180.

Mackie, T. R., Holmes, T., Swerdloff, S., Reckwerdt, P., Deasy, J. O., Yang, J., Paliwal, B. & Kinsella, T. (1993). Tomotherapy: a new concept for the delivery of dynamic conformal radiotherapy. *Medical physics*, *20*(6), 1709-1719.

Maleki, L. A., Baradaran, B., Majidi, J., Mohammadian, M. & Shahneh, F. Z. (2013). Future prospects of monoclonal antibodies as magic bullets in immunotherapy. *Human antibodies*, *22*(1-2), 9-13.

Malik, D., Kaul, D. (2018). Human cellular mitochondrial remodelling is governed by miR-2909 RNomics. *PLoS ONE*, 13(9), e0203614.

Malik, D., Kaul, D. (2015). KLF4 Genome: A double edged sword. *J Solid Tumors*, 5, 49-64

Malik, D., Kaul, D., Chauhan, N., Marwaha, R.K. (2014). miR-2909-mediated regulation of KLF4: a novel molecular mechanism for differentiating between B-cell and T-cell pediatric acute lymphoblastic leukemias. *Molecular Cancer*, 13 (1), 175.

Malik D, Sharma A, Raina A, Kaul D (2015). Deregulated blood cellular miR-2909 RNomics observed in Rhematoid Arthritis Patients. *Archives of Medicine*, 7:1:1.

Mani, H. & Elaine, S. J. (2009). "Hodgkin Lymphoma: An Update On Its Biology With Newer Insights Into Classification." *Clinical Lymphoma and Myeloma*, *9* (3), 206–16.

Marginean, C. O., Lorena, E. M., Emoke, H., Horea, G. & Mihaela, I. C. (2018). "Non-Hodgkin Lymphoma, Diagnostic, and Prognostic Particularities in Children – a Series of Case Reports and a Review of the Literature (CARE Compliant)." *Medicine*, *97* (8), e9802.

Matasar, M. & Andrew, Z. (2008). "Overview of Lymphoma Diagnosis and Management." *Radiologic Clinics of North America*, *46*, 175–98, vii.

Matloob, S. A., Nasir, H. A. & Choi, D. (2016). Proton beam therapy in the management of skull base chordomas: systematic review of indications, outcomes, and implications for neurosurgeons. *British journal of neurosurgery*, *30*(4), 382-387.

Mátrai, J., Chuah, M. K. & VandenDriessche, T. (2010). Recent advances in lentiviral vector development and applications. *Molecular therapy*, *18*(3), 477-490.

McCormick, B. & Hunt, M. (2011, January). Intensity-modulated radiation therapy for breast: is it for everyone? In *Seminars in radiation oncology*, (Vol. *21*, No. 1, 51-54). WB Saunders.

Mead, G. M. & Jacobs, C. (1982). Changing role of chemotherapy in treatment of head and neck cancer. *The American Journal of Medicine*, *73* (4), 582–595.

Mohan, R. & Grosshans, D. (2017). Proton therapy–present and future. *Advanced drug delivery reviews*, *109*, 26-44.

Morgan-Fletcher, S. L. (2001). Prescribing, recording and reporting photon beam therapy (Supplement to ICRU Report 50), *ICRU Report* 62. ICRU, pp. ix+ 52, 1999 (ICRU Bethesda, MD) $65.00 ISBN 0-913394-61-0.

Mouw, K. W., Goldberg, M. S., Konstantinopoulos, P. A. & D'Andrea, A. D. (2017). DNA damage and repair biomarkers of immunotherapy response. *Cancer discovery*, *7*(7), 675-693.

Mroz, P., Yaroslavsky, A., Kharkwal, G. B. & Hamblin, M. R. (2011). Cell death pathways in photodynamic therapy of cancer. *Cancers*, *3* (2), 2516–2539.

Mukesh, M. B., Barnett, G. C., Wilkinson, J. S., Moody, A. M., Wilson, C., Dorling, L., Chan Wah Hak, C., Qian, W., Twyman, N., Burnet, N. G. & Wishart, G. C. (2013). Randomized controlled trial of intensity-modulated radiotherapy for early breast cancer: 5-year results confirm superior overall cosmesis. *Journal of clinical oncology*, *31*(36), 4488-4495.

Mukhtar, E., Adhami, V. M. & Mukhtar, H. (2014). Targeting Microtubules by Natural Agents for Cancer Therapy. *Molecular Cancer Therapeutics*, *13* (2), 275–284.

Narayanasamy, G., Saenz, D., Cruz, W., Ha, C. S., Papanikolaou, N. & Stathakis, S. (2016). Commissioning an Elekta Versa HD linear accelerator. *Journal of applied clinical medical physics*, *17*(1), 179-191.

Neumann, T., Schneidewind, L., Thiele, T., Schulze, M., Klenner, A. F., Busemann, C., Pink, D., Greinacher, A., Dölken, G. & Krüger, W. H., (2016). Reduced platelet transfusions and earlier platelet engraftment using alemtuzumab-based conditioning regimen in allogeneic stem cell transplantation. *Journal of cancer research and clinical oncology*, *142*(5), 1091-1097.

Oak, E. & Bartlett, N. L. (2015). Blinatumomab for the treatment of B-cell lymphoma. *Expert opinion on investigational drugs*, *24*(5), 715-724.

Otto, K. (2008). Volumetric modulated arc therapy: IMRT in a single gantry arc. *Medical physics*, *35*(1), 310-317.

Pardoll, D. (2015, August). Cancer and the immune system: basic concepts and targets for intervention. In *Seminars in oncology*, (Vol. *42*, No. 4, 523-538). WB Saunders.

Park, T. S., Rosenberg, S. A. & Morgan, R. A. (2011). Treating cancer with genetically engineered T cells. *Trends in biotechnology*, *29*(11), 550-557.

Passegue, E., Jamieson, C. H., Ailles, L. E. & Weissman, I. L. (2003). "Normal and Leukemic Hematopoiesis: Are Leukemias a Stem Cell Disorder or a Reacquisition of Stem Cell Characteristics?" *Proceedings of the National Academy of Sciences*, *100* (Supplement 1), 11842–49.

Pignol, J. P., Olivotto, I., Rakovitch, E., Gardner, S., Sixel, K., Beckham, W., Vu, T. T. T., Truong, P., Ackerman, I. & Paszat, L. (2008). A multicenter randomized trial of breast intensity-modulated radiation therapy to reduce acute radiation dermatitis. *Journal of Clinical Oncology*, *26*(13), 2085-2092.

Pivot, X., Aulagner, G., Blay, J. Y., Fumoleau, P., Kaliski, A., Sarkozy, F. & Limat, S. (2015). Challenges in the implementation of trastuzumab biosimilars: an expert panel's recommendations. *Anti-cancer drugs*, *26*(10), 1009-1016.

Pommier, Y. (2006). Topoisomerase I inhibitors: camptothecins and beyond. *Nature Reviews Cancer*, *6* (10), 789–802.

Potters, L., Kavanagh, B., Galvin, J. M., Hevezi, J. M., Janjan, N. A., Larson, D. A., Mehta, M. P., Ryu, S., Steinberg, M., Timmerman, R. & Welsh, J. S. (2010). American Society for Therapeutic Radiology and Oncology (ASTRO) and American College of Radiology (ACR) practice guideline for the performance of stereotactic body radiation therapy. *International Journal of Radiation Oncology• Biology• Physics*, *76*(2), 326-332.

Ralhan, R. & Kaur, J. (2007). Alkylating agents and cancer therapy. *Expert Opinion on Therapeutic Patents*, *17* (9), 1061–1075.

Ramamurthy, R., Hughes, M., Morris, V., Bolouri, H., Gerbing, R.B., Wang, Y.C., Loken, M. R., Raimondi, S. C., Hirsch, B.A., Gamis, A.S., Oehler, V. G., Alonzo, T.A. & Meshinchi, S. (2016). miR-155 expression and correlation with clinical outcome in pediatric AML: A report from Children's Oncology Group. *Pediatr Blood Cancer*. 63(12): 2096–2103.

Ramadoss, M. & Mahadevan, V. (2018). Targeting the cancer epigenome: synergistic therapy with bromodomain inhibitors. *Drug Discovery Today*, *23* (1), 6–89.

Raty, J. K., Pikkarainen, J. T., Wirth, T. & Yla-Herttuala, S. (2008). Gene therapy: the first approved gene-based medicines, molecular mechanisms and clinical indications. *Current molecular pharmacology*, *1*(1), 13-23.

Reid, T., Warren, R. & Kirn, D. (2002). Intravascular adenoviral agents in cancer patients: lessons from clinical trials. *Cancer gene therapy*, *9*(12), 979-986.

Restifo, N. P., Dudley, M. E. & Rosenberg, S. A. (2012). Adoptive immunotherapy for cancer: harnessing the T cell response. *Nature Reviews Immunology*, *12*(4), 269-281.

Ringborg, U., Bergqvist, D., Brorsson, B., Cavallin-Ståhl, E., Ceberg, J., Einhorn, N., Frödin, J. E., Järhult, J., Lamnevik, G., Lindholm, C. & Littbrand, B. (2003). The Swedish Council on Technology Assessment in Health Care (SBU) systematic overview of radiotherapy for cancer including a prospective survey of radiotherapy practice in Sweden 2001--summary and conclusions. *Acta Oncologica*, *42*(5-6), 357-365.

Rogers, S. & Pfuderer, P. (1968). Use of viruses as carriers of added genetic information. *Nature*, *219*(5155), 749-751.

Rogers, S., Lowenthal, A., Terheggen, H. G. & Columbo, J. P. (1973). Induction of arginase activity with the *Shope papilloma* virus in tissue culture cells from an argininemic patient. *Journal of Experimental Medicine*, *137*(4), 1091-1096.

Rosenberg, S. A., Aebersold, P., Cornetta, K., Kasid, A., Morgan, R. A., Moen, R., Karson, E. M., Lotze, M. T., Yang, J. C., Topalian, S. L. & Merino, M. J. (1990). Gene transfer into humans—immunotherapy of patients with advanced melanoma, using tumor-infiltrating lymphocytes modified by retroviral gene transduction. *New England Journal of Medicine*, *323*(9), 570-578.

Roskoski, R. Jr. (2019). Properties of FDA-approved small molecule protein kinase inhibitors. *Pharmacological Research*, *144*, 19–50.

Sagar, J., Chaib, B., Sales, K., Winslet, M. & Seifalian, A. (2007). Role of stem cells in cancer therapy and cancer stem cells: a review. *Cancer Cell International*, *7* (1), 9.

Sandoval, M. & Harris, L. (2014). Cancer stem cells. *Oncology (Williston Park, N.Y.)*, *28* (12), 1110–1114.

Sathyanarayanan, V. & Neelapu, S. S. (2015). Cancer immunotherapy: Strategies for personalization and combinatorial approaches. *Molecular oncology*, *9*(10), 2043-2053.

Sauane, M., Su, Z. Z., Gupta, P., Lebedeva, I. V., Dent, P., Sarkar, D. & Fisher, P. B. (2008). Autocrine regulation of mda-7/IL-24 mediates cancer-specific apoptosis. *Proceedings of the National Academy of Sciences*, *105*(28), 9763-9768.

Saultz, J. N. & Ramiro, G. (2016). "Acute Myeloid Leukemia: A Concise Review." *Journal of Clinical Medicine*, *5* (3), 33.

Schmitt, T. M., Stromnes, I. M., Chapuis, A. G. & Greenberg, P. D. (2015). New strategies in engineering T-cell receptor gene-modified T cells to more effectively target malignancies. *Clinical Cancer Research*, *21*(23), 5191-5197.

Schreiber, R. D., Old, L. J. & Smyth, M. J. (2011). Cancer immunoediting: integrating immunity's roles in cancer suppression and promotion. *Science*, *331*(6024), 1565-1570.

Scott, J. G., Berglund, A., Schell, M. J., Mihaylov, I., Fulp, W. J., Yue, B., Welsh, E., Caudell, J. J., Ahmed, K., Strom, T. S. & Mellon, E. (2017). A genome-based model for adjusting radiotherapy dose (GARD): a retrospective, cohort-based study. *The Lancet Oncology*, *18*(2), 202-211.

Seita, J. & Irving, L. W. (2010). "Hematopoietic Stem Cell: Self-Renewal versus Differentiation." *Wiley Interdisciplinary Reviews. Systems Biology and Medicine*, *2* (6), 640–53.

Shanbhag, S. & Richard, F. A. (2018). "Hodgkin Lymphoma: A Review and Update on Recent Progress." *CA: A Cancer Journal for Clinicians*, *68* (2), 116–32.

Sharma, S., Kaul, D., Arora, M., Malik, D., (2015). Oncogenic nature of a novel mutant AATF and its interactome existing within human cancer cells. *Cell Biol Int.*, 39 (3):326-333.

Shawver, L. K., Slamon, D. & Ullrich, A. (2002). Smart drugs: Tyrosine kinase inhibitors in cancer therapy. *Cancer Cell*, *1* (2), 117–123.

Slade, D. (2020). PARP and PARG inhibitors in cancer treatment. *Genes and Development*, *34* (5-6), 360–394.

Shirley, S. A., Heller, R. & Heller, L. C. (2014). Electroporation gene therapy. In *Gene Therapy of Cancer* (93-106). Academic Press.

Su, Z., Emdad, L., Sauane, M., Lebedeva, I. V., Sarkar, D., Gupta, P., James, C. D., Randolph, A., Valerie, K., Walter, M. R. & Dent, P., (2005). Unique aspects of mda-7/IL-24 antitumor bystander activity: establishing a role for secretion of MDA-7/IL-24 protein by normal cells. *Oncogene*, *24*(51), 7552-7566.

Speiser, D. E. & Flatz, L. (2014). Cancer immunotherapy drives implementation science in oncology. *Human vaccines & immunotherapeutics*, *10*(11), 3107-3110.

Springfeld, C., Hackert, T., Jäger, D., Büchler, M. W. & Neoptolemos, J. P. (2020). Neoadjuvante und adjuvante Therapie beim Pankreaskarzinom [Neoadjuvant and adjuvant treatment of pancreatic cancer]. *Der Chirurg; Zeitschrift fur alle Gebiete der operativen Medizen*, 10.1007/s00104-020-01169-9. Advance online publication.

Sterling, C. & Webster, J. (2020). Harnessing the immune system after allogeneic stem cell transplant in acute myeloid leukemia. *American Journal of Hematology*, *95* (5), 529–547.

Stone, J. D., Chervin, A. S., Aggen, D. H. & Kranz, D. M. (2012). T cell receptor engineering. In *Methods in enzymology*, (Vol. *503*, 189-222). Academic Press.

Sun, J., Wei, Q., Zhou, Y., Wang, J., Liu, Q. & Xu, H. (2017). A systematic analysis of FDA-approved anticancer drugs. *BMC Systems Biology*, *11*(Suppl 5), 87.

Teillaud, J. L. (2012). From whole monoclonal antibodies to single domain antibodies: think small. In *Single Domain Antibodies*, (3-13). Humana Press, Totowa, NJ.

Terheggen, H. G., Lowenthal, A., Lavinha, F., Colombo, J. P. & Rogers, S. (1975). Unsuccessful trial of gene replacement in arginase deficiency. *European Journal of Pediatrics*, *119*(1), 1-3.

Terwilliger, T. & Abdul-Hay, M. (2017). "Acute Lymphoblastic Leukemia: A Comprehensive Review and 2017 Update." *Blood Cancer Journal*, *7* (6), e577.

Thill, M. (2015). New frontiers in oncology: biosimilar monoclonal antibodies for the treatment of breast cancer. *Expert review of anticancer therapy*, *15*(3), 331-338.

Thoma, C., Bachy, V., Seaton, P., Green, N. K., Greaves, D. R., Klavinskis, L., Seymour, L. W. & Morrison, J. (2013). Adenovirus serotype 11 causes less long-term intraperitoneal inflammation than serotype 5: implications for ovarian cancer therapy. *Virology*, *447*(1-2), 74-83.

Thomas, A., Teicher, B. A. & Hassan, R. (2016). Antibody–drug conjugates for cancer therapy. *The Lancet Oncology*, *17*(6), e254-e262.

Timon, G., Ciardo, D., Bazani, A., Garioni, M., Maestri, D., De Lorenzo, D., Pansini, F., Cambria, R., Rondi, E., Cattani, F. & Marvaso, G. (2016). Rationale and protocol of AIRC IG-13218, short-term radiotherapy for early prostate cancer with concomitant boost to the dominant lesion. *Tumor Journal*, *102*(5), 536-540.

Tipton, K., Launders, J. H., Inamdar, R., Miyamoto, C. & Schoelles, K. (2011). Stereotactic body radiation therapy: scope of the literature. *Annals of internal medicine*, *154*(11), 737-745.

Tong, A. W., Nemunaitis, J., Su, D., Zhang, Y., Cunningham, C., Senzer, N., Netto, G., Rich, D., Mhashilkar, A., Parker, K. & Coffee, K. (2005). Intratumoral injection of INGN 241, a nonreplicating adenovector expressing the melanoma-differentiation associated gene-7 (mda-7/IL24): biologic outcome in advanced cancer patients. *Molecular therapy*, *11*(1), 160-172.

Tucker, M. A., Meadows, A. T., Boice, J. D., Jr. Stovall, M., Oberlin, O., Stone, B. J., Birch, J., Voûte, P. A., Hoover, R. N. & Fraumeni, J. F. Jr. (1987). Leukemia after therapy with alkylating agents for childhood cancer. *Journal of the National Cancer Institute*, *78* (3), 459–464.

Vassilev, L. T. (2007). MDM2 inhibitors for cancer therapy. *Trends in Molecular Medicine*, *13* (1), 23–31.

Ventola, C. L. (2017). Cancer immunotherapy, part 3: challenges and future trends. *Pharmacy and Therapeutics*, *42*(8), 514.

Vicini, F. A., Sharpe, M., Kestin, L., Martinez, A., Mitchell, C. K., Wallace, M. F., Matter, R. & Wong, J. (2002). Optimizing breast cancer treatment efficacy with intensity-modulated radiotherapy. *International Journal of Radiation Oncology* Biology* Physics*, *54*(5), 1336-1344.

Visconti, R., Della Monica, R. & Grieco, D. (2016). Cell cycle checkpoint in cancer: a therapeutically targetable double-edged sword. *Journal of Experimental and Clinical Cancer Research: CR*, *35* (1), 153.

Viseur, C. le., Marc, H., Simon, B., Kerrie, W., Silja, R., André, S., Annegret, R., Julie, I., Ronald, W. S., Leonard, D. S., Jochen, H., Heribert, J., Martin, S., Rob, P. & Josef, V. (2008). "In Childhood Acute Lymphoblastic Leukemia, Blasts At Different Stages Of Immunophenotypic Maturation Have Stem Cell Properties." *Cancer Cell*, *14* (1), 47–58.

Wahl, D. R. & Lawrence, T. S. (2017). Integrating chemoradiation and molecularly targeted therapy. *Advanced Drug Delivery Reviews*, *109*, 74–83.

Wahida, F., Shehzada, A., Khanb, T., Kima, Y.Y. (2010). MicroRNAs: Synthesis, mechanism, function, and recent clinical trials. *Biochimica et Biophysica Acta - Molecular Cell Research*, 1803(11), 1231-1243.

Waldum, H. L., Arne, K. S., Eiliv, B., Reidar, F., Gunnar, Q. & Jun, S. (2008). "Classification of Tumours." *Journal of Experimental and Clinical Cancer Research : CR*, *27* (1), 70.

Wang, J., Faust, S. M. & Rabinowitz, J. E. (2011). The next step in gene delivery: molecular engineering of adeno-associated virus serotypes. *Journal of molecular and cellular cardiology*, *50*(5), 793-802.

Weiskopf, K., Peter, J. S., Wendy, W. P., Mark, P. C., Akanksha, C., Jun S., Mingye, F. & Irving, L. W. (2016). "Myeloid Cell Origins, Differentiation, and Clinical Implications." *Microbiology Spectrum*, *4* (5).

Westphal, M., Ylä-Herttuala, S., Martin, J., Warnke, P., Menei, P., Eckland, D., Kinley, J., Kay, R., Ram, Z. & ASPECT Study Group, (2013). Adenovirus-mediated gene therapy with sitimageneceradenovec followed by intravenous ganciclovir for patients with operable high-grade glioma (ASPECT): a randomised, open-label, phase 3 trial. *The Lancet Oncology*, *14*(9), 823-833.

Whittaker, S. R., Mallinger, A., Workman, P. & Clarke, P. A. (2017). Inhibitors of cyclin-dependent kinases as cancer therapeutics. *Pharmacology and Therapeutics*, *173*, 83–105.

Wirth, T. & Ylä-Herttuala, S. (2014). Gene therapy used in cancer treatment. *Biomedicines*, *2*(2), 149-162.

Woo, S. R., Corrales, L. & Gajewski, T. F. (2015). Innate immune recognition of cancer. *Annual review of immunology*, *33*, 445-474.

Yamashita, M., Paul, V. D., Oakley, C. O. & Emmanuelle, P. (2020). "Dysregulated Haematopoietic Stem Cell Behaviour in Myeloid Leukaemogenesis." *Nature Reviews Cancer*, 1–18.

Yan, L. X., Huang, X. F., Shao, Q., Huang, M.Y., Deng, L., Wu, Q.L., Zeng, Y.X. & Shao, J.Y. (2008). MicroRNA miR-21 overexpression in human breast cancer is associated with advanced clinical stage, lymph node metastasis and patient poor prognosis. *RNA*, 14(11), 2348–2360.

Yang, Y. (2015). Cancer immunotherapy: harnessing the immune system to battle cancer. *The Journal of clinical investigation*, *125*(9), 3335-3337.

Yang, Y., Sun, M., Wang, L. & Jiao, B. (2013). HIFs, angiogenesis, and cancer. *Journal of Cellular Biochemistry*, *114* (5), 967–974.

Ye, Z., Qian, Q., Jin, H. & Qian, Q. (2018). Cancer vaccine: learning lessons from immune checkpoint inhibitors. *Journal of Cancer*, *9*(2), 263.

In: An Introduction to Cancer Therapy
Editor: Neville Charron
ISBN: 978-1-53618-450-1

Chapter 2

KINASES INHIBITORS IN CANCER THERAPY

Ana Bela Sarmento Ribeiro[1,2,3,4,5], Ana Cristina Gonçalves[1,2,3,4], Carolina Afonso[5], Raquel Alves[1,2,3,4], Inês Gois[6,7], Joana Jorge[1,2,3,4], João Eduardo Casalta[2,3,4,6,7], Lenka Ruzickova[5], Marília Dourado[2,3,4], Marília Gomes[1,5] and José Manuel Nascimento Costa[2,3,4,5]

[1]University of Coimbra, Faculty of Medicine (FMUC), Laboratory of Oncobiology and Hematology and University Clinic of Hematology, Coimbra, Portugal

[2]University of Coimbra, Coimbra Institute for Clinical and Biomedical Research (iCBR) – Group of Environment, Genetics and Oncobiology (CIMAGO), FMUC, Coimbra, Portugal

[3]University of Coimbra, Center for Innovative Biomedicine and Biotechnology (CIBB), Coimbra, Portugal

[4]Clinical Academic Center of Coimbra (CACC), Coimbra, Portugal

[5]Clinical Hematology Department, Centro Hospital e Universitário de Coimbra (CHUC), Coimbra, Portugal

[6] University of Coimbra, FMUC, University Clinic of Oncology, Coimbra, Portugal

[7]Radiotherapy Service, CHUC, Coimbra, Portugal

ABSTRACT

Cancer is a major human health problem, worldwide. Significant progress has been achieved over the past 35 years in understanding the molecular basis of cancer, contributing to the development of new targeted therapies.

Kinases - receptor tyrosine kinases (RTK) and non-receptor tyrosine kinases (NRTKs), play a fundamental role in cell proliferation, survival, and migration. They are constitutively overexpressed and/or activated in several solid and hematological malignant disorders, associated with cancer development, progression and metastasis constituting, therefore, a potential treatment target.

Therapies against deregulated RTKs comprise the targeting of the intracellular tyrosine kinase domain by reversible or irreversible tyrosine kinase inhibitors (TKIs) as well as, binding to extracellular domains. A considerable number of small molecule inhibitors have been developed, and many are already on clinical practice such as, TKIs inhibitors (*Gefitinib, Lapatinib*), and several monoclonal antibodies that bind to extracellular regions, including antibodies against EGFR (*Cetuximab and Panitumumab*), HER2 (*Trastuzumab and Panitumumab*), VEGFR1/R2 (*Bevacizumab, Ramucirumab*) and PDGFRα (*Olaratumab*).

Non-receptor tyrosine kinases (NRTKs) are cytoplasmic proteins or proteins anchored to cell membrane that trigger intracellular signals derived primarily from RTK and from other growth factor receptors. Several specific kinase inhibitors have also been developed to target mutated kinases and inhibit their activity playing a central role on the control of carcinogenesis.

In general, TKIs exhibit excellent clinical results as they are efficacious and well tolerated. Imatinib (IMA), a BCR-ABL inhibitor, was the first TKI approved, initially indicated for chronic myeloid leukemia (CML), and later for acute lymphoblastic leukemia (ALL), Philadelphia positive. It is also a useful therapeutic agent for gastrointestinal stromal tumors (GIST), due to the well-recognized oncogenic mutations seen in the RTK, KIT. Although IMA remains one of the gold standards for first-line CML treatment, the emergence of IMA resistance led to the development and use, in this setting, of second and third-generation TKIs, *Nilotinib, Dasatinib, Bosutinib* and *Ponatinib*, respectively.

Ibrutinib is the first approved Bruton's tyrosine kinase (BTK) inhibitor that has shown clinical activity against B-cell malignancies. *Ruxolitinib* is the first JAK inhibitor approved for the treatment of intermediate and high-risk myelofibrosis. Other TKIs that target tyrosine kinase receptors including, *Midostaurin* (FLT3 F691), *Erlotinib and Gefitinib* (EGFR T790) and *Sunitinib*, were approved for treatment of newly diagnosed

FLT3-mutated AML, advanced systemic mastocytosis, non-small-cell lung cancer (NSCLC) and renal cell carcinoma (RCC), respectively.

Vemurafenib and *Dabrafenib* are BRAF inhibitors which approved for melanoma treatment, in cases exhibiting the specific BRAF/V600E mutation. Although, 75% of patients with this BRAF mutation respond to *Vemurafenib*, resistance to this drug occurs, leading to de development of novel BRAF inhibitors such as, *Regorafenib* and *Encorafenib,* to overcome this condition.

Vandetanib has been approved for the treatment of medullar thyroid cancer exhibiting RET kinase activity and, *Crizotinib* is currently used to treat patients with ALK-positive non-small cell lung cancer.

Sorafenib, a multi-kinase inhibitor is indicated in the treatment of hepatocellular carcinoma, renal cell carcinoma, and thyroid carcinoma. This drug inhibits several tyrosine kinases, and the serine/threonine kinases RAF, MEK1/2 and ERK1/2 kinases.

Activation of the phosphoinositide 3-kinase (PI3K) signaling pathway is frequently observed in breast cancer and in some hematological cancers. The delta PI3K inhibitors, *Idelalisib* and *Duvelisib*, have been approved for the treatment of indolent B cell neoplasias. *Copanlisib* extends existing treatment options for indolent non-Hodgkin lymphoma (NHL) and shows promising response rates in aggressive NHL, especially in DLBCL of the activated B-cell type.

Other kinases, as Aurora A kinase (AAK), Cyclin-Dependent Kinases (CDK) and Polo-like kinases (PLK), play a pivotal role in cancer cells mitosis and activates EMT during the metastatic process (Figure 2). The development of AAK inhibitors including *Alisertinib, Danusertib, Barasertib, Tozasertib, Hesperidin* and *Radotinib,* has been promoted. Several CDK inhibitors entered clinical trials such as, *Roscovitine (Seliciclib*) and the natural product derivative flavopiridol (*Alvocidib*). The clinical response evaluation to the CDK inhibitor *Alvocidib* in hematological tumors was limited and was associated with non-acceptable toxicities. *Palbociclib, Abemaciclib and Ribociclib*, which are CDK4/6-selective inhibitors have been already approved for the treatment of metastatic breast cancer (HR+, HER2-) in combination with endocrine therapy. Clinical trials with PLK1 inhibitors, *Rigosertib, Volasertib* and *Poloxin*, are ongoing to evaluating their potential clinical benefit in sensitizing tumors to chemotherapy.

Twenty-eight kinase inhibitors deserved FDA approval since the initial development of Imatinib; *Brigatinib* and *Osimertinib*, were the latest and they are indicated to treat metastatic NSCLC ALK-positive. Despite a such considerable number of already approved kinase inhibitors, more than three thousand of new kinase inhibitors are still under ongoing phase I-III clinical trials. Yet and so far, one may consider that only a small fraction of the *kinome* is currently being targeted.

Protein kinase inhibitors, currently in clinical practice and under research for potential clinical usefulness, will be reviewed in this chapter.

INTRODUCTION

Noncommunicable diseases (NCDs) are now responsible for the majority of global deaths. Cancer is becoming the leading cause of death, being a major public health problem. GLOBOCAN estimates that about 18.1 million of new cancer cases and 9,6 million of cancer-related deaths occurred in 2018 worldwide (Bray et al., 2018).

The survival rates of different types of malignant neoplasias remained low in the last decade, despite considerable improvements in diagnostic and therapeutic interventions. Currently, most commonly used anti-tumor drugs are cytotoxic molecules, usually with high acute toxicity, poor selectivity, strong side effects and easily developing drug resistance (Jiao et al., 2018).

Novel cancer treatment approaches, directed to specific targets on cancer, has been one of the main focus of research. These targeted therapies rely on drugs that inhibit biological pathways involved in cancer proliferation and survival (Ke & Shen, 2017).

Recent advances in the knowledge of the molecular mechanisms involved in cancer cell signaling have depicted a crucial role for kinases in the carcinogenesis of various cancer types (Bhullar et al., 2018).

Most protein kinases, when constitutively overexpressed or active, promote cell proliferation, survival and migration, and are associated with cancer development, progression and metastasis (Bhullar et al., 2018; Sarmento-Ribeiro et al., 2019). Over the last three decades, dysfunction of protein and lipid kinases (tyrosine, serine or threonine kinases), and deactivated phosphatases, resulting from chromosomal alterations, genetic and/or epigenetic alterations, have been identified in multiple human malignancies (Table 1). This kinome, has since become an attractive target for the treatment of numerous types of cancers. There are at least 518 kinases (Manning et al. 2002) and 156 phosphatases (Shi, 2009) in the human genome, and despite intensive research in this area, the underlying biology of many of these enzymes remains to be fully elucidated (Gross et al., 2015).

Table 1. Mechanisms of kinase activation in cancer

Activation mechanism	Kinases
Point mutations	ACVR1B, ACVR2B, AKT1, ALK, ALPK2, ATM, BRAF, CDK12, CDK4, EGFR, EPHA2, ERBB2, ERBB3, FGFR1, FGFR2, FGFR3, FGFR4, FLT3, JAK2, KIT, MAP2K1, MAP3K1, MAP4K3, MET, MTOR, PIK3CA, SGK1, STK19, TGFBR2
Gene amplification	CDK4, CDK6, CRKL, EGFR, ERBB2, FGFR1, FGFR2, FGFR3, FLT3, IGF1R, KIT, MET, PAK1, PDGFRA, PIK3CA, PRKC
Gene amplification or fusion of a kinase ligand	FGF19 (FGFR4), HGF(MET), NRG1 (ERBB3), VEGFA (VEGFR)
Gene fusions	ALK, ABL1, BRAF, EGFR, FGFR1, FGFR2, FGFR3, FGR, JAK2, MET, NTRK1, NTRK2, NTRK3, PDGFRA, PDGFRB, PIK3CA, PRKACA, PRKCA, PRKCB, RAF1, RET, ROS1, SYK

Adapted from Gross et al. 2015.

Single and multiple kinase inhibitors, both synthetic and natural molecules, became targeted therapeutic strategies used in clinical practice for treatment of human malignancies (Bhullar et al., 2018). These kinase inhibitors (KI), include target kinome members such as PIK3CA, BRAF, epidermal growth factor receptor (EGFR), ERBB2, VEGFRs, KIT, PDGFRs, ABL, SRC and mTOR, among others. These kinases activate significant tumor cell signaling pathways; their inhibition by KI, have provided benefits to patient' clinical outcome and health status (Hanahan & Weinberg, 2011; Knowles et al., 2006; Zhang, Yang & Gray, 2009).

The first tyrosine kinase inhibitor (TKI), imatinib, for treatment of chronic myeloid leukemia (CML) was approved by FDA in 2001 inaugurating new opportunities to cancer treatment. So far, more than 20 kinds of TKI have been approved by the FDA. These drugs have high selectivity, high efficacy, low side effects, easy preparation, and have demonstrated clinical superiority when compared to traditional cytotoxic antineoplastic agents, in the treatment of chronic myeloid leukemia (CML), non-small cell lung cancer (NSCLC), renal cell carcinoma (RCC) (Torkamani, Verkhivker & Schork 2009) becoming, some of them, the first-line drug choice for the treatment of cancer (Gross et al., 2015).

Kinase inhibitors have, in this context, played an increasingly prominent role in the treatment of cancer and other diseases and since the initial development of Imatinib, FDA approved 28 kinase inhibitors, small-molecule inhibitors (Table 2) and monoclonal antibodies for cancer therapy (Bhullar et al., 2018, Roskoski, 2019).

Table 2. FDA-approved kinase inhibitors and respective targets

Drug target	Protein substrate	Drug
ALK	Tyrosine	Crizotinib, Ceritinib, Alectinib, Brigatinib, Lorlatinib
BCR-ABL	Tyrosine	Bosutinib, Dasatinib, Imatinib, Nilotinib, Ponatinib, Radotinib
B-Raf	Serine/threonine	Vemurafenib, Dabrafenib
BTK	Tyrosine	Acalabrutinib, Ibrutinib, Zanubrutinib
CDK family	Serine/threonine	Abemaciclib, Palbociclib, Sorafenib, Ribociclib
c-Met	Tyrosine	Crizotinib, Cabozantinib
EGFR family	Tyrosine	Cetuximab, Gefitinib, Erlotinib, Lapatinib, Vandetanib, Afatinib, Osimertinib, Panitumumab, Necitumumab
JAK family	Tyrosine	Fedratinib, Ruxolitinib, Tofacitinib, Baricitinib
MEK1/2	Dual specificity	Binimetinib, Cobimetinib, Selumetinib, Trametinib
PDGFR α/β	Tyrosine	Axitinib, Gefitinib, Imatinib, Lenvatinib, Nintedanib, Pazopanib, Regorafenib, Sorafenib, Sunitinib, Olaratumab
RET	Tyrosine	Vandetanib, Lenvatinib, Cabozantinib, Regorafenib, Sunitibib, Selpercatinib
Src family	Tyrosine	Bosutinib, Dasatinib, Ponatinib, Vandetanib
VEGFR family	Tyrosine	Axitinib, Lenvatinib, Nintedanib, Ramucirumab, Regorafenib, Pazopanib, Sorafenib, Sunitinib

Adapted de Bhullar et al., 2018.

In this chapter, a review on the protein kinase inhibitors currently in clinical practice and under research for potential clinical usefulness will be presented.

CELL SIGNALING AND DRUG TARGETS

Cancer is a multifactorial disease derived from genetic and epigenetic alterations, marked by signal transduction pathways dysregulation that are involved in the control of essential cell processes such as, growth factor, differentiation and survival. This complex information is transmitted through protein-protein interactions (PPIs) in an interactome network which knowledge opens a new way towards a personalized and precision medicine (Kanhaiya et al., 2017).

A number of hormones, growth factors and cytokines regulate cell proliferation and differentiation. These molecules interact with cellular receptors and communicate with the nucleus of the cell through a network of intracellular signaling pathways (Figure 1) (Adjei & Hidalgo, 2005). In cancer cells, key components of these pathways may be altered by oncogenes through overexpression or mutation, leading to dysregulated cell signaling, inhibition of apoptosis, metastasis, and cell proliferation. The components of these abnormal signaling pathways, which are specific to neoplastic cells, represent potential selective targets for new anticancer therapies (Adjei & Hidalgo, 2005). These potential targets include ligands (typically growth factors), cellular receptors, intracellular second messengers, and nuclear transcription factors. The intracellular signaling molecules that play a critical role in carcinogenesis and the maintenance of the malignant phenotype are, in majority, protein kinases (Tsintarakis & Zafiropoulo, 2017).

Protein kinases are enzymes that covalently attach phosphates to the side chain of either serine, threonine, or tyrosine residues of specific proteins inside cells. In addition, a few members of the phosphatidylinositol kinase family also exhibit protein-serine/threonine kinase activity (Adjei & Hidalgo, 2005). Such phosphorylation of proteins can control their enzymatic activity, their interaction with other proteins and molecules, their location in the cell, and their propensity for degradation by proteases. Their activity is normally tightly controlled and regulated. Perturbation of protein kinase signaling by mutations and other genetic alterations results in deregulated kinase activity and malignant transformation. Among the approximately 32,000 coding genes identified in the human genome are more than 520 protein kinases exerting tight and reversible control on protein phosphorylation (Tsintarakis & Zafiropoulo, 2017). Examples include, proteins involved in signaling pathways that are commonly activated in many physiological responses, such as growth factor receptor tyrosine kinases (RTKs; e.g., the epidermal growth factor receptor, EGFR), small GTPases (e.g., RAS), serine/threonine kinases (e.g., RAF and AKT), cytoplasmic tyrosine kinases (NRTKs; e.g., SRC, SYK and ABL), lipid kinases (e.g., phosphoinositide 3-kinases, PI3Ks), as well as nuclear receptors (e.g., the estrogen receptor, ER) and cell cycle effectors (e.g., cyclins dependent kinases, CDK).

Many of the genes commonly mutated in cancer encode components or targets of the RAS/RAF/MAPK, PI3K/AKT/mammalian target of rapamycin (mTOR), PLC-γ/protein kinase C (PKC) and Janus kinase (JAK)/STAT pathways (Yarden & Pines, 2012) (Figure 1). The PI3K-AKT pathway can be activated through amplification or activating mutations affecting several PI3K-Akt-pathway proteins, in particular the type I PI3K isoform PIK3CA, AKT, and the adaptor protein PIK3R, or through deletion or inactivating mutations in the phosphatases that hydrolyze PI3K products such as PTEN and INPP4B tumor suppressors. (Laplante & Sabatini 2012). Similarly, the RAS-ERK pathway is activated by RAS mutations, or its downstream target RAF, that cause constitutive activation of these proteins or by inactivation of GTPase-activating proteins (GAPs), such as NF1, DAB2IP, and RASAL2, that stimulate the hydrolysis of GTP bound to RAS, leading to its inactivation. (Sever & Brugge, 2015) Moreover, several lines of evidence implicated the RTK, B-cell receptor (BCR), as a key survival molecule for normal B cells and for most B-cell malignancies (Burger & Wiestner, 2018). Antigen-mediated BCR activation generates a cascade of intracellular signaling that involves the activation of kinases, culminating in the activation of transcription factors such as NF-kB and the activated nuclear factor of T cells (NFAT), essential for proliferation, survival, differentiation and migration of normal B cells (Burger & Wiestner, 2018; Sarmento-Ribeiro et al., 2013).

Cytokine binding to the extracellular domain of receptors, induces conformation changes that enable cross-phosphorylation and activation of the associated JAK (Vainchenker et al., 2018; Muller, 2019). As a result, JAK phosphorylate tyrosine residues on the intracellular part of the receptor, which then can serve as docking sites for SH2 domain of signaling molecules, such as the signal transducer and activator of transcription (STAT) (Vainchenker et al., 2018).

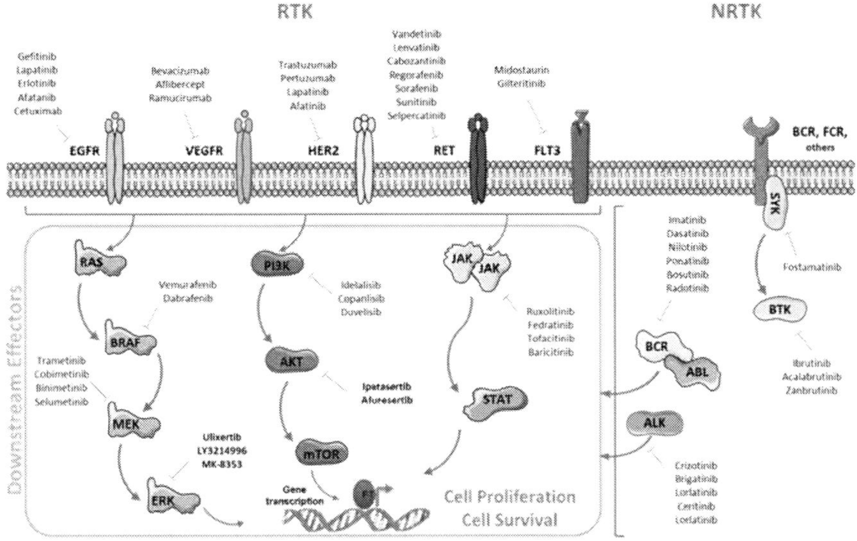

Figure 1. Cancer signaling pathways. Growth factors (GF) binding to a membrane receptor, with tyrosine kinase activity (RTK). Upon activation of the first type receptors, several intracellular effector pathways can be activated, such as the Phosphatidyl Inositol-3-kinase (PI3K), the RAS/MAPK pathway, the phospholipase C g pathway (PLCg) and less often the JAK/STAT pathway, culminating in the activation of genes important in the regulation of proliferation, cell cycle and cell survival. The biding of GF binds to the extracellular portion of the RTK and causes dimerization of the intracellular part of the receptor and association with adaptor proteins, Son of Sevenless (SOS), and growth factor receptor binding protein 2 (GRB 2). These proteins interact through SRC-homology (SH) domains SH2 and SH3, respectively. Then, the SOS-GRB 2 complex activates RAS which induces an intracellular cascade of kinases to promote proliferation. Once activated, RAS transmits the growth signal the serine/threonine kinase, RAF. RAF initiates a cascade of mitogen-induced protein kinases (MAPKs), which culminate in the nucleus with the activation of transcription factors. Another RAS effector gene is phosphoinositol 3-kinase (PI-3K), which initiates a signaling pathway for cell survival through phosphorylation of the protein kinase B, AKT/PKB, on serine and threonine residues. This kinase phosphorylates BAD, a pro-apoptotic protein, that became inactivated, inhibiting apoptosis and promoting cell survival and activate mTOR complex promoting cell proliferation, angiogenesis and metastization. Antigen binding leads to the formation of a complex of kinases and phosphorylation of the immunoreceptor tyrosine–based activation motifs in the C-terminal tail of BCR-associated Ig, CD79A and CD79B, by the SRC-family kinase LYN. This recruit and activate the tyrosine kinase SYK, which further propagated the BCR signal via association with the adaptor molecule B-cell linker protein (BLNK) and its downstream signaling components Bruton tyrosine kinase (BTK) and phospholipase Cγ2 (PLC-γ2). Activation of PLC-γ2 leads to the generation of the downstream second messenger's inositol-1,4,5-triphosphate (IP3) and diacylglycerol (DAG), which induce the release of intracellular Ca2+ and activate protein kinase C (PKC), respectively. PKC subsequently induces the activation of transcription factors, including NF-kB and nuclear factor of activated T cells, NFAT. Activation of mitogen-activated protein kinase pathways (MAPK), including the extracellular signal-regulated kinase 1/2 (ERK1/2), can also be regulated by PLC-γ2 and RAS/RAF signaling. The third phase of events mediate changes in cell proliferation, survival, and migration, through modulation of multiple downstream regulators.

STATs are latent transcription factors that reside in the cytoplasm until activated (Rawlings, Rosler & Harrison, 2004). The STAT family consists of seven members (named STAT1 to STAT4, STAT5A, STAT5B, and STAT6), which share highly conserved homology regions, including a DNA-binding domain and SH2 domain (Recio, 2018). The STAT proteins are recruited to the receptor complex through their SH2 domain, being phosphorylated by receptor associated JAK (Babon et al., 2014). Phosphorylated STATs form dimers and translocate into the nucleus; once in the nucleus, dimerized STATs bind specific regulatory sequences to activate or repress transcription of target genes (Rawlings, Rosler & Harrison, 2004).

JAK/STAT pathway is known to be activated by more than 50 different cytokine receptors, and is the main signaling mechanism for a wide array of cytokines and growth factors, including pro-inflammatory cytokines (Interleukin (IL)-6, tumor necrosis factor (TNF) α, IL-12, IL-23), anti-inflammatory cytokines (IL-4, IL-10), hematopoietic cell growth factors (granulocyte colony-stimulating factor (G-CSF), erythropoietin (EPO), thrombopoietin (TPO)) and metabolic cytokines (Muller, 2019; Rawlings, Rosler & Harrison, 2004). The effects of hematopoietic cell growth factors are mainly mediated by JAK2 (Bousoik & Aliabadi, 2018).

Most of these intracellular signaling pathways culminate in cell cycle progression from G0/G1 into S phase, in which DNA replication occurs. The cyclin-dependent kinases (CDKs) are a large conserved family of serine/threonine kinases highly implicated in cell-cycle regulation (Lee & Nurse, 1987). CDKs are small proteins, with a molecular weight of around 35 to 40 kDa, constituted mainly by its kinase domain (Crosby, 2007). The function as an active kinase depends on its prior binding to regulatory proteins cyclins, forming the cyclin-CDK complex. Most cyclin-CDK complexes are responsible for the progression through the cell-cycle phases via phosphorylation of target genes, such as the retinoblastoma tumor suppressor protein (Rb). The interaction between Cyclin D and CDK4/6 facilitates the hyperphosphorylation of the Rb gene product, leading to progression to the S phase through the G1 checkpoint (Figure 2).

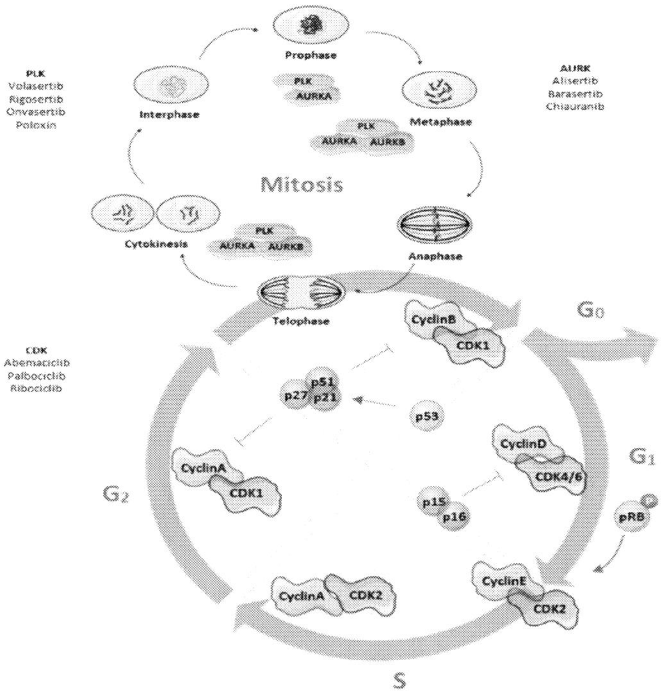

Figure 2. Cell cycle regulation and major regulatory proteins.
Mitogenic signals activate complexes of cyclins and cyclin-dependent kinases (CDKs), namely CDK4,6 that promote progression from the G1 phase into S phase mainly by phosphorylating the retinoblastoma protein (RB) and subsequent activation of transcription by the E2F family of transcription factors. The major cell cycle regulators are p53 and pRB and the activity of CDK4 and CDK6 is also controlled by several mechanisms: positively by association with D-type cyclins (D1, D2 and D3) and negatively by binding to CDK inhibitors of the INK4 family (p16INK4A, p15INKB, p18INK4C and p19INK4D) and CIP/KIP (p21CIP, P27INK1 and p57INK2) families (). Progression through S phase and from G2 phase into mitosis (M phase) is also controlled by cyclin-CDK complexes, together with a variety of other proteins, such as Polo-like kinase 1 (PLK1) and Aurora kinases (Aurora A/B). All of these kinases can be targeted as represented in figure.

Changes in this pathway resulting in the loss of the Rb checkpoint have been associated with BC endocrine resistance (Finn, Aleshin & Slamon, 2016).

The complexity of the cancer signaling network presents a enormous challenge to develop targeted anticancer drugs. These are related with the redundancy of the pathways that control cell proliferation and survival, crosstalk between pathways, and feedback inhibition mechanisms that cause pathway reactivation. As the pathways, such as RAS-ERK and AKT-PI3K, control so many cancer cells characteristics, and components of these pathways, or upstream receptors, are mutated commonly in a variety of cancers, provides a rational approach to target these pathways successfully. However, the efficacy of these targeted therapies could be limited by multiple factors, including factors from the tumor microenvironment that may stimulate alternative pathways that maintain cell viability, despite the inhibition of these pathways (Castells et al., 2012; Muranen et al., 2012). Otherwise, mutations in other pathways that circumvent the targeted pathway, and epigenetic or stochastic changes in the state of cancer cells can also activate intrinsic resistance pathways (Holohan et al., 2013; Holzel, Bovier & Tuting et al., 2013; Sever & Brugge, 2015), leading to drug resistance development and therapeutic failure.

Tyrosine Kinase Inhibitors

The tyrosine kinases inhibitors (TKI) are a class of drugs that target tyrosine kinases belonging to two categories of proteins according to their structures, receptor tyrosine kinases (RTK) and non-receptor tyrosine kinases (NRTK). These enzymes transfer a phosphate group from ATP to tyrosine residues of specific proteins and together with phosphatases regulate cell growth, differentiation, and death (Bhullar et al., 2018; Jiao et al., 2018), (Sarmento-Ribeiro et al., 2019).

RTKs comprised an extracellular domain which contains the ligand-binding site and defines its specificity, a single transmembrane region and a cytosolic domain that contains the tyrosine kinase domain (Yamaoka et al., 2018). Members of the RTKs family are the receptors of the epidermal (EGF), platelet derived (PDGF), vascular endothelial (VEGF), fibroblast (FGF) and hepatocyte (HGF) (MET) growth factors, as well as the leukocyte tyrosine kinase (LTK) (ALK) (Yamaoka et al., 2018) and FLT3 a cytokine receptor that belongs to the class III RTKs. Therapies against deregulated RTKs include targeting of the intracellular tyrosine kinase domain by reversible or irreversible tyrosine kinase inhibitors (TKIs) or binding to extracellular domains. Thus, a number of small molecule inhibitors, such as multikinase inhibitors (in the case of VEGFR, PDGF/kit and FGFR) or specific TKIs, along with several monoclonal Abs, including antibodies against EGFR (cetuximab, panitumumab and necitumumab), HER2 (trastuzumab, emtansine and panitumumab), VEGFR2 (ramucirumab) and PDGFRα (olaratumab) that bind to extracellular regions leading to prevention of downstream signaling have been developed (Yamaoka et al., 2018; Ana Bela Sarmento-Ribeiro et al., 2019).

NRTKs are cytoplasmic proteins or proteins anchored to cell membrane that trigger intracellular signals mediated by RTK and other growth factor receptors (Jiao et al., 2018; Siveen et al., 2018). These tyrosine kinases can be subclassified into nine subfamilies according to kinase domains sequence similarities: ABL, FES, JAK, ACK, SYK, TEC, FAK, SRC, and CSK (Du and Lovly, 2018; Siveen et al., 2018; Sarmento-Ribeiro et al., 2019) Given the central role of NRTKs on carcinogenesis, several specific kinase inhibitors have been developed to target mutated kinases and inhibit their activity, which had revolutionized cancer therapy.

RECEPTOR TYROSINE KINASE (RTK)

FLT3 Inhibitors

Fms-Like Tyrosine kinase 3 (*FLT3*), is a type III receptor tyrosine kinase, expressed on hematopoietic stem and progenitor cells, regulating cellular differentiation and proliferation through multiple activation pathways. *FLT3* acts as a cytokine receptor for the ubiquitously expressed FLT3 ligand (FL). Upon binding to FL, *FLT3* dimerizes and undergoes a conformational change to allow auto-phosphorylation of the ATP-binding pocket. The resulting FLT3 receptor activation leads to increased cell proliferation, decreased apoptosis, and reduced differentiation of hematopoietic cells via PI3K/AKT, MAPK/ERK, and STAT signaling cascades (Figure 1) (Scholl, Gilliland & Fröhling, 2008).

Mutation in the *FLT3* gene, located on chromosome 13q12, is the most frequent genetic alteration in acute myeloid leukemia (AML) and is well known as an important driver mutation for the development of myeloid malignancies.

AML carrying internal tandem duplication (ITD) of *FLT3* gene is associated with high risk of relapse and poor clinical outcome upon treatment with conventional chemotherapy. Conversely, the role of tyrosine kinase domain (TKD) point mutation D835 is still controversial.

Identification of *FLT3* mutations enables targeted treatment that may help to achieve longer and more durable remissions. First-generation FLT3 inhibitors developed for clinical use are broad-spectrum multikinase inhibitors. Next-generation FLT3 inhibitors are more specific, more potent, and have fewer toxicities associated with off-target effects. Primary and secondary acquired resistance to FLT3 inhibitors remains a challenge and provides a rationale for combining FLT3 inhibitors with other therapies. Two FLT3 inhibitors have been approved for the treatment of *FLT3*-mutated AML subtype: Midostaurin in combination with conventional induction and consolidation chemotherapy in newly diagnosed patients and gilteritinib in monotherapy for relapsed/refractory (R/R) *FLT3*-mutated patients (Perl et al., 2019).

Characteristics of FLT3 Inhibitors and Principles of Use

Mutations in the *FLT3* gene are present in 30% of adults with newly diagnosed AML. Approximately three quarters of these patients have a *FLT3*-ITD mutation, which occurs in the juxtamembrane domain of the FLT3 receptor (a substitution of tyrosine for aspartic acid at codon 835, D835Y, in the TKD), responsible for the auto-inhibitory function. ITD mutations are associated with a poor prognosis owing to a high relapse rate, particularly when there is a high ratio of mutant to wild-type *FLT3* alleles. However, in approximately 5% to 10% of patients with newly diagnosed AML a point mutation in *FLT3* gene, is most common. The effect of these TKD mutations on prognosis is uncertain (Bacher et al., 2008).

Two generations of FLT3 tyrosine kinase inhibitors (TKI) with variable kinase inhibitory properties, pharmacokinetics and toxicity profiles, have been developed and explored so far in preclinical and clinical settings. The first generation includes a broad-spectrum TKI (sorafenib, midostaurin) with a cascade activity involving the proto-oncogene receptor tyrosine kinase c-KIT, the platelet derived growth factors (PDGF), and the vascular endothelial growth factor (VEGF). This characteristic has led the use of these compounds also in systemic mastocytosis and non-hematological cancers, but the off-target mechanisms may contribute to a higher toxicity profile. Second generation FLT3 inhibitors (quizartinib, gilteritinib) refer to new inhibitors with higher specificity and potency against *FLT3*.

Another general classification based on the conformation of the targeted kinase divides FLT3 inhibitors into Type I and Type II. Type I inhibitors including sunitinib, midostaurin, lestaurtinib, crenolanib and gilteritinib, bind to the ATP-binding site when the receptor is in the active conformation. Type II inhibitors, like sorafenib and quizartinib, interact with a hydrophobic region directly adjacent to the ATP-binding domain that is only accessible when the receptor is in its inactive conformation and they prevent receptor activation. Type I inhibitors prevent activity in AML cells against both ITD and TKD with generally stronger binding to the *FLT3*-ITD-mutated kinase, while Type II inhibitors target ITD but lack efficiency against TKD mutations. Nevertheless, the development of TKD mutations, in particular D835, in AML cells with ITD, could be a mechanism of acquired resistance to Type II FLT3 inhibitors.

Clinical Efficacy

These agents have been evaluated in phase II–III clinical trials and midostaurin and gilteritinib have obtained US Federal Drug Administration (FDA) and European Medicines Agency (EMA) approval.

Midostaurin

Midostaurin, a first-generation multi-kinase inhibitor, was originally developed as a protein kinase C inhibitor for treatment of patients with solid tumors. This agent is the first FLT3 inhibitor shown to improve survival in *FLT3*-mutated AML based on the RATIFY trial (Stone et al., 2017). It is approved for patients with newly diagnosed AML and *FLT3*-ITD or

FLT3-TKD mutation (defined by an AR $\geq$ 0.05) in combination with induction chemotherapy.

The RATIFY trial was a multicenter phase III pivotal trial of 717 patients (age 18–59 years) with newly diagnosed *FLT3*-mutated AML. The study showed a significant benefit in event-free survival (EFS) (8.2 months for midostaurin *vs* 3 months for placebo) and 4-year overall survival (OS) (51.4% for midostaurin *vs* 44.2% for placebo).

Maintenance treatment with midostaurin is approved only in patients who are in complete remission (CR) after induction and consolidation chemotherapy, but not after allogeneic hematopoietic stem cell transplantation (alloHCT). Exploratory analysis of the RATIFY trial failed to clarify whether midostaurin maintenance contributes to the OS benefit of midostaurin (Larson et al., 2017). Importantly, midostaurin maintenance should not replace alloHCT in transplant candidates.

As a multikinase inhibitor, midostaurin inhibits D816V-mutated KIT, a primary driver of pathogenesis of systemic mastocytosis (SM). Two single-arm, open-label multicenter trials evaluated the safety of midostaurin at a dose of 100 mg twice daily as a single agent in adult patients with advanced systemic mastocytosis (ASM), SM with an associated hematologic neoplasm (SM-AHN), or mast cell leukemia (MCL). The first small study has followed-up 26 patients with ASM for more than 10 years (median duration of follow-up 124 months). During the first 12 cycles of therapy, the overall response rate was 69% (major/partial response: 50%/19%). Median overall survival (mOS) for the entire cohort was 40 months, and 18.5 months for MCL patients (DeAngelo et al., 2018). The second trial studied 116 patients, including 89 with organ damage due to mastocytosis and 16 with mast cell leukemia. They were treated continuously in four-week cycles. The median duration of treatment was 11.4 months. There was a response in 60% of patients which lasted for a median of 24.1 months (Gotlib et al., 2016).

Gilteritinib

Gilteritinib is an oral, selective type I FLT3 inhibitor, approved by FDA and EMA as a single-agent in R/R *FLT3*-mutated AML. This approval is based on results from the Phase III ADMIRAL trial, which investigated gilteritinib versus salvage chemotherapy in 371 adult patients with R/R *FLT3*-mutated AML. The mOS in the gilteritinib group was significantly longer than that in the chemotherapy group (9.3 months *vs* 5.6 months; hazard ratio (HR) for death, 0.64; 95% confidence interval (CI), 0.49 to 0.83; P<0.001). The median EFS was 2.8 months in the gilteritinib group and 0.7 months in the chemotherapy group (HR for treatment failure or death, 0.79; 95% CI, 0.58 to 1.09). Rates of one-year survival were 37% for patients who received gilteritinib, compared to 17% for patients who received salvage chemotherapy (Perl et al., 2019).

Other Selective FLT3 Inhibitors

Quizartinib is another oral, highly potent and selective type II FLT3 inhibitor, which also showed a survival benefit in R/R *FLT3*-ITD-mutated patients compared to investigator choice salvage chemotherapy (mOS 6.2 versus 4.7 months) in QuANTUM-R phase 3 study (Cortes et al., 2019), but was not approved by FDA's Oncologic Drugs Advisory Committee (ODAC) and EMA due to the risk of QT interval prolongation, modest survival results, and methodologic concerns. Phase III randomized trial (QuANTUM-First), comparing the effect of quizartinib versus placebo (administered with standard induction and consolidation chemotherapy, then administered as continuation therapy for up to 36 cycles) on event-free survival in patients with FLT3-ITD positive AML is underway.

Crenolanib is also potent type I selective FLT3 inhibitor, although it retains activity against TKD mutations, overcoming the known mechanism of resistance of the previous second generation drug. Crenolanib has been studied alone in the R/R AML setting with an overall response rate (ORR) of 50% and is now on study in combination with standard induction chemotherapy also compared to other FLT3 inhibitors such as midostaurin (Stone et al., 2019).

Adverse Effects and Resistance

There are several important considerations to keep in mind when employing the FLT3 inhibitors in clinical practice. In the RATIFY study, the observed adverse events were comparable between the midostaurin and placebo treatment groups. The most frequent grade 3 or higher adverse events were hematologic toxicities, febrile neutropenia, infection, diarrhea, hypokalemia, pain, and increased alanine aminotransferase. Drug-drug interactions mediated via cytochrome P450 (CYP) 3A4 are of particular interest, as the use of interacting supportive care medications (azole antifungals for prophylaxis of fungal infections) is common during induction and consolidation. Concomitant administration of strong CYP3A4 inhibitors leads to increased exposure to midostaurin and its active metabolites. In phase I study in healthy volunteers, the inhibition of CYP3A4 by ketoconazole resulted in a significant increase in midostaurin maximum concentration and delayed formation and excretion of its active metabolites (Dutreix et al., 2013).

Gilteritinib is also a CYP3A4 substrate, and pharmacokinetic study demonstrated that concomitant administration with CYP3A4 inhibitors (itraconazole and fluconazole) increases gilteritinib exposure (Levis et al., 2017). There is still little information available addressing management of these interactions in terms of dose adjustments or timing of administration.

Metabolism and interaction information on the newer FLT3 inhibitors (e.g., quizartinib, crenolanib) is not readily available, although these agents are still being evaluated in clinical trials.

A major limitation in the treatment of *FLT3*-mutated AML by FLT3 inhibitor is disease relapse related to development of drug resistance. The mechanisms are heterogeneous, both inherent and acquired, they are likely to vary between patients and multiple mechanisms may co-exist.

The primary cause of resistance is the acquisition of point mutations in the ATP binding region of the FLT3 kinase domain, thereby altering the conformational state and weakening the binding affinity to specific FLT3 inhibitors. Mutations may occur at the activation loop (e.g., D835, I836) or gate-keeper site (e.g., F691), and the frequencies and mutation sites depend on the specific FLT3 inhibitors being used. Nonmutational mechanisms of resistance include upregulation of parallel prosurvival pathways and signal transducer and activator of transcription pathways, upregulation of the FLT3 ligand or FLT3 receptor, mutations in other kinases, activation of antiapoptotic proteins and bone marrow microenvironment-mediated resistance (Daver et al., 2015). New strategies have been developed to improve the treatment outcome of *FLT3*-ITD patients.

Planned and ongoing studies are investigating the utility of combining different agents that inhibit key signaling pathways through different modes of action or by using two or more agents that target different leukemic cell survival signaling pathways. There are findings suggesting that resistance to type I FLT3 inhibitor may be overcome by an alternate type FLT3 inhibitor or by combining FLT3 inhibitors. Thus, combinations of FLT3 inhibitors or switching FLT3 inhibitors may overcome mutational resistance and this strategy should be further evaluated (Daver et al., 2015). Combinations of FLT3 inhibitors with approved antileukemic therapies, such as hypomethylating agents, low-dose cytarabine, CPX-351, and investigational agents (e.g., BCL-2 and CYP3A4 inhibitors) are currently being evaluated in clinical trials (Daver et al., 2019).

EGFR/HER2/VEGFR/PDGFR Inhibitors

Carcinogenesis occurs after a cell acquires several characteristics that confer advantages, such as in survival and cell proliferation, as well as the possibility of evading cell death and immune modulation, rewiring metabolic mechanisms and providing a favorable microenvironment. (Hanahan & Weinberg, 2000; Hanahan & Weinberg, 2011; Fouad & Aanei, 2017). Some of these advantages are achieved when genetic alterations change the activity of some growth factors (GF) and their transmembrane receptors, such as the family of tyrosine kinase receptors (RTK). These receptors are implied in several cellular processes as cell survival, proliferation, apoptosis, angiogenesis and migration, through the activation of several intracellular signaling pathways (Du & Lovly, 2018; Lemmon & Schlessinger, 2010).

The RTK family includes 58 types of receptors grouped into 20 subfamilies based on their kinase domain sequence, as epidermal growth factor receptor (EGFR/HER2), vascular endothelial growth factor receptor (VEGFR) and platelet-derived growth factor receptor (PDGFR). All RTKs contain an extracellular domain (holding the ligand-binding site), a single transmembrane region and a cytosolic domain, which includes the region with protein tyrosine kinase activity (Yamaoka et al., 2018.) Binding of GF to each extracellular RTK region leads to self-association and dimerization, producing activated tyrosine kinases (Du & Lovly, 2018; Lemmon & Schlessinger, 2010; Yamaoka et al., 2018.). These activated kinases stimulate their corresponding signaling pathways cascades, including the KRAS/BRAF/MEK/ERK, the PI3K/AKT/mTOR, the PLC-gamma, and the JAK/STAT, which leads to cell proliferation, angiogenesis, migration, survival, and adhesion (Figure 1). Owing the several mutations harbored in various genes involved in these pathways, these cellular processes are often deregulated in malignant cells (Seshacharyulu et al., 2012), being targets to treat cancer.

The EGFR is a transmembrane glycoprotein member of the ErbB receptor tyrosine kinase superfamily. The ErbB family of receptors comprises four known members namely ErbB1/EGFR/HER1, ErbB2/HER2/Neu, ErbB3/HER3 and ErbB4/HER4. These receptors can be activated by 13 known ligands, which include EGF, transforming growth factor alpha (TGF-α), amphiregulin (AR), betacellulin (BTC), heparin binding EGF-like growth factor (HB-EGF), epiregulin (EPR), epigen (EPG) and neuregulins (NRG). Among these ligands, EGF, TGF-α, AR, BTC and EPR bind specifically to HER1 (Seshacharyulu et al., 2012).

The PDGF/KIT, fibroblastic growth factor (FGF) and VEGF receptors family have been implicated in vascular development, being the VEGF family (VEGF-A, -B, -C, -D and placenta growth factor, PlGF) the major regulators of tumor angiogenesis. VEGF is expressed in most human cancers such as breast, kidney and colon and transfer the angiogenesis signal via two

VEGF receptors, VEGFR-2 (KDR/FLK-1) and VEGFR-1 (FLT-1). The PDGFR family, are a class III RTKs, that includes PDGFRα, PDGFRβ, KIT (CD117, stem cell factor receptor, SCFR), colony-stimulating factor 1 receptor (CSFR) and Fms-like tyrosine kinase 3 (FLT3). Mutations in PDGFR family genes, particularly PDGFRα and c-KIT, are most frequently found in gastrointestinal stromal tumors (GISTs) (Seshacharyulu et al., 2012).

Aberrant activation of RTKs can be caused by ligand-dependent or ligand-independent mechanisms. In colorectal cancer, epidermal growth factor receptor (EGFR) ligand aberrations, with amphiregulin, epiregulin and transforming growth factor (TGF)-α may act as prognostic indicators and predictive biomarkers of the response to anti-EGFR antibodies, such as cetuximab or panitumumab, even when wild-type KRAS is present. EGFR mutation in non-small cell lung cancer (NSCLC), RET mutation in medullary thyroid carcinoma, ALK translocation and ROS1 translocation in NSCLC and HER2 amplification in breast cancer have been reported and therapies have been established (Yamaoka et al., 2018).

Some mechanisms of resistance in cancer treatments have also been correlated with the expression of RTK by tumor cells, with an association of the expression of epidermal growth factor receptor (EGFR) to radiotherapy resistance in head and neck squamous cell carcinoma (HNSCC) and non-small cell lung cancer (NSCLC) (Bhattacharya et al., 2018). Given the importance of these receptors in many aspects of carcinogenesis, they constitute a major target in anti-cancer treatment. Several antibodies have been developed and approved for treatments in oncology, such as cetuximab for targeting EGFR, bevacizumab for targeting VEGFR, oralatumab targeting platelet-derived growth factor receptor (PDGFR) and trastuzumab and pertuzumab for HER2 receptor blockade. Some of these drugs and their clinical use will be discussed below.

EGFR Inhibitors

Following the functional involvement concept of EGFR role in diverse cellular processes, several EGFR inhibitors have been developed for cancer treatment. Two distinct therapeutic approaches are currently employed for targeting EGFR in various human malignancies: monoclonal antibodies and small molecule tyrosine kinase inhibitors (TKIs) (Figure 1, Table 2). While anti-EGFR antibodies bind to extracellular domains and are administered intravenously, the TKIs target the intra cellular TK domain and are given orally. Recent studies have indicated the use of various chemopreventive agents in downregulating EGFR at gene level. Moreover, several studies have validated and conferred significant benefits of anti-EGFR agents in the treatment of several types of solid tumors including, colorectal cancer (CCR), head and neck cancer (HNSCC), non-small cell lung cancer (NSCLC) and pancreatic cancer (PC) showing clear benefits in terms of overall survival (OS), progression free survival (PFS) and overall response rate (ORR) (Seshacharyulu et al., 2012).

Cetuximab

Cetuximab is a chimeric monoclonal antibody that inhibits EGFR by binding to its extracellular domain (Goldstein et al., 1995). One international recommendation for its use in oncology is in the treatment of K-RAS wild-type metastatic colorectal cancer (mCRC) with overexpression of EGFR (Van Cutsem et al., 2014). This recommendation was approved by US FDA and EMA in 2004.

Numerous trials have assessed the efficacy of cetuximab in this setting. The phase II OPUS trial included patients with mCRC treated either with a fluorouracil, oxaliplatin and leucovorin regimen (FOLFOX) alone or in combination with weekly cetuximab. The combination regimen was associated with a higher objective response rate (61% vs. 37%) and a slightly lower risk for disease progression for the subgroup of patients with K-RAS wild-type tumors (Bokemeyer et al., 2009). In a phase III trial, the benefit of adding cetuximab to a fluoropyrimidine and oxaliplatin based regimen (either FOLFOX or CAPEOX) was assessed in patients with mCRC. Although no benefit was observed in OS or PFS, an increase in response rate was observed in K-RAS wild-type patients (Maughan et al., 2011). On the other hand, the phase III TAILOR trail showed a significant benefit of adding cetuximab to the FOLFOX regimen, with an increase median in PFS (9.2 versus 7.4 months), OS (20.7 versus 17.8 months) and overall response rate (ORR) (Qin et al., 2018).Another clinical trial confirmed the benefit of adding cetuximab to FOLFIRI in patients with mCRC, with an increase in both median PFS (9.9 versus 8.4 months, HR 0.70) and OS (23.5 versus 20.0 months, HR 0.80) (Van Cutsem et al., 2011). Another randomized phase III trial aimed to compare the addition of cetuximab or bevacizumab, an anti-VEGF antibody, to chemotherapy regimens as first-line treatment for patients with mCRC. With the inclusion of 1137 patients, there was no difference between these two antibodies for patients with K-RAS wild-type tumors (Venook et al., 2017).

Cetuximab is also used for treatment of head and neck squamous cell carcinoma (HNSCC). In a phase III multinational trial, 424 patients with locally advanced HNSCC of the oropharynx, hypopharynx and larynx were randomized for treatment with radiotherapy alone *versus* concomitant radiotherapy and cetuximab treatment. Cetuximab was initially administered in an initial dose of $400mg/m^2$ of body surface area, one week before radiotherapy, with a concomitant weekly dose of $250mg/m^2$. Radiotherapy was administered using either conventional or hyperfractionation schedules, with an equivalent dose in 2Gy per fraction of around 70Gy. Patients who underwent concomitant treatment experienced a significantly prolonged PFS (with a hazard ratio [HR] of 0.70) and median OS (49.0 months versus 29.3 months, HR 0.74) (Bonner et al., 2006). This benefit was maintained for longer follow-up (Bonner et al., 2010). For recurrent or metastatic HNSCC, the phase III randomized EXTREME trial compared a chemotherapy regimen with cisplatin (or carboplatin) with fluorouracil to the same regimen with the addition of weekly cetuximab, for a maximum total of 6 cycles, with a maintenance of cetuximab treatment until progression or unacceptable adverse effects for the latter arm. An increased median OS (7.4 months versus 10.1 months, HR 0.80), median PFS (3.3 months versus 5.6 months, HR 0.54) and response rate (20% versus 36%) was obtained for the cetuximab group (Vermorken et al., 2008). With these results, cetuximab was approved by the FDA for treatment of HNSCC in these contexts, and it is included in international guidelines for treatment of this cancer (Grégoire et al., 2013). Another treatment option for locally advanced HNSCC is the use of induction chemotherapy, followed by radiotherapy ± systemic therapy. TREMPLIN phase II trial was designed aiming to comparing the use of chemoradiotherapy with cisplatin versus bioradiotherapy with cetuximab after induction chemotherapy with docetaxel, cisplatin and fluorouracil in locally advanced larynx or hypopharynx HNSCC. No differences in PFS and OS were observed between those to regimens, although no comparison with radiotherapy alone was performed (Lefebvre et al., 2013). As adjuvant treatment of HNSCC there is no current guideline for using cetuximab containing regimens. However, the RTOG-0234 trial combined a chemoradiation schedule with conventional fractionated radiotherapy in a total dose of 60Gy with the addition of weekly cetuximab associated with either cisplatin or docetaxel, showing a favorable outcome for PFS and OS in the docetaxel regimen (Harari et al., 2014). RTOG-1216 (NCT01810913) is further investigating the use of adjuvant chemoradiotherapy with docetaxel and cetuximab. For NSCLC treatment, a large phase III trial assessed the addition of cetuximab to cisplatin and vinorelbine for patients with advanced disease. An increase in median OS was observed (11.3 versus 10.1 months, HR 0.87), but associated with a significantly higher rate of grade 4 side-effects (Pirker et a., 2009).

Panitumumab

Panitumumab is another monoclonal antibody against EGFR, which differs from cetuximab for being a fully human monoclonal antibody. In 2006, US FDA and EMA approved panitumumab for use in the same patient's population were cetuximab was approved (mCRC without K-RAS mutation).

The addition of these antibody to a FOLFOX regimen in patients with K-RAS wild-type mCRC was assessed in the PRIME trial, showing a significant increase from the addition of panitumumab in both median PFS (10.1 versus 7.9 months, HR 0.72) and median OS (19.3 versus 15.5 months, HR 0.77) (Douillard et al., 2010; Douillard et al., 2013) A meta-analysis including seven randomized controlled trials with the use of EGFR inhibitors for mCRC showed a significant increase in PFS (HR 0.77) and OS (HR 0.81) in patients with K-RAS wild-type tumors (Pietrantonio et al., 2016). Another meta-analysis showed no significant benefit of adding these inhibitors to chemotherapy regimens for patients with K-RAS mutations (Sorich et al., 2015). Regarding all the results described above, there is an international recommendation for the use of these monoclonal antibodies against EGFR in association with chemotherapy regimens for the treatment of mCRC (Van Cutsem et al., 2014).

Bardelli et al. suggest that CRCs lacking oncogenic alterations in KRAS, BRAF, PIK3CA, and PTEN genes have the highest probability of response to anti-EGFR therapies and are defined as "quadruple negative." The rapid and effective translation of these findings into predictive biomarkers to couple EGFR-targeted antibodies to the patients who benefit from them is a paradigm of modern clinical oncology (Bardelli et al., 2010).

Erlotinib and Gefitinib

Other EGFR inhibitors have been evaluated for metastatic NSCLC treatment, namely erlotinib and gefitinib.

Gefitinib is an EGFR inhibitor, anilinoquinazoline derived, orally active with low-molecular-weight and selective tyrosine kinase activity. Gefitinib has a 200-fold greater affinity for EGFR relative to the other ErbB family members. Due to the overexpression of EGFR, gefitinib is approved for the treatment of patients with NSCLC after failure of both platinum-based or docetaxel chemotherapies. The IPASS phase III trial compared gefitinib to carboplatin plus paclitaxel regimen as first line treatment in metastatic NSCLC. Increased response rate (71.2% versus 47.3%) and PFS (HR 0.74 for all patients, 0.48 for patients with EGFR mutations) were reported (Mok et al., 2009), but with similar OS (Fukuoka et al., 2011).

Erlotinib hydrochloride is another FDA-approved low molecular weight molecule similar to gefitinib, that is orally given, being a potent and selectively reversible inhibitor of EGFR tyrosine kinase. Like gefitinib, erlotinib functions by competing with ATP binding pockets within the RTKs. Erlotinib is currently approved in patients with relapsed NSCLC and for maintenance therapy in advanced NSCLC patients whose disease had not progressed after four cycles of platinum-based first line chemotherapy. It is also approved for use in locally advanced, unresectable or metastatic pancreatic cancer patients in combination with a gemcitabine.

Erlotinib for the treatment of metastatic NSCLC with EGFR sensitizing mutations was assessed in both the EURTAC and OPTIMAL phase III trials. These trials show a longer PFS for patients receiving erlotinib in monotherapy comparing to patients receiving chemotherapy (EURTAC: median 9.7 versus 5.2 months, HR 0.37; OPTIMAL 13.1 versus 4.6 months, HR 0.16) (Zhou et al., 2011; Rosell et al., 2012). WGOG 5108L phase 3 trial compared the efficacy of erlotinib and gefitinib for patients previously treated with chemotherapy, reporting no differences in PFS for both regimens in patients with lung adenocarcinoma and EGFR sensitizing mutations (Urata et al., 2016). The association of erlotinib with other drugs for NSCLC was also addressed in different trials. CALGB 30406 compared erlotinib to its association with chemotherapy, identifying no differences between these regimens (Jänne et al., 2012). The RELAY phase III trial assessed treatment with erlotinib ± ramucirumab, with a longer median PFS (19.4 versus 12.4 months, HR 0.59) for the combination of both drugs, but an increase in the rate of grade 3-4 side effects (Nakagawa et al., 2019). Association of erlotinib with bevacizumab also showed a significant increase in median PFS in the phase III NEJ026 randomized trial (16.9 versus 13.3 months, HR 0.61) (Saito et al., 2019). These results lead to FDA approval for both gefitinib and erlotinib for treatment of metastatic NSCLC with EGFR sensitizing mutations (Cohen et al., 2005; Cohen et al., 2003).

The efficacy of erlotinib was also evaluated in patients with advanced pancreatic cancer. In a phase III trial, 569 patients were randomized to treatment with gemcitabine ± erlotinib. 53% of these patients had a positive expression of EGFR. The authors reported a significant longer median OS (6.24 versus 5.91 months, HR 0.82) and median PFS (3.75 versus 3.55 months, HR 0.77) for patients treated with the combination regimen, regardless of EGFR status (Moore et al., 2007).

HER2 Inhibitors

One of the major breakthroughs in breast cancer (BC) was identifying prognostic subgroups using molecular markers (Dai et al., 2015). HER-2 is a transmembrane receptor of the EGFR family, which is overexpressed on some of BC cells. The first recombinant antibody approved by the FDA to target HER2-positive breast cancers was trastuzumab or Herceptin (1998) followed by other agents like pertuzumab and lapatinib. (Masoud et al., 2017). More recently (2019), FDA approved a conjugated monoclonal antibody, TDM1 (trastuzumab emtansine, a microtubule inhibitor) (Markham et al., 2020).

Trastuzumab is a humanized monoclonal antibody that blocks the HER-2 receptor by binding to its extracellular domain (Burstein, 2005), in the juxtamembrane region of the HER2 receptor tyrosine kinase. This results in the uncoupling of the HER2/HER3 heterodimers and consequent inhibition of downstream signaling and cytotoxicity (Masoud e al., 2017).

Several randomized clinical trials have assessed the use of this antibody in treating HER-2 positive BC. Two of these trials, NSABP B-31 and NCCTG N9831, were analyzed together in order to assess the benefit of adjuvant chemotherapy with paclitaxel with trastuzumab. With the inclusion of 4045 patients, an increased PFS and OS were observed for patients treated with trastuzumab at four an eight-year follow-up periods (Perez et al., 2011; Perez et al., 2014; Romond et al., 2005). All HER-2 positive patients benefited from trastuzumab, regardless of other tumor characteristics, and the most relevant side-effect was cardiac toxicity (Perez et al., 2014).

Another trial (HERA) included 5081 patients with HER-2 positive BC, testing the benefit of the addition of trastuzumab to chemotherapy. With a median follow-up of 11 years, it showed a disease-free survival (DFS) and OS benefit with a one-year treatment with trastuzumab regarding DFS (Piccart-Gebhart et al., 2005) and OS, the latter after 2-year follow-up, with no differences between 1 and 2 years of treatment with trastuzumab (Cameron et al., 2017). Also, the BCIRG 006 clinical trial showed a significant benefit in DFS for patients with HER-2 positive node-positive or high risk node negative BC treated with trastuzumab, with an HR of 0.64 (Smith et al., 2007).

Another monoclonal antibody against HER-2 receptor is pertuzumab. The CLEOPATRA phase III trial included 808 patients with metastatic HER-2 positive BC. The addition of pertuzumab to docetaxel and trastuzumab showed a benefit regarding median PFS (18.7 versus 12.4 months, HR 0.69) and median OS (57.1 versus 40.8 months, HR 0.69), with a median follow-up of 99.9 months. (45,46) With these results, there is an international recommendation for adjuvant treatment with trastuzumab for one-year, and it should be started during chemotherapy, although not during anthracycline treatment due to cardiotoxicity (Cardoso et al., 2017). For metastatic breast cancer, the use of chemotherapy with dual blockade with trastuzumab and pertuzumab was recommended in an international consensus guideline (Cardose et al., 2018).

Trastuzumab emtansine (T-DM1) is a conjugated monoclonal antibody that links the biologic drug trastuzumab (anti-HER2, T) with the chemotherapy drug emtansine (a microtubule inhibitor, DM1). This nanoparticle transports the DM1 drug directly into the breast cancer cells inhibiting its growth. T-DM1 allows for selective delivery of the chemotherapy drug into HER2-overexpressing cells, resulting in cell cycle arrest and apoptosis (Masoud et al., 2017; Markham et al., 2020).

FDA approved T-DM1 in 2019 for adjuvant (postoperative) treatment of patients with residual invasive disease after neoadjuvant (preoperative) treatment with a regimen that included a taxane and trastuzumab. This approval of adjuvant T-DM129 came in response to the phase III KATHERINE trial (ClinicalTrials.gov identifier NCT01772472) which included nearly 1,500 patients. All patients had residual invasive disease following neoadjuvant treatment with taxane- and trastuzumab-based regimens. Those who received adjuvant T-DM1 had a 50% lower risk of recurrence of invasive disease or death compared with those who received postoperative trastuzumab (Markham et al., 2020).

Anti-HER-2 targeted therapies have also been tested for gastric cancer. The ToGA phase III trial included 594 patients with HER-2 positive gastric or gastroesophageal junction tumors, treated with fluoropyrimidine + cisplatin ± trastuzumab. An increase in median PFS (6.7 versus 5.5 months, HR 0.71) and median OS (13.8 versus 11.1 months, HR 0.60) was obtained for trastuzumab treated patients (Bang et al., 2010), and this combination is now included in international guidelines for treatment of inoperable or metastatic HER-2 positive gastric or gastroesophageal junction cancer (Smyth et al., 2016).

EGFR and HER-2 Dual Blockade

Lapatinib is a quinazoline derivative that reversibly blocks both EGFR and HER-2 receptors (Rusnak et al., 2001). A phase III randomized clinical trial that included 399 patients with locally advanced or metastatic HER-2 positive BC previously treated with chemotherapy plus trastuzumab. It compared treatment with capecitabine plus lapatinib versus capecitabine alone. The interim analysis showed an increased median PFS (8.4 versus 4.4 months, HR 0.49), although no differences in OS were observed (Geyer et al., 2006). Based on these results, accrual was suspended and arm cross-over was proposed to all patients treated with capecitabine alone. Updated analysis was published, confirming better median PFS (6.2 versus 4.3 months, HR 0.57) and a non-significant OS benefit, with a lower frequency of central nervous system metastasis when first progression was reported (Cameron et al., 2008). This lead to FDA approval in this setting, and combination of lapatinib and capecitabine is considered as an option for advanced BC after progression on trastuzumab-based treatment in international guidelines (Cardoso et al., 2018).

Afatinib is another oral dual receptor inhibitor for both EGFR and HER-2 (Nelson et al., 2013). The LUX-Lung 3 phase III trial tested EGFR mutation-positive patients to afatinib or chemotherapy with cisplatin plus pemetrexed, with a longer median PFS for afatinib (11.1 versus 6.9 months, HR 0.58) (Sequist et al., 2013). This lead to FDA approval of afatinib in patients with NSCLC with EGFR sensitizing mutations (Dungo & Keating, 2013).

VEGF Inhibitors

Another RTK target is the VEGF receptor. The most known drug to inhibit its activation is bevacizumab, a humanized recombinant monoclonal antibody that binds to VEGF, preventing the activation of the corresponding receptor. As shown for cetuximab and panitumumab, bevacizumab has also an important role for the treatment of mCRC, has shown in several trials. One of the first trials showing the benefit of bevacizumab in mCRC revealed a significant increase in median PFS (10.6 versus 6.2 months, HR 0.54) and median OS (20.3 versus 15.6 months, HR 0.66) when associated with FOLFIRI (Hurwitz et al., 2004). A combined analysis of the results of three clinical trials, comparing patients treated with fluorouracil ± bevacizumab, showed an increased median PFS (8.8 versus 5.6 months, HR 0.74) as well as an increased median OS (17.9 versus 14.6 months, HR 0.74) (Kabbinavar et al., 2005). Another large phase III trial, with 1401 patients with mCRC, compared the use of capecitabine and oxaliplatin (CAPEOX) ± bevacizumab with FOLFOX ± bevacizumab, which resulted in a significant increase in median PFS for bevacizumab group (9.4 versus 8.0 months, HR 0.83), although not achieving statistical significance for median OS (21.3 versus 19.9 months) (Saltz et al., 2008). Several meta-analysis assessing the role of bevacizumab for first-line treatment of mCRC have been published so far. One included nine clinical trials with a total of 3914 patients, comparing chemotherapy for mCRC, with or without bevacizumab. It was shown that adding bevacizumab to chemotherapy treatment lead to better response rates (HR 0.89), PFS (HR 0.69) and OS (HR 0.87) (Botrel et al., 2016). Another meta-analysis confirmed the value of adding bevacizumab to chemotherapy in first-line treatment, with HR of 0.56 for PFS and 0.83 for OS (Zhang et al., 2015). In a subgroup analysis of a meta-analysis it has been suggested that this benefit might be restricted to irinotecan containing regimens (Macedo et al., 2012). As described before, the addition of either bevacizumab or cetuximab to FOLFOX or FOLFIRI for treatment for patients with mCRC showed no significant difference among patients with K-RAS wild-type tumors, with both regimens being suitable for first-line treatment in this context (Van Cutsem et al., 2014; Venook et al., 2017).

The role of maintenance treatment with inclusion of bevacizumab has also been assessed in clinical trials. The phase III CAIRO3 study evaluated the role of capecitabine and bevacizumab as maintenance treatment versus observation after chemotherapy for mCRC. There was a significant increase in PFS (11.7 versus 8.5 months, HR 0.67), but no for OS (21.6 vs. 18.1 months) (Simkens et al., 2015). The results of PRODIGE 9 phase III trial showed no benefit of maintaining treatment with bevacizumab after a regimen containing FOLFIRI + bevacizumab (Aparicio et al., 2018).

The use of bevacizumab in patients with nonsquamous NSCLC was addressed in ECOG 4599 phase III trial, which randomized 878 patients for treatment with paclitaxel and carboplatin ± bevacizumab. An increase in median OS (12.3 versus 10.3 months, HR 0.79), PFS (6.2 versus 4.5 months, HR 0.66) and response rate (35% versus 15%) was observed. (66) FDA approval was obtained for this regimen in NSCLC treatment (Cohen et al., 2007).

In the treatment of metastatic BC, several phase III clinical trials showed benefit of its use in association with different chemotherapy regimens. The association of bevacizumab with paclitaxel showed a higher median PFS (11.8 versus 5.9 months, HR 0.60) comparing to paclitaxel alone (Miller et al., 2007). When assessing the combination of docetaxel ± bevacizumab in HER-2 negative metastatic BC patients, an increase in median PFS (10.1 versus 8.2 months, HR 0.77) was observed (Miller et al., 2007). The RIBBON-1 trial, enrolling 1237 patients with HER-2 negative metastatic BC, in which the administration of bevacizumab with different chemotherapy regimens was tested, showed a significant increase of PFS for the association scheme with capecitabine, taxanes and anthracyclines (Robert et al., 2011).

Systemic first-line treatment recommendations for patients with good or intermediate risk clear cell renal cell carcinoma include a combination of bevacizumab with interferon (Escudier et al., 2019). A randomized phase III trial that included 641 patients with metastatic renal cell carcinoma that was not previously treated, showed an advantage of combining both drugs comparing to interferon treatment alone, with a longer median PFS (10.2 versus 5.4 months, HR 0.63) (Escudier et al., 2007).

Novel anti-VEGFR agents are emerging and some of them have been approved for second-line treatment of CRC. Aflibercept is a VEGFR-1 and VEGFR-2 extracellular domain recombinant fusion protein that acts as a ligand trap targeting VEGF-A, VEGF-B, and PIGF. Aflibercept has a stronger affinity for VEGF-A than bevacizumab.

Ramucirumab, is a fully humanized monoclonal antibody anti- VEGFR-2, also FDA-approved for second-line treatment of metastatic CRC based on the phase III RAISE trial. In this second-line-setting trial, a combination of ramucirumab and FOLFIRI significantly prolonged PFS (5.7 vs. 4.5 months; HR = 0.79, $p < .0005$) and OS (13.3 vs. 11.7 months, HR = 0.84, $p = 0.022$) compared with FOLFIRI-placebo. Similar to the findings with aflibercept, a phase II trial showed that the FOLFOX regimen may not benefit from addition to ramucirumab in terms of PFS (Xie et al., 2020).

PDGFR Inhibitors

Oralatumab is a monoclonal antibody that targets PDGFRa and has shown a lower proliferation rate in *in vivo* models of several tumor cell lines (Papadopoulos et al., 2018). In a phase II trial, 133 patients with soft-tissue sarcoma were randomized for treatment with doxorubicin ± oralatumab, and a significant increase in median OS was observed for the combination treatment (26.5 versus 14.7 months; HR 0.46) (Tap et al., 2016). This lead its approval by the FDA in this setting (Shirley, 2017). A phase III trial (ANNOUNCE – NCT02451943) was designed in order to confirm this described benefit. However, after a negative results interim report of this trial, FDA withdrew the approval of oralatumab for soft-tissue sarcoma treatment. A new phase I/II trial has been initiated in June 2017, testing the effect of oralatumab in combination with nab-paclitaxel and gemcitabine in patients with metastatic pancreatic cancer (NCT03086369).

RET Inhibitors

The RET proto-oncogene is located on chromosome 10q11.2 and plays an important role in the development of several human cancers. This gene encodes a transmembrane tyrosine-kinase glycoprotein with a relevant role in the embryogenic development of several organs and tissues, such as the enteric nervous system and the kidneys (de Graaff et al., 2001; Drilon et al., 2018), being responsible for the activation of several intracellular signaling cascades, such as the MAPK, JAK-STAT and PI3K pathways (Arighi, Borrello & Sariola, 2005). Its activation during carcinogenesis can result from germline mutations, such as those present in multiple endocrine neoplasia (MEN) syndromes type 2A and 2B, or from somatic mutations. (Arighi, Borrello & Sariola, 2005; Drilon et al., 2018; Shaw et al., 2013). RET activation was initially identified in papillary thyroid cancer, with later recognition of its involvement in other endocrine neoplasms, such medullary thyroid carcinoma (both sporadic and associated with familial syndromes). Less frequently, it was also identified in a small portion of non-small cell lung cancer, mainly in adenocarcinomas (Ferrara et al., 2018; Lin et al., 2015). As the deregulated activity of RET contributes to the development of several cancers, targeting RET have proven to be an advantage in the treatment of these neoplasms (Drilon et al., 2018; Gainor & Shaw, 2013; Jhiang, 2000; Kato et al., 2017; Mulligan, 2014; Shaw et al., 2013).

RET inhibition can be achieved by using several kinases inhibitors as shown in Figure (Chau & Haddad, 2013; Kato et al., 2017; Yoh et al., 2017), all of these with FDA approval for different malignant tumors treatment.

Table 3. RET inhibition using multiple kinase inhibitors

Kinase inhibitors	Target
Vandetanib	RET/EGFR/VEGFR2
Lenvatinib	RET/FGFR/ VEGFR/KIT/PDGFR
Cabozantinib	RET/MET/VEGFR2
Regorafenib	RET/VEGFR/KIT/BRAF/CRAF
Sorafenib	RET/VEGFR/KIT/ BRAF/CRAF
Sunitinib	RET/VEGFR/KIT/ PDGFR/FLT3
Ponatinib	RET/ FGFR/VEGFR/KIT/PDGFR/BCR-ABL

Vandetanib

Vandetanib is approved by the FDA for treatment of medullary thyroid carcinoma. A randomized double-blinded phase 3 trial that included 331 patients with locally advanced or metastatic medullary thyroid cancer showed an increase in progression-free survival (PFS) for patients who underwent treatment with vandetanib, comparing to the placebo group (hazard ratio [HR] 0.46, $p<0.001$), with an increase in side effects, namely diarrhea, hypertension, nausea, rash and headache. (13) Two phase II randomized clinical trials assessed the role of vandetanib in non-small cell lung cancer (NSCLC) with RET rearrangements and negative for EGFR mutations. In LURET trial, 1536 patients were screened for RET rearrangements, with a positivity rate of 2% and with an enrollment of 19 patients for 300mg of oral vandetanib. A median PFS of 4.7 month was obtained, with hypertension, skin rash and diarrhea as the most common grade 3 or 4 side effects (Yoh et al., 2017). Lee and colleagues also included NSCLC patients with RET rearrangements treated with the same dose of vandetanib in a phase II trial. In a total of 18 patients, a disease control rate of 65% was observed, with a median PFS of 4.5 months and a median overall survival (OS) of 11.6 months. As for grade 3 side effects, hypertension and QT prolongation were the most reported effects (Lee et al., 2017).

To assess the safety profile of vandetanib, a systematic review with metanalysis included 11 trials evaluated the increased risk of hypertension in cancer patients treated with this compound, confirming an increased risk of hypertension with an HR of 5.1 (Qi et al., 2013). An increased risk of diarrhea and cutaneous rash were also demonstrated in two metanalysis (Rosen et al., 2012; Yang et al., 2018).

Lenvatinib

Lenvatinib is another multiple tyrosine kinase inhibitor for oral administration. The corresponding molecular targets are PDGF, FGF and VEGF receptors, as well as the proto-oncogenes KIT and RET.

The assessment of this drug efficacy and safety in thyroid cancer was performed in several studies. A phase II trial assessed the efficacy of lenvatinib in 55 patients with a diagnosis of medullary thyroid cancer, with an ORR of 36% and disease control rate of 80%, with a median PFS of 9.0 months. Side effects were manageable, with grade 3-4 for hypertension, diarrhea, fatigue and decreased appetite (Schlumberge et al., 2016). The SELECT phase III trial (NCT01321554) was a multicentric and randomized (2:1) study designed to evaluate the role of lenvatinib in the treatment of thyroid cancer patients with progressive disease refractory to iodine-131. With a dose of 24 mg per day, a significantly increase in median PFS was observed for lenvatinib (18.3 months versus 3.6 months), together with an increased rate of side effects, being the commoner, hypertension and diarrhea (Schlumberge et al., 2015). This significant difference was maintained for a longer follow-up, with a median PFS of 19.4 months versus 3.7 months. Patients who showed a response to treatment with lenvatinib had also a higher median PFS when compared to non-responders (33.1 months versus 7.9 months) (Gianoukakis et al., 2018).

Regarding advanced or metastatic renal cell carcinoma, a phase I trial tested the safety profile of the association of lenvatinib with everolimus, which appeared to be well tolerated, with a manageable side effect profile (Matsubara et al., 2018). A phase II randomized multicentric three-arm trial compared treatment with lenvatinib, everolimus or a combination of both in this context. In which concerns PFS, both the association of lenvatinib with everolimus (median PFS of 14.6 months) and the treatment with lenvatinib alone (median PFS of 7.4 months) showed a significant benefit when compared to everolimus alone (median PFS of 5.5 months) (Motzer et al., 2015).

Levantinib also showed an acceptable anti-tumor effect in other malignant tumors, including hepatocellular carcinoma, metastatic adenoid cystic carcinoma and advanced endometrial cancer in phase II trials, (Ikeda et al., 2017; Makker et al., 2019; Tchekmedyian et al., 2019) with a phase III trial showing a non-inferiority effect of this drug on OS when comparing to sorafenib in the treatment of hepatocellular carcinoma (Kudo et al., 2018).

Cabozantinib

Cabozantinib is an inhibitor of multiple TKI, namely RET, hepatocyte growth factor receptor (HGFR) and vascular endothelial growth factor receptor 2 (VEGFR2). In a phase I dose-escalation trial, 85 patients with a diagnosis of medullary thyroid cancer were treated with cabozantinib, which presented an acceptable safety profile and activity (Kurzrock et al., 2011). A subsequent randomized (2:1) double-blinded phase II trial evaluated the efficacy of 140mg daily cabozantinib in 330 patients with metastatic thyroid cancer. A significantly increased PFS was observed (median of 11.2 months vs. 4.0 months), with an HR of 0.28, although an increase in side effect rates was also registered, namely palmar-plantar erythrodysesthesia, diarrhea, nausea and fatigue (Elisei et al., 2013). Another phase II trial enrolled 26 patients with metastatic or unresectable NSCLC with RET rearrangements for assessment of overall response rate (ORR) using cabozantinib in a dose of 60mg per day. An ORR of 28% was observed, with manageable side effects and no drug-related deaths, although a dose reduction was needed for 73% of these patients (Drilon et al., 2016).

Other RET Inhibitors

Other non-specific RET inhibitors have also been approved for the treatment of malignant tumors: sorafenib has been approved for treating differentiated thyroid carcinoma, renal cell carcinoma and hepatocellular carcinoma, ponatinib for chronic myeloid leukemia and Philadelphia chromosome–positive acute lymphoblastic leukemia, sunitinib for renal cell carcinoma and imatinib-resistant gastrointestinal stromal tumor (GIST), and regorafenib for colorectal cancer and GIST (Chau & Haddad, 2013; Kato et al., 2017; Yoh et al., 2017).

Some selective RET kinase inhibitors are also being assessed for cancer treatment. Selpercatinib (LOXO-292) proved to be effective in inhibiting RET hyperactivation, resulting from fusion proteins or missense mutations. It was recently approved by FDA (May, 2020) for oral treatment of metastatic RET fusion-positive non-small cell lung cancer, for advanced or metastatic RET-mutant medullary thyroid cancer in adults and children aged 12 years or more, as well as for advanced or metastatic RET fusion-positive thyroid cancer refractory to radioactive iodine therapy (Guo et al., 2019; Markham, 2020; Seoane & Capdevila, 2018; Wirth et al., 2019). Also, this selective RET inhibitor is under study in a phase I/II trail (NCT03899792), aiming to recruit pediatric patients with advanced solid or primary central nervous system tumor with RET-alterations.

Another novel and selective another RET inhibitor, RXDX-105, is being tested in a phase I clinical trial to assess the benefit of continued treatment with this drug in patients with NSCLC or ovarian cancer, with an estimated completion date on December 2020 (Drilon et al., 2019; Li et al., 2017;).

Pralsetinib (BLU-667), another selective oral RET inhibitor about 100 times more potent than other RET inhibitors in preclinical research, is being studied in patients with thyroid cancer, NSCLC and other advanced solid tumors in a phase I/II trial (ARROW, NCT03037385), in order to define safety, tolerability and preliminary antitumor activity (Ackermann et al., 2019; Subbiah et al., 2018).

NON-RECEPTOR TYROSINE KINASE (NRTK)

BCR-ABL Inhibitors

Due to the importance of the Non-Receptor Tyrosine Kinase (NRTK) in cancer, BCR-ABL was the first target explored in the development of targeted therapies inhibitors. Imatinib was the first tyrosine kinase inhibitor approved by the FDA and EMA in 2001 and change dramatically the course of CML (Cohen et al., 2002). Currently, six BCR-ABL inhibitors are approved for CML treatment, namely Imatinib, Dasatinib, Nilotinib, Bosutinib, Ponatinib, and Radotinib (this last one is only approved by Korean authorities). All these molecules are orally administrated and competitively inhibit BCR-ABL TK by binding at the ATP-binding site. Consequently, blocking the phosphorylation of several substrates shutting of the oncogenic signal for downstream pathways.

Imatinib, a first-generation TKI, can bind to the inactive form of BCR-ABL, preventing its activation by switching to the active conformation. In addition to this target, this TKI is also able to inhibit PDGFR and c-KIT tyrosine kinases (Manley et al., 2002; Savage & Antman, 2002). Due to this multiple targets, Imatinib is currently approved for different diseases associated with *BCR-ABL1* fusion gene (CML and Ph+ ALL), *PDGFR* gene re-arrangements (MDS/MPN) or involved in fusion genes (hypereosinophilic syndrome or chronic eosinophilic leukemia), and with *c-KIT* mutations as in case of GIST tumors KIT positive. Regarding BCR-ABL activity, Imatinib was approved firstly for CML patients at accelerated phase or in blast crisis and for those in chronic phase that failure IFN-α treatment (O'Brien et al., 2003). The results of the IRIS trial, where Imatinib 400 mg once daily was compared with IFN-α plus cytarabine, reveal an improvement on CCyR at 18 months in imatinib arm (76.2% for Imatinib vs. 14.5% for IFN-α/ara-C) associated with lower progression rate (O'Brien et al., 2003). This lead to the approval of Imatinib 400 mg as the gold standard for CML-CP patients, and currently, this is used as a reference arm in multiple BCR-ABL clinical trials. The introduction of this TKI in CML treatment increased unquestionably the overall survival to 83% comparing to available treatment (IFN plus cytarabine) on 10-years follow-up (Hochhaus et al., 2017). However, at this same time point, 11% of patients presented unsatisfactory therapeutic effects, and a total of 52% of patients discontinue treatment due to lake of response, intolerance, or adverse effects (Hochhaus et al., 2017). One approach to overcome a lack of response or to more aggressive forms of the disease is dose-escalation until 800 mg daily (Liu et al., 2016). With extended use in clinical practice, the Imatinib safety profile is very well known, and the most common adverse effects are fluid retention, edema, nausea, vomiting, diarrhea, fatigue, and some skin disorders. This adverse events are aggravated with dose escalation (Caldemeyer et al., 2016). Particularly for the pediatric population, the recommended dose range from 260-340 mg/sqm/ day, and this can be associated with growth deceleration and lower bone mineral density (Giona et al., 2013).

Despite the good results in several diseases, approximately 20 to 30% of patients do not achieve the best results with Imatinib and need to change the therapeutic protocol (Patel, O'Hare, & Deininger, 2017; Yang & Fu, 2015). The most common cause of resistance to BCR-ABL TKIs is the occurrence of a point mutation in *BCR-ABL1,* and each TKI presents a different sensitivity profile to the different mutations identified (Table 4). Imatinib presents an intermediated sensitivity to Q252H, F317L, F359V/C and to H396R/P mutations, but is completely resistant to G250E, Y253H/F, E255K/V, V299L and to the most aggressive mutations the T315I (Meenakshi Sundaram et al., 2019; Redaelli, et al. 2012; Soverini, et al. 2011). In addition to *BCR-ABL1* point mutations, mechanisms associated with drug transporters are crucial for TKI efficacy. OCT1 is the main uptake drug transporter that mediates the TKI entrance in cells, where ABC transporters, as P-gP and BCRP, are involved in the extrusion of TKI from the cells (Alves et al., 2015; Eadie et al., 2014; Neul et al., 2016). An unbalance in drug transporters expression and activity are associated with TKI resistance (Ben Hassine et al., 2017; de Lima et al., 2014; White et al., 2007). All the next-generation TKI approved were developed with aim to overcome resistance and intolerance observed in patients treated with Imatinib, especially the point mutations identified as a key factor for TKI success. Dasatinib, Nilotinib, Bosutinib, and Radotinib are second-generation TKI (2nd TKI), where Ponatinib is a 3rd generation TKI.

Table 4. Most frequent BCR-ABL1 mutation and the sensitivity degree to the different approved TKIs

BCR-ABL1 Mutation	Imatinib	Dasatinib	Nilotinib	Bosutinib	Radotinib	Ponatinib
Wild-Type	Sen	Sen	Sen	Sen	Sen	Sen
M244V	Sen	Sen	Sen	Sen	Sen	Sen
G250E	Res	Sen	Int	Int	Int	Sen
Q252H	Int	Int	Sen	Sen	Sen	Sen
Y253H/F	Res	Sen	Res	Sen	Res	Sen
E255K/V	Res	Int	Res	Int	Res	Int
V299L	Res	Res	Sen	Int	Sen	Sen
T315I	Res	Res	Res	Res	Res	Sen
F317L	Int	Int	Sen	Int	Sen	Sen
M351T	Sen	Sen	Sen	Sen	Sen	Sen
F359V/C	Int	Sen	Int	Sen	Int	Sen
H396R/P	Int	Sen	Int	Sen	Sen	Int

Sen: Sensitive; Int: intermediate sensitivity; Res: Resistant. Data derived from the following references: Meenakshi Sundaram et al., 2019; Redaelli et al.; 2012; Soverini et al. 2011; Eskazan & Keskin, 2017.

Dasatinib can bind to BCR-ABL TK in active and inactive conformation. This dual SRC/ABL inhibitor showed *in vitro* over 300-fold more potency than Imatinib and is also able to inhibit SRC family kinases, c-KIT, EPHA2, and PDGFRβ (Aguilera & Tsimberidou, 2009). Currently, dasatinib is approved to treat CML patients in any phase of disease and to ALL patients Ph+ with resistance or intolerance to prior therapy, and for pediatric cases of CML in chronic phase or Ph+ ALL. Based on DASISION trial results, the use of this 2nd TKI upfront reveals higher CCyR and molecular responses compared to Imatinib. Despite no differences in overall survival between the two TKIs, dasatinib was associated with deeper molecular responses and lower progression to CML-AP and CML-BC (Jabbour, 2016; Kantarjian et al., 2012). The prescribing dose for chronic phase is 100 mg once daily and, for CML-AP or CML-BC dose increases to 140 mg once daily, and for pediatric cases the dose is 60 mg/sqm once daily (Pushpam & Bakhshi, 2020). In terms of toxicity for adults, dasatinib presents similar low-grade adverse events as other TKIs, like vomiting, rash, fluid retention, fatigue. However, it is also associated with pleural effusion and pulmonary hypertension (Caldemeyer et al., 2016). The last two types of adverse events were not observed in pediatric cases, where dasatinib is associated with bone growth impairment (Gore et al., 2018). Resistance to this TKI is also observed as result of target point mutations (Table 4), particularly V299L and T315I, and unbalance of efflux drug transporters (Eadie, et al. 2014; Meenakshi Sundaram, et al. 2019; Redaelli, et al. 2012; Soverini, et al. 2011). In the case of dasatinib, the entrance in cells is not dependent on OCT1 since this molecule passively diffuses over the plasmatic membrane (Giannoudis et al., 2008; Hiwase et al., 2008).

Nilotinib results from a chemical modification of Imatinib, and *in vitro* has approximately 30-fold higher potency than 1st generation TKI. Nilotinib binds to inactive conformation of BCR-ABL as Imatinib, but also targets PDGFR and c-KIT (Sacha & Saglio, 2018). The ENESTnd trial results pointed out an improvement in response rates of newly diagnosed CML patients treated with 300 mg of Nilotinib twice daily when compared to Imatinib. However, as described to other 2nd TKI, the upfront of Nilotinib does not impact the overall survival of these patients, being very similar to the ones obtained with Imatinib (Saglio et al., 2010). Nilotinib is approved for newly diagnosed CML patients at chronic phase with a 300 mg twice daily, for patients in chronic or accelerated phase resistant or intolerants to previously treatment at dose of 400mg twice daily, and for CML pediatric cases with a recommended dose of 230 mg/sqm twice daily (Pushpam & Bakhshi, 2020). The principal toxicities associated with Nilotinib are prolongation in cardiac electrical conductivity, pancreatitis, hyperglycemia, hepatotoxicity, and vascular events (Caldemeyer et al., 2016). One important aspect for nilotinib absorption is the interaction with food, and because of that is advised to avoid food intake 2 hours before and 1 hour after this TKI intake (Cuellar et al., 2018). Resistance pattern to Nilotinib is very similar to observed for Imatinib regarding drug transporters, but this 2nd TKI presented a different resistance profile to *BCR-ABL1* point mutations. Nilotinib is resistant to Y253H/F, E255K/V, and T315I (Eadie, et al. 2014;

Meenakshi Sundaram, et al. 2019; Redaelli, et al. 2012; Soverini, et al. 2011) (Table 4).

In 2012, FDA approved Bosutinib, a 2nd TKI, for the treatment of CML cases previously treated with one or more TKI and for those patients where Imatinib, Nilotinib, and Dasatinib was not considered appropriate, at the dose of 500 mg once daily (Khoury et al., 2012). This drug is a dual ABL/SRC kinase inhibitor able to bind to BCR-ABL in both conformations. LYN, HCK, SRC are some of the other kinases targeted by bosutinib, but no effect is observed in PDGFR and c-KIT inhibition (Cortes et al., 2011; Puttini et al., 2006). Later, this TKI was approved for newly diagnosed CML-CP patients with a recommended dose of 400 mg once daily. The approval was based on BFORE trial, where a lower dose of bosutinib (400 mg) provides the right balance between efficacy and toxicity (Cortes et al., 2017). In terms of side effects, gastrointestinal and hepatic toxicity are the most severe ones described (Pushpam & Bakhshi, 2020). The resistance to this drug could results from the development of V299L and T315I *BCR-ABL1* point mutations and, as with the other TKI, influx and efflux drug transporters are also involved in this TKI efficacy (Meenakshi Sundaram et al., 2019; Redaelli et al., 2012; Soverini et al., 2011) (Table 4).

Only approved by Korea authorities, Radotinib is a 2nd TKI very similar to Nilotinib, that have been developed for CML treatment and show *in vitro* an IC_{50} of 34 nM. With different sensitivity, Radotinib is also able to inhibit PDGFR, LYN, and aurora kinases (AK) (Eskazan & Keskin, 2017; Zabriskie et al., 2014). Firstly approved for CML resistant and intolerant to other TKI with a dose of 400 mg/ twice daily and in 2015, this TKI can be used in newly diagnosed patients (using 300 mg/twice daily, following RERISE trial) (Kim et al., 2014; Kwak et al., 2017). The higher dose could be applied in CML patients in advanced phase, but is not approved for pediatric use (Pushpam & Bakhshi, 2020). Radotinib presented so far similar response levels to those achieved with other 2nd TKI in front-line, however a longer follow-up is needed to confirm efficacy (Kwak et al., 2017). Besides, for this TKI is extremely important to perform new clinical trials that involve different populations rather than only Asian to prove the efficacy of this inhibitor. Skin rash, nausea, thrombocytopenia, and neutropenia were the most common adverse effects for Radotinib treatment (Kwak et al., 2017). The resistance cases to this 2nd TKI have been associated with *BCR-ABL1* point mutations, namely Y235H, E255V, T315I, and T315M (Eskazan & Keskin, 2017) (Table 4).

Ponatinib is a 3rd generation TKI designed to overcome the most aggressive point mutations identified in *BCR-ABL1*, T315I. This TKI binds to the inactive conformation of BCR-ABL and *in vitro* presented 500 times more potency than Imatinib (O'Hare et al., 2009). SRC, VEGFR, PDGFR, c-KIT, and FLT3 are other kinases inhibited by this TKI (Cuellar et al., 2018). The results obtained in PACE Trial conducted to Ponatinib approval to all adults CML and ALL Ph+ patients with T315I mutations or for patients resistant to 2nd TKI (Cortes et al., 2012; Cortes et al., 2013). The prescribing dose is 45 mg once daily, but dose adjustments should be considered to proper management of adverse effects (Jabbour & Kantarjian, 2018). Consequently, this TKI is not recommended for newly diagnosed adult patients and pediatric use. The toxicity profile of Ponatinib is similar to other TKIs except for adverse vascular effects (Rea, 2015). Resistance to this 3rd TKI has been associated with *BCR-ABL1* mutation, even those including T315I, and with influx and efflux drug transporters, as P-gP and BCRP (Braun, Eide & Druker, 2020; Zabriskie et al., 2014).

In addition to the six approved molecules that target BCR-ABL, other drugs are currently under clinical trials with the purpose to improve this kinase inhibition, as the case of Asciminib, PF-114, HQP1351, and K0706 (Cortes et al., 2019; Özgür Yurttaş & Eşkazan, 2020). The most promising inhibitor in test is Asciminib because the different mechanisms of action. This TKI is the first allosteric inhibitor that binds to myristoyl site of ABL kinase, with an *in vitro* IC_{50} of 1-20 nM (Schoepfer et al., 2018; Wylie et al., 2017). The myristoyl group is involved in autoregulation of ABL activity, but with BCR fusion becomes constitutively activated (Nagar et al., 2003). In a phase 1 trial (NCT02081378), Asciminib was administered once or twice daily (10 to 200 mg) in patients heavily treated (Hughes et al., 2019). In terms of safety, asymptomatic elevations in the lipase levels, rash, fatigue, and nausea were the most common adverse effects. The efficacy of this treatment was measured by major molecular response (MMR), where 48%

of patients achieved or maintained MMR at 12 months of treatment (Hughes et al., 2019). By targeting different portions of ABL kinase, Asciminib may be very useful to overcome TKI resistance mediated by point mutations previously mentioned. However, for this TKI, mechanisms that could lead to resistance were already identified, namely point mutation at myristoylation pocket (V468F and I502L) and the function of ABC transporters (Eadie et al., 2018; Zhan, Ma & Zheng, 2019). The other molecules under clinical trials inhibit competitively the BCR-ABL TK at the ATP-binding site. PF-114 and HQP1351 present a higher potency against a wide-range of *BCR-ABL1* mutations, with an *in vitro* IC_{50} of 0.78 nM and 0.68 nM for T315I (Ivanova et al., 2019; Liu et al., 2019; Mian et al., 2014; Ren et al., 2013). Also, these TKIs affect FGFR, PDGFR, DDR1, and are currently involved in several clinical trials, as NCT02885766 and NCT04260022.

To overcome TKI resistance or improve discontinuation rate, new approaches have been tested in the clinical trial scenario, as drug combination of TKI with immunomodulators and other kinase inhibitors (Özgür Yurttaş & Eşkazan, 2020). Due to different mechanisms of action on the same kinase, the combination of approved TKI with Asciminib has been explored to reduce the possible appearance of *BCR-ABL1* mutant clones (NCT03595917, NCT03578367) (Eide et al., 2019; Westerweel et al., 2019). Drug combination between BCR-ABL TKI and Ruxolitinib (JAK2 inhibitor) is under study in the NCT03654768 trial, with the goal of target two different signaling pathways essential for tumor growth (Sweet et al., 2018). Other approaches have investigated the use of immune modulation associated with BCR-ABL TKI. The effect of Interferon-α (IFN) and immune checkpoint inhibitor has been studied since CML is a disease sensitive to immunological control (Brauer et al., 2006). The combination of approved TKI with pegylated forms of IFN was well-tolerated, reducing substantially the toxicity of non-pegylated form of IFN previously described in other trials (Westerweel et al., 2019). The interest in IFN therapy increased when it was associated with a higher chance of durable TKI discontinuation (Saussele et al., 2018). In the same line, PD-L1 inhibitors as Nivolumab and Avelumab have been combined with TKI (NCT02011945,

NCT02767063) with the potential to increase immunoreactivity against leukemic cells. Few results are available to evaluate the potential efficacy of these strategies, but all of them try to target BCR-ABL additional mechanism that could justify loss of response.

Bruton's Tyrosine Kinase Inhibitors

The Bruton's Tyrosine Kinase (BTK) is a cytoplasmatic protein of the B-cell Receptor (BCR) signaling pathway, critical for the development, proliferation and survival of normal B-cells. This kinase is expressed at all stages of B-cell development, except in the terminally differentiated plasma cells. It is also expressed in marrow-derived stem cells and developing myeloid cells, but not in T cells or nonhematopoietic cells (Castillo, Treon & Davids, 2016).

BTK´s loss of function is responsible for the inhibition of B-cells maturation, and consequently for the lack of production of immunoglobulins. This was first observed in the primary immunodeficiency X-linked agammaglobulinemia, due to mutations of BTK`s kinase domain, characterized by a profound hypogammaglobulinemia and markedly defective antibody response, associated with scarce lymphoid tissue and recurrent infections, predominantly by encapsulated bacteria (Aalipour & Advani, 2014; Aw & Brown, 2017; Thomas, Rodgers & Reagan, 2018).

The activation of BCR, and consequently of BTK pathways, also plays an important role in the pathophysiology of several heterogeneous mature B-cell neoplasms, namely Chronic Lymphocytic Leukemia (CLL), Mantle Cell Lymphoma (MCL), Waldenström`s Macroglobulinemia (WM) and Activated B-cell Type of Diffuse Large B Cell Lymphoma (ABC-DLBCL) (Castillo, Treon & Davids, 2016).

The knowledge of BTK role in the pathogenesis of B-cell malignancies, led to the development of novel drugs that target BTK, changing their treatment paradigm. Early clinical studies in several B-cell malignancies have shown that this therapeutic strategy was effective, with significant clinical responses, and with a tolerable safety profile, leading to the introduction of BTK inhibitors (BTKi) in the clinical practice. Ibrutinib was the first BTK inhibitor (BTKi) to be developed and tested in clinical trials.

Characteristics of BTK Inhibitors

Several molecules targeting BTK have been developed for the treatment of mature B-cell neoplasms. Ibrutinib was the first BTK inhibitor (BTKi) to be approved by US Food and Drug Administration (US FDA), for relapsed refractory (R/R) MCL in 2013. This oral drug is an irreversible BTKi by binding covalently to the cysteine residue (Cys-481) of the ATP binding site, leading to inhibition of its enzymatic activity, and also, by inhibiting BTK autophosphorylation at Tyr-223, blocking the full activation of BTK (Kim, 2019). However, ibrutinib also inhibits multiple related TEC family kinases, including endothelial growth factor receptor (EGFR), interleukin-2-inducible T cell kinase (ITK), tyrosine kinase expressed in hepatocellular carcinoma (TEC), and bone marrow tyrosine kinase on chromosome X (BMX), that are in part responsible for off-target effects, namely adverse events (AEs), and eventually for its clinical limitations (Bond & Woyach, 2019; Kim, 2019). Encouraging clinical data led to the development of second generation BTKi, acalabrutinib and zanubrutinib, which have been also approved for clinical use by US FDA. These oral drugs also inhibit BTK irreversibly by a covalent binding to its ATP binding site. Acalabrutinib is a more potent and highly selective BTKi, consequently with less off-target inhibition of EGFR and ITK, when compared to ibrutinib. Zanubrutinib in comparison to ibrutinib, displays a greater selectivity for BTK relative to ITK, but less global kinase selectivity for BTK in comparison to acalabrutinib. Although, covalent and irreversible binding of BTKi to Cys-481 results in high BTK selectivity, it also renders more susceptibility to resistance due to C481S mutation. Currently, are being developed novel inhibitors acting through a non-covalent reversible bond to BTK, that don`t rely upon interaction with Cys-481, representing a promising treatment in patients with ibrutinib resistance due to C481S mutation (Table 5).

Table 5. Characteristics of approved and novel BTK inhibitors

BTK inhibitor	Binding mechanism	Target position	Selectivity	Inhibition of other kinases
Ibrutinib (PCI-32765)	Covalent, irreversible	Cys-481; Tyr-223	Moderate	EGFR, ITK, TEC
Acalabrutinib (ACP-196)	Covalent, irreversible	Cys-481	High	ERK, IKB, ATK
Zanubrutinib (BGB-311)	Covalent, irreversible	Cys-481	Moderate	ITK
Tirabrutinib (ONO/GS-4059)	Covalent, irreversible	Tyr-223	High	TEC
Vecabrutinib (SNS-062)	Non-covalent, reversible	Cys-481	High	ITK

Data derived from the following references: Kim, 2019; Neuman et al., 2016; Pula et al., 2019; Wu et al., 2016.

Clinical Experience with BTK's Inhibitors

Prominent clinical trial data supporting the use of BTKi in hematological malignancies, leading to the approval of the first and second generation BTKi in several indications, like CLL, MCL, WM and Marginal Zone Lymphoma (MZL), which are summarized below.

Ibrutinib

Ibrutinib is currently approved by FDA and the European Medicines Agency (EMA) for the treatment of CLL in any line of therapy, R/R MCL, and of WM. In addition, approval for MZL following at least one prior anti-CD20-based therapy was granted. It was first evaluated in a phase Ia trial that enrolled relapsed/refractory (R/R) B-cell non-Hodgkin Lymphoma (B-NHL) patients with diverse histologies, including CLL/small lymphocytic lymphoma (SLL), MCL, follicular lymphoma (FL), DLBCL, MZL, and WM. This study demonstrated that ibrutinib had a substantial activity across all B-cell histologies in a 560 mg oral daily (Aw & Brown, 2017), inducing significant objective responses. The objective response rate (ORR) was 60%, including a complete response (CR) rate of 16%. The highest response rate was observed in patients with MCL (78%) and CLL/SLL (69%). The responses were durable, with the majority maintaining their responses for at least 10 months (Advani et al., 2013). In patients with CLL was observed a transient lymphocytosis, a characteristic pattern of response, reported with other agents affecting BCR signaling pathway. This reflects the disruption of BCR-mediated stromal chemotaxis and adhesion, resulting in an egress of tissue-resident malignant lymphocytes (Aalipour & Advani, 2014).

Ibrutinib for Mantle Cell Lymphoma

The US FDA accelerated approval for ibrutinib use in monotherapy at a daily dose of 560 mg for R/R MCL, based on the results of a phase II registration study. An ORR of 68% and a CR of 21% were obtained. Transient lymphocytosis was observed in 34% of patients. Prior treatment with bortezomib had no impact in ORR. The median duration of response was 17.5 months, and after a median follow-up of 15.3 months, the estimated median Progression-Free Survival (PFS) was 13.9 months (Wang et al., 2013). The results were updated after 26.7 months of follow-up, confirming the durable responses and a favorable safety profile (Wang et al., 2015). Posteriorly, a phase III randomized trial was developed comparing single-agent ibrutinib with temsirolimus, a mammalian target of rapamycin (mTOR) pathway inhibitor (Dreyling et al., 2016; Hess et al., 2009). After a median follow-up of 20 months, ORR was superior in the ibrutinib arm (72% vs 40%; $p<0{\cdot}0001$)), with a median duration of response not reached (vs 7.0 months in the temsirolimus arm). PFS was significantly better for ibrutinib (median PFS 14.6 vs. 6.2 months). Ibrutinib was associated with a non-significant trend towards Overall Survival (OS) benefit, despite 23% crossover from the temsirolimus group. Median treatment duration was four times longer for the ibrutinib group (14.4 vs 3.0 months) (Dreyling et al., 2016).

Despite the unprecedented clinical activity of ibrutinib as a single agent in R/R MCL, the majority of patients continue to experience disease progression, particularly in the high-risk MIPI subgroup or in blastoid histology. To overcome primary disease resistance and minimize development of acquired treatment-emergent resistance, research efforts are focus in defining combination treatments that include other agents that have demonstrated significant clinical activity in MCL, namely rituximab, bendamustine, lenalidomide or venetoclax, in the relapsed/refractory setting (Table 6), but also in naïve patients.

Table 6. Combination regimens with ibrutinib in R/R MCL patients

Regimen	N	Median age, years (range)	Intermediate and high risk MIPI (%)	Median prior therapies, n (range)	ORR (CR), %	PFS	OS
Ibrutinib Rituximab	50	67 (45–86)	56	3 (1–9)	88 (44)	68% @3y	69% @3y
Ibrutinib Venetoclax	23	68 (47-81)	96	2 (1–6)	71 (71)	57% @18m	74% @18m
Ibrutinib Palbociclib	27	65 (42-81)	NR	NR	67 (37)	59% @2y	61% @2y
Ibrutinib Lenalidomide Rituximab	50	69 (45-85)	76	2 (1–7)	76 (56)	Median, 16 m	Median, 22 m

ORR: overall response rate; CR: complete response rate, PFS: progression-free survival; OS: overall survival; m: months; y: years. Data derived from the following references: Jerkeman et al., 2018; Martin et al., 2019; Ruan et al., 2019; Tam et al., 2018; Wang et al., 2016.

In order to overcome primary ibrutinib resistance in MCL expressing wild-type BTK, an association between ibrutinib and palbociclib was developed. Palbociclib, an orally available specific Cyclin-dependent Kinase 4/6 (CDK4/6) inhibitor, induces a prolonged early G1 cell cycle arrest and sensitizes MCL killing by ibrutinib. In a phase I trial in R/R MCL, this combination demonstrated to be safe and effective with an ORR of 67%, a CR rate of 37%, and a 2-year PFS rate of 59%. A phase II intergroup multicenter clinical trial (AFT-32; NCT03478514) is ongoing (Martin et al., 2019; Ruan, 2019; Tam et al., 2018; Wang et al., 2016).

Ibrutinib in Waldenström's Macroglobulinemia

Ibrutinib was approved in monotherapy for the therapy of Waldenström's Macroglobulinemia (WM) in any line of treatment in January 2015 by the US FDA, based in a phase II study for R/R WM. The ibrutinib dose was 420 mg once daily, administered until disease progression or unacceptable toxicity. The rationale was the identification of an activating somatic mutation in MYD88 (MYD88 L265P) in WM tumor cells, that triggers activation of NF-κB through two divergent pathways involving BTK and the interleukin-1 receptor–associated kinases (IRAK1 and IRAK4). The ORR was 91%, with 73% of responding patients achieving a major response (MR), defined as a CR or at least 50% reduction in IgM. The IgM flare, a complication observed with rituximab therapy, was not associated with ibrutinib (Treon et al., 2015). The influence of MYD88 and CXCR4 mutation status in response was evaluated, with a higher ORR among patients with MYD88 L265P and wild-type CXCR4 (100%), followed by patients with MYD88 L265P CXCR4 WHIM (85.7%), and finally by patients with both wild-type MYD88 and CXCR4 (71.4%). The median PFS was not reached, and the 24-month estimated PFS was 69% (Treon et al., 2017). After a median follow-up of 47.1 months, it was confirmed that ibrutinib is highly active in symptomatic R/R WM patients, producing durable responses. Ibrutinib as a single-agent in treatment-naïve WM with the MYD88 L265P mutation was also evaluated. Rates of MR were higher (94% vs 71%) and time to major responses more rapid (1.8 vs 7.3 months; P = 0.01) in patients with wild-type CXCR4 versus those with CXCR4MUT, respectively. The 18-month PFS and OS rates achieved were 92% and 100%, respectively, including in patients with high tumor and serum IgM burden, and those with intermediate- and high-risk disease (Treon et al., 2018). Preclinical studies have shown a synergistic activity between ibrutinib and rituximab and in a phase III trial (iNNOVATE study). Both treatment-naïve and R/R patients were included. The rate of MR was higher with ibrutinib-rituximab (72% vs.32%, P<0.001). But complete remissions were infrequent, as with ibrutinib in monotherapy. At 30 months, the PFS rate was significantly superior in the ibrutinib–rituximab arm (82% vs 28%; P<0.001). The benefit observed in the ibrutinib-rituximab group was independent of the MYD88 or CXCR4 genotype. This combination induced a more rapid decrease of median IgM levels, which could be a strategy to prevent rituximab-related IgM flare (Dimopoulos et al., 2018).

Ibrutinib in CLL/SLL

Initially, ibrutinib was evaluated in a phase Ib/II trial that enrolled 85 patients with R/R CLL/SLL, that determined 420 mg daily as the standard CLL dose in monotherapy. It was a heavily pre-treated population, and with high-risk disease. After a median follow-up of 20.9 months, the ORR was 71%. Partial response (PR) with lymphocytosis (PR-L), defined as patients achieving a PR by conventional criteria, except for the lack of a 50% reduction in blood lymphocyte count, was 20% for patients receiving a dose of 420 mg (Byrd et al., 2013). In the 5-year update the median duration of response (DOR) was 57 months, and an improvement of CR rate with time was observed in a small proportion of patients, demonstrating a deepening of responses induced by ibrutinib. The median PFS was of 51 months, demonstrating long-term efficacy and durable responses (O'Brien et al., 2018). The RESONATE study, a phase III randomized trial between single-agent ibrutinib and ofatumumab, corroborated the efficacy of Ibrutinib in R/R setting and provided justification for full regulatory approval of ibrutinib in previously treated CLL in 2014. This trial enrolled 391 patients with R/R CLL/SLL, most with advanced disease (57%) and heavily pre-treated (almost half had at least 3 prior treatments). In respect of high-risk features, del(17p) and del(11q) were present in about one third of all patients, respectively, and IGHV gene was unmutated in 98/134 patients of the ibrutinib arm and in 84/133 patients of the ofatumumab arm. With a median follow-up of 44 months, of the 68% of patients in the ofatumumab arm initiated ibrutinib on crossover. The ORR was 91% for ibrutinib, with CR rate increasing over time (Byrd et al., 2014). Ibrutinib significantly improved PFS compared with ofatumumab (median not reached vs. 8.1 months) and, in multivariate analysis, the independent factors associated with the decrease of PFS were greater number of prior lines (2 or more) and elevated β-2Microglobulin. No difference in PFS was observed in the several genomic subgroups, including del(17p), del(11q) or unmutated IGHV. Median OS remained not reached in both arms, with 74% of patients on the ibrutinib arm and 65% on the ofatumumab arm (irrespective of crossover to ibrutinib) alive at 3 years of follow-up after randomization (Byrd et al., 2019). The RESONATE-2 trial, a phase III randomized study compared ibrutinib to chlorambucil in treatment-naïve patients aged 65 years or older without del(17p), allowed the expansion of ibrutinib`s label by the US FDA in March 2016 to include frontline treatment of CLL.

Several trials have been developed in frontline and in R/R setting combining ibrutinib with other CLL-directed therapies with distinct mechanisms of action, in order to achieve deeper responses, namely CR and undetectable MRD, to reduce discontinuation rates, either due to toxicity or progression related to the emergence of BTK mutations, and to reduce de financial burden of continuous therapy. In April 2020 the US FDA expanded the indication of ibrutinib to include its combination with rituximab for the initial treatment of adult patients with CLL/SLL. ORR was higher in de ibrutinib-rituximab arm (95.8% vs. 81.1%). However, CR rate and MDR in PB at 12 months were lower than in the FCR arm, 17.2% vs. 30.3% and 8.3% vs. 59.2%, respectively. At a median follow-up of 33.6 months, the results of the analysis of PFS and OS favored significantly ibrutinib–rituximab over FCR, 89.4% vs. 72.9% and 98.8% vs. 91.5% at 3 years, respectively. In a subgroup analysis of 281 patients, out of 395 patients tested, that had unmutated IGHV, ibrutinib–rituximab resulted in better PFS at 3 years than FCR (90.7% vs. 62.5%) (Shanafelt et al., 2019). Other trials addressed the benefit of combining ibrutinib with chemoimmunotherapy, with other monoclonal anti-CD20 antibodies than rituximab, like ofatumumab or obinutuzumab, and with venetoclax, in frontline and R/R patients.

Acalabrutinib

Acalabrutinib is a highly selective irreversible second-generation BTK inhibitor, approved by the US FDA for the treatment of adults with MCL who have received at least one prior therapy, and for the treatment of CLL or SLL.

Acalabrutinib in Mantle Cell Lymphoma

A phase 2 trial (ACE-LY-004) evaluated acalabrutinib, 100mg twice daily, in R/R MCL until disease progression or unacceptable toxicity. This study showed an ORR of 81% with CR of 40%, after a median follow-up of 15.2 months. The median PFS and OS were not reached, and the estimated rates at 12 months were 67% and 87%, respectively (Wang et al., 2018a). An update to the study was presented at the ASH 2018. After a median follow-up of 26.3 months, 40% of patients remained on treatment. The ORR was not significantly different from the original publication. The median DOR was 25.7 months, and the median PFS and OS were 19.5 months and not reached, respectively. The estimated 24-month OS rate was 72% (Wang et al., 2018b). However, an additional phase III trial is required to confirm clinical meaningful benefits for patients in this setting. The focus of future studies with acalabrutinib will be improving the depth and duration of response in R/R MCL through novel combinations, like venetoclax (NCT03946878).

In the frontline setting, a large phase III trial is evaluating regimens combining acalabrutinib with BR (NCT02972840) with the goal of improving outcomes in transplant ineligible patients. Other ongoing studies are testing the combination with lenalidomide-rituximab (NCT03863184) (Girard et al., 2019).

Acalabrutinib in CLL/SLL

Acalabrutinib obtain approval in 2019 by US FDA for CLL and SLL treatment based initially in a phase I/II trial, in a cohort of 61 patients with R/R CLL. After a median follow-up of 14.3 months, the ORR was 95% including 85% of PR and 10% of PR-L. The ORR among the 31% of patients with del(17p) was 100% (Bryd et al., 2016; Kim, 2019). Two randomized phase III controlled trials, ELEVATE-TN (NCT02475681) and ASCEND (NCT02970318) (Ghi et al., 2019; Tam et al., 2019) lead to this drug approval. The ASCEND trial evaluated the efficacy and safety of acalabrutinib vs. investigator's choice of idelalisib/rituximab (idR) or bendamustine/rituximab (BR) in patients with R/R CLL. The ORR was not significantly different with acalabrutinib vs idR or BR (81% vs 75%). At a median follow-up of 16.1 months, acalabrutinib significantly prolonged median PFS vs idR or BR (not reached vs 16.5 months; P< .0001). The PFS was also improved with acalabrutinib across subgroups including del(17p), TP53 mutation, and Rai stage. OS at 12 months were 94% and 91% for acalabrutinib and investigator`s choice, respectively (Ghia et al., 2019). The ELEVATE-TN evaluated the efficacy and safety of acalabrutinib in combination with obinutuzumab vs acalabrutinib alone vs obinutuzumab in combination with chlorambucil (CHL) in treatment-naïve CLL patients. ORR was higher with acalabrutinib-obinutuzumab arm (94%; 95% CI, 89.3%-96.5%) vs. obinutuzumab-CHL arm (94% vs. 79%; P<0.0001); the ORR with acalabrutinib monotherapy was 85%. Also, CR rates were higher with acalabrutinib-obinutuzumab vs. obinutuzumab-CHL (13% vs. 5%). In the acalabrutinib monotherapy arm only one patient attained CR. At a median follow-up of 28 months, it was shown that both acalabrutinib-obinutuzumab and acalabrutinib in monotherapy significantly improved PFS vs obinutuzumab-CHL even in high-risk subgroups including del(17p). Estimated 30 months PFS rates with acalabrutinib-obinutuzumab, acalabrutinib, and obinutuzumab-chlorambucil were 90%, 82%, and 34%, respectively. Median OS was not reached in any arm, although a trend toward improved OS was observed in both acalabrutinib arms, despite 45% of patients crossed over, for disease progression, in obinutuzumab-CHL arm (Bryd et al., 2019), A head-to-head phase III trial comparing acalabrutinib with ibrutinib in previous treated high-risk R/R CLL patients is open for accrual (NCT02477696), and the results of this trial are eagerly awaited. Similarly, to MCL, studies evaluating acalabrutinib in combination with venetoclax, with or without obinutuzumab, in treatment-naïve or R/R CLL patients are ongoing (NCT04169737; NCT03580928).

Zanubrutinib

Zanubrutinib is highly potent, selective, irreversible BTK inhibitor, that obtained an accelerated approval by the US FDA in November 2019 for the treatment of adult patients with MCL who have received at least one prior therapy, based on two trials: BGB-3111-AU-003 (NCT02343120) and BGB-3111-206 (NCT03206970). The efficacy of zanubrutinib was assessed in a phase I/II dose-escalation, single-arm trial BGB-3111-AU-003 (NCT02343120) that enrolled patients with multiple B-cell malignancies, including 37 previously treated MCL patents. The ORR of MCL cohort was 86.5%, with a CR of 29.7%, with a median DOR of 14.7 months. The recommended dose was determined to be 160 mg administered twice daily (Tam et al., 2019). A phase II multicenter single-arm trial (NCT03206970) enrolled 86 patients with MCL who received at least one prior therapy to receive zanubrutinib orally at 160 mg twice daily until disease progression or unacceptable toxicity. The ORR was 84.7%, with a CR of 76.5% and a median DOR of 14.0 months. The ORR was generally consistent across subgroups analyzed (MIPI, previous therapy, blastoid variant, etc). The median PFS was 16.7 months (Song et al., 2019). Zanubrutinib was also evaluated in CLL/SLL in monotherapy, 160 mg twice dally, until disease progression (PD) or unacceptable toxicity, in a single-arm, multicenter phase 2 study (NCT03206918), that included 91 patients with R/R CLL/SLL. The ORR was 91.2%, with 4.4% CR. In patients with del(17p) or TP53 mutation, ORR was 95.5%. Among responders, the median time to first response was 2.79 months. The estimated 1-year PFS rate was 80.9% (Xu et al., 2019). In the nonrandomized arm of the open-label phase III SEQUOIA trial (NCT03336333), after a median follow-up of 7.0 months, in 90 treatment-naïve and del(17p) mutated CLL/SLL patients, zanubrutinib treatment was associated with an ORR of 92.2% (Syed, 2020).

Several trials are ongoing with zanubrutinib, either in monotherapy or in combination, namely the following phase III clinical trials: zanubrutinib plus rituximab versus bendamustine plus rituximab in previously untreated patients with MCL who are not eligible for stem cell transplantation (NCT04002297); zanubrutinib versus ibrutinib in patients with RR CLL/SLL (NCT03734016; ALPINE); zanubrutinib with or without venetoclax versus bendamustine plus rituximab in patients with previously untreated CLL/SLL (NCT03336333; SEQUOIA) (Syed, 2020).

Other BTK Inhibitors in Development

Tirabrutinib

Tirabrutinib is a highly selective inhibitor of BTK, blocking reversibly the BCR signaling by a covalent binding. It displays a higher selectivity for BTK compared to ibrutinib (Kim, 2019). In a phase I trial, that included patients with diverse R/R B-cell malignancies, in the CLL group 96% of patients responded to tirabrutinib with a median treatment duration of 80 weeks; and all evaluable patients with del 17p or TP53 mutations without del 17p responded. In the MCL group the ORR was 92%. In the DLBCL group consisting of non-germinal center B-cell (non-GCB) DLBCL (89%) and GCB DLBCL patients (6%), 35% of non-GCB patients responded with about CR/CRu of 9%. None of the GCB patients responded. The majority of AEs (75%) were grade 1 or 2, with those occurring in less than 10% of patients. Grade 3 or 4 AEs were mainly hematologic, occurred early during therapy and recovered spontaneously. Only 1 case of new onset atrial fibrillation was observed but it was not thought to be related to the drug. Further investigations of tirabrutinib are ongoing, focusing on combination therapies in CLL and other B-cell malignancies, including with other BCR inhibitors such as idelalisib (PI3K inhibitor) or entospletinib (SYK inhibitor), with the aim to overcome some mechanisms of resistance in the BTK signaling. Additionally, comparison with or without anti-CD20 monoclonal antibody are involved in those combination studies.

Vecabrutinib (SNS-062)

Vecabrutinib is the only noncovalent second-generation BTK inhibitor, with high selectivity. As opposed to ibrutinib and acalabrutinib, it is active against both WT BTK and C481S-mutated BTK, rendering it a good candidate for patients carrying BTK C481S mutations associated with ibrutinib resistance (Neuman et al., 2016). A phase 1b study is ongoing in patients with B-cell malignancies with and without the BTK C481S mutation (NCT03037645).

Spebrutinib (CC-292; AVL-292)

Spebrutinib`s efficacy and safety were evaluated in a phase I study in patients with R/R B-cell malignancies. The ORR in CLL/SLL patients was 60% at all dosing regimens, with no case of CR and 63% of those receiving twice-daily dosing responded, including a PR of 50% and a PR-L of 13%. Although the administration of spebrutinib achieved high BTK occupancy, it showed inferior clinical efficacy compared to other BTK inhibitors. The reasons for this suboptimal efficacy are not completely clear. The hematologic grade 3 or 4 AEs were neutropenia and thrombocytopenia (Kim, 2019).

M7583, CB1763, GNE-431 and LOXO-305

M7583 is another irreversible, highly selective and second-generation inhibitor that binds covalently to BTK. A phase I/II trial is ongoing to evaluate its safety, tolerability, PK, BTK occupancy and preliminary antitumor activity in patients with R/R B-cell malignancies (NCT02825836) (Kim, 2019).

CB1763 is a novel noncovalent BTKi, that as also a potent inhibitory activity for C481S-mutant BTK in preclinical models, suggesting that CB1763 has the potential to treat ibrutinib-resistant patients (Asami et al., 2018; Kim, 2019).

GNE-431 is another novel noncovalent BTKi showing higher selectivity for BTK than any of the covalent or noncovalent inhibitors (Kim, 2019).

LOXO-305 is a non-covalent BTKi with equivalent strong inhibitory potency against wild-type and C481 mutated BTK, with potential to overcome acquired resistance to covalent BTK inhibitors. Currently is being evaluated in a multicenter phase I/II trial in patients with previously treated B-cell malignancies (NCT03740529) (Kim, 2019).

Adverse Events, Drug Interactions, Resistance Mechanisms

Safety and Adverse Events

Single-agent ibrutinib is associated with a particular adverse events (AEs) profile, that in the clinical trials were transient, manageable and generally decreased over time, for patients remaining on ibrutinib therapy, with few exceptions (hypertension and bruising), with limited treatment discontinuations, dose reductions, or deaths due to AEs (Aw & Brown, 2017; Munir et al, 2019; O'Brien et al., 2018). However, the use of ibrutinib outside clinical trials had a higher frequency of discontinuation due to AEs (16.9-51.2%) (Broccoli et al., 2018; Mato et al., 2017; Sharman et al., 2018). The exception is the real data collected from 715 patients with MCL from 26 countries enrolled in the named patient program (NPP) that had a discontinuation rate due to AEs of 1.3% (Rule et al., 2016). In a pooled safety population of 1,476 patients with B-cell malignancies, ibrutinib`s most common AEs (≥30%) were thrombocytopenia, diarrhea, fatigue, musculoskeletal pain, neutropenia, rash, anemia, and bruising. Ibrutinib has been associated with an increased risk of any grade bleeding which is related to BTK`s relevant role in glycoprotein VI signaling. BTKi has been shown to prevent collagen-mediated platelet aggregation (Gribben et al., 2018). Most bleeding AEs observed in the clinical studies were grade 1–2, occurred early, required no dose interruption or dose modification, improved and frequently disappeared over time. The incidence of new emergent bleeding AEs also decreased significantly over time, being less frequent after the first 6 months of therapy (Gribben et al., 2018). The most common bleeding AEs are petechia, contusion, epistaxis and bruising, and are seen in patients both with and without thrombocytopenia Major hemorrhage (grade ≥3), including intracranial and gastrointestinal bleeding, has also occurred in ibrutinib-treated patients in clinical trials., ranging from 1% to 10% in CLL trials, and 4.5 to 10% in MCL trials (Aw & Brown, 2017; Dreyling et al., 2016; Wang et al., 2013; Wang et al., 2015; Wang et al., 2016). Whenever an association between a major bleeding and ibrutinib is suspected, it is recommended withholding ibrutinib (Gribben et al., 2018). The individual risk of each patient should be evaluated before starting ibrutinib. Concomitant use of antiplatelet agents, nonsteroidal anti-inflammatory drugs, anticoagulants, and supplements associated with bleeding (such as fish oils, vitamin E), should be avoided in patients receiving ibrutinib (Aw & Brown, 2017). Experts recommend avoiding ibrutinib in patients with a history of major or potentially life-threatening hemorrhage owing to an irreversible cause. Similarly, an alternative therapy for B-cell malignancy should be considered in patient requiring long-term anticoagulation or dual antiplatelet therapy (Brown, 2018; Gribben et al., 2018). Ibrutinib should be held 3-7 days prior to and after any invasive procedures owing to the risk of periprocedural bleeding (Brown, 2018; Gribben et al., 2018). Infection is a common complication in ibrutinib treated patients (Brown, 2018; Gribben et al., 2018). The most frequent infections in clinical trials included pneumonia, upper respiratory tract infections, sinusitis and urinary tract infections (Byrd et al., 2014; Burger et al., 2015; Dreyling et al., 2016; Wang et al., 2013; Wang et al., 2015; Wang et al., 2016). Most infections occur early after initiation of ibrutinib therapy and decrease with time (Byrd et al., 2014; Burger et al., 2015; Wang et al., 2015). A large meta-analysis of ibrutinib-treated patients in published clinical trials found that 56% of patients had an infectious complication and 1 of every 5 patients developed pneumonia. In a real-world retrospective analysis of ibrutinib-treated patients, infection led to treatment discontinuation in 11%. The median time to ibrutinib discontinuation for infection was 6 months (Stephens & Byrd, 2019). Other infections are being reported, for example invasive aspergillosis, cryptococcus infections, varicella-zoster virus (VZV) reactivation, and mild cases of pneumocystis jiroveci pneumonia (PJP) (Brown, 2018). Universal infectious prophylaxis for both VZV and PJP is not consensual. Some experts recommend a case-by-case decision, depending on factors such as prior therapy, immune status, splenectomy and prior infections (Brown,

2018; Gribben et al., 2018). However, prior to starting ibrutinib treatment, patients should be strongly encouraged to have relevant vaccinations (e.g., for influenza and pneumonia) (Brown, 2018). Atrial fibrillation (AF) has been reported in 6-16% of ibrutinib-treated patients in clinical trials (Byrd et al., 2014; Burger et al., 2015; Chanan-Khan et al., 2016; Dreyling et al., 2016). Pathophysiologic mechanisms of ibrutinib-induced AF have not been well elucidated but may be related to inhibition of the PI3K-Akt pathway in cardiac myocytes, an "off-target effect" (Aw & Brown, 2017; Stephens & Byrd, 2019). In a pooled analysis of 1505 patients across four ibrutinib clinical trials (ibrutinib alone or in combination with BR), most AF events typically occurred within the first 6 months of therapy. At the initial follow-up at 16.6 months, the incidence of AF was 6.5% in the ibrutinib arm versus 1.2% in the comparator arm, however, at the later follow-up (36 months), it increased to 10.4% in the ibrutinib arm. The events were generally manageable, with 14.3% of patients who developed AF discontinuing therapy, which subsequently decreased to 9% with extended follow-up (<1% of total population). Approximately 50% of patients needed no change in dose or dose interruption (Brown et al., 2017). On multivariable analysis, independent risk factors for developing AF included ibrutinib use, age over 65 years, and a prior history of AF (Aw & Brown, 2017). Outside the clinical trial setting, incidence of AF may be slightly higher due to increased comorbidities and a less tightly controlled setting, and a common cause of ibrutinib discontinuation (Aw & Brown, 2017; Gribben et al., 2018). Patients who develop AF should have a cardiac evaluation for rate or rhythm control, and the role of anticoagulation for stroke prevention should be carefully weighed given the bleeding risk associated with ibrutinib (Aw & Brown, 2017; Mato et al., 2016).

The prevalence for grade 3 or greater hypertension was 4% (year 0-1), 6% (year 1-2), 8% (year 2-3), 9% (year 3-4), and 9% (year 4-5). The incidence for the 5-year period was 11%. The underlying mechanism for hypertension is unclear (Stephens & Byrd, 2019). Prior to initiation, or during ibrutinib`s treatment, hypertension should be vigorously managed (Brown, 2018; Gribben et al., 2018).

Acalabrutinib is a highly selective irreversible BTKi with significantly less off-target kinase inhibition, which impacts the AEs profile. The most common AEs of any grade in patients treated with acalabrutinib were anemia, neutropenia, thrombocytopenia, headache, upper respiratory tract infection, and diarrhea (Bryd et al., 2016; Ghia et al., 2019; Sharman et al., 2019; Wang et al., 2018a). Grade≥ 3 infections occurred in 19% of 1029 patients treated with acalabrutinib in clinical trials, most often respiratory tract infections (11%). These infections predominantly occurred in the absence of grade 3 or 4 neutropenia, with neutropenic infection reported in 1.9% of all patients. Opportunistic infections included hepatitis B virus (HBV) reactivation, fungal pneumonia, PJP pneumonia, Epstein-Barr virus reactivation, cytomegalovirus, and progressive multifocal leukoence-phalopathy have been reported. Prophylaxis should be considered in patients who are at increased risk for opportunistic infections. Acalabrutinib does not induce major platelet dysfunction, as has been associated with ibrutinib. Dysfunctional aggregation suggests that acalabrutinib inhibits platelet Btk and Tec at physiological concentrations and justifies the occurrence bleeding events of any grade in 22% of patients (Girard et al., 2019). Major hemorrhage (grade≥ 3 or any central nervous system bleeding) occurred in 3.0% of patients, with fatal hemorrhage occurring in 0.1% of 1029 patients in clinical trials Consider the benefit-risk of withholding acalabrutinib for 3-7 days pre-and post-surgery depending upon the type of surgery and the risk of bleeding. Grade 3 or 4 cytopenias, including neutropenia, anemia and thrombocytopenia occurred in 23%, 8% and 7% respectively. Grade 4 neutropenia developed in 12% of patients. Atrial fibrillation or flutter was reported in 4.1% of 1029 patients treated in clinical trials, with grade 3 occurring in 1.1%. The risk may be increased in patients with cardiac risk factors, hypertension, previous arrhythmias, and acute infection. Second primary malignancies, including skin cancers and other solid tumors, occurred in 12% patients exposed to acalabrutinib in clinical trials. The most frequent second primary malignancy was skin cancer, reported in 6% of patients. Dose reductions and discontinuation due to any adverse reaction were reported in 1.6% to 7% and 6.5% to 11%, of patients treated in clinical trials, respectively (Bryd et al., 2016; Ghia et al., 2019; Tam et al., 2019; Wang et al., 2018a).

Zanubrutinib is a potent, selective and irreversible BTKi inhibitor, with minimal inhibition of off-target kinases such as EGFR, ITK, JAK3, HER2, and TEC, which relates to a specific toxicity profile (Kim, 2019; Pula et al., 2019; Wu et al., 2016). The most common AEs (≥20%) included neutropenia, thrombocytopenia, upper respiratory tract infection, anemia, rash, bruising, diarrhea, and cough. The most common serious AEs were pneumonia in 11% and hemorrhage in 5% of patients. Grade ≥3 infections occurred in 23% of patients treated with zanubrutinb, being pneumonia the most common. HBV reactivation has been reported. Prophylaxis for herpes simplex virus, PJP pneumonia, and other infections should be considered, according to standard of care in patients who are at increased risk for infections. Bleeding events of any grade, including purpura and petechiae, occurred in 50% of patients. Two percent of patients had grade≥3 bleeding events including intracranial and gastrointestinal hemorrhage, hematuria, and hemothorax. Withholding zanubrutinib for 3-7 days pre-and post-surgery, should be considered depending upon the type of surgery and the bleeding risk. Hematological toxicity is a common AE. Grade 3-4 neutropenia, thrombocytopenia and anemia, occurred in 27%, 10% and 8% of zanubrutinib-treated patients, respectively. Second primary malignancies have occurred in 9% of patients treated with zanubrutinib monotherapy, being skin cancer (basal cell carcinoma and squamous cell carcinoma of skin) the most frequent, reported in 6% of patients. Atrial fibrillation and atrial flutter were also reported in 2% of zanubrutinib-treated patients in monotherapy, of which 0.6% were grade ≥3. Treatment discontinuation due to AEs occurred in 8.8% to 10.5% patients (Song et al., 2019; Xu et al., 2019).

Drug Interactions

BTKi ibrutinib, acalabrutinib and zanubrutinib, are primarily metabolized in the liver, by cytochrome P450 enzyme 3A4 (CYP3A4), which increases the potential for drug interactions. Ibrutinib, in a minor extent, is also metabolized by CYP2D6, and acalabrutinib by glutathione conjugation and amide hydrolysis (Gribben et al., 2018). Co-administration of BTKi with strong CYP3A inhibitors (for example: clarithromycin, itraconazole, ketoconazole, indinavir, nelfinavir and ritonavir) or moderate CYP3A inhibitors (for example: ciprofloxacin, erythromycin, amiodarone, diltiazem, verapamil, aprepitant, fluconazole, voriconazole, imatinib, amprenavir, atazanavir, darunavir, grapefruit juice), increase BTKi`s plasma concentrations, and consequently their toxicity. Co-administration should be avoided. If the CYP3A inhibitor is used, interrupt acalabrutinib and reduce ibrutinib and zanubrutinib dose, according to the prescribing information (Gribben et al., 2018). The co-administration of BTKi with strong CYP3A inducers (for example: rifampicin, carbamazepine, phenytoin, St John's Wort) may decrease their plasma concentrations, and therefore reducing their efficacy. Avoidance of strong CYP3A inducers co-administration is recommended (Gribben et al., 2018).

Resistance Mechanisms

Two important secondary resistance mechanisms have been identified in CLL patients who lose response to ibrutinib (Aw & Brown, 2017; Pula et al., 2019; Zhang et al., 2015). Resistance often involves a cysteine-to-serine mutation in BTK at position 481 (C481S) where drug binding occurs, disrupting covalent binding, allowing for reversible inhibition, instead of strong irreversible binding to BTK by ibrutinib, reducing its clinical activity (Zhang et al., 2015). The C481S mutation isn`t present prior to ibrutinib exposure, can be found in CLL cells up to one year before the clinical relapse occurs and is associated with clinical progression (Pula et al., 2019). Additional mutations at the T474 (T474I and T474S) locus lead to diminished ibrutinib selectivity and affinity. A substitution mutation T316A coding the non-kinase SH2 domain was identified, probably resulting in diminished BTK interactions with BLNK and other proteins leading to ibrutinib resistance (Pula et al., 2019). Three distinct PLCG2 mutations were found in CLL patients with secondary resistance to ibrutinib therapy: arginine-to-tryptophan mutation at position 665 (R665W), leucine-to-phenylalanine at position 845 (L845F), and a serine-to-tyrosine mutation at position 707 (S707Y) (Martin et al., 2019). Aberrations in PLCG2, downstream from BTK, may act as gain-of-function mutations in which BCR activity is maintained, despite adequate drug binding (Aw & Brown, 2017). Further understanding of resistance mechanisms is of ongoing importance as next-generation BTK inhibitors are developed and alternate treatment strategies post ibrutinib failure are considered (Aw & Brown, 2017). New and more specific BTKi are being developed, and that have shown the potential to overcome C481S mutation, like Vecabrutinib or LOXO-305. Other kinases inhibitors, like Entospletinib a Spleen tyrosine kinase (SYK) inhibitor or Cerdulatinib, a dual SYK/JAK kinase inhibitor, are being evaluated in ibrutinib resistance patients, due to their potential to overcome PLCG2 and C481S mutations, respectively (Pula et al., 2019).

JAK Inhibitors

The Janus Kinase (JAK) family of non-receptor tyrosine kinases play a central role in signal transduction initiated by a wide range of cytokine receptors (Babon et al., 2014; Bousoik & Aliabadi, 2018). JAK activation stimulates cell proliferation, differentiation, cell migration and apoptosis (Rawlings, Rosler & Harrison, 2004). In mammals, the JAK family has four members: JAK1, JAK2, JAK3 and Tyrosine kinase 2 (TYK2) (Yamaoka et al., 2004). JAK1, JAK2 and Tyk2 are ubiquitously expressed; in contrast JAK3 is predominantly expressed in hematopoietic cells (Yamaoka et al., 2004). Each JAK protein contains seven conserved sequence regions, called JAK homology (JH) domains (JH1–JH7) (Recio, 2018). JH1 is located in the C-terminal end of the molecule and is catalytically active; the upstream pseudokinase domain JH2 is structurally analogous to JH1 but lacks catalytic activity; JH3 and JH4 domains constitute an SRC homology 2 (SH2-like) domain, which mediates interactions with signaling proteins; JH5–JH7 domains are located in the N-terminus and contain a FERM (band

4.1, ezrin, radixin, moesin) motif, which mediates interactions with cytokine receptors (Recio, 2018; Vainchenker et al., 2018).

JAK proteins are bound to the cytoplasmic regions of cytokine receptors (Fragoulis, McInnes & Siebert, 2019). In contrast to receptor tyrosine kinases, such as c-KIT, this cytokine receptor lacks the intrinsic protein tyrosine kinase domain and, consequently, rely on the catalytic activity of constitutively-associated JAKs to mediate signal transduction to the nucleus trough the signal transducer and activator of transcription (STAT) (Babbon et al., 2014; Vainchenker et al., 2018).

The JAK/STAT pathway is frequently dysregulated in malignant diseases and in disorders with an abnormal immunological response (Vainchenker et al., 2018). Genetic alterations targeting this signaling pathway are associated mainly with hematologic malignancies; the paradigm is represented by myeloproliferative neoplasms (MPNs) *BCR-ABL1*–negative as they are all related to mutations activating JAK2 (Vainchenker et al., 2018). At present, small-molecules namely JAK inhibitors (JAKi), are considered as a novel category of drugs in the treatment of cancer and immune-mediated diseases (Elli et al., 2019). Currently, 3 JAKi are approved by the FDA (Food and Drugs Administration) and the EMA (European Medicines Agency): ruxolitinib for treatment of patients with myelofibrosis (MF) and hydroxyurea (HU)-resistant and intolerant polycythemia vera (PV); tofacitinib for treatment of patients with rheumatoid arthritis (RA) and psoriatic arthritis; baricitinib for treatment of RA (Muller, 2019; Vainchenker et al., 2018).

Ruxolitinib

Ruxolitinib is a potent and selective oral inhibitor of both JAK1 and JAK2 kinases [10]. It was approved by the FDA in 2011 for the treatment of patients with intermediate- or high-risk MF, including Primary MF (PMF), post-PV MF, and MF post-essential thrombocythemia (ET) (Elli et al., 2019). On 2012, the EMA approved the drug for the treatment of splenomegaly and/or constitutional symptoms of MF, irrespective of the patient risk group (Cervantes & Pereira, 2017). On December 2014, ruxolitinib received approval from the FDA for the treatment of patients with PV who have had an inadequate response to or are intolerant to cytoreductive therapy with hydroxyurea (Raedeller, 2015). Ruxolitinib also received approval for PV by the EMA in 2015. More recently, on May 2019, the FDA approved ruxolitinib for steroid-refractory acute graft-versus-host disease (aGVHD) in adult and pediatric patients 12 years and older (Gomez et al., 2012).

Mechanism of Action

Ruxolitinib is a potent JAK1 and JAK2 inhibitor, that exerts its anti-JAK activity by competitive inhibition of the ATP-binding catalytic site of the kinase domain (Elli et al., 2019; Mascarenhas & Hoffman, 2012). Ruxolitinib is not specific for the mutated form of JAK2 and inhibits both the wild type and JAK2V617F (Elli et al., 2019; Mascarenhas & Hoffman, 2012). Given the complexity of the signaling pathways modulated by JAK1 and JAK2, and the wide range of immune system components affected, it is therefore not surprising that therapeutic JAK/STAT pathway targeting will have both direct and indirect immunological consequences (Elli et al., 2019; McLornan, Khan, & Harrison, 2015). Available evidence suggests that ruxolitinib acts on cellular components of both innate and adaptive immunity; it impairs several cytokines, modulates dendritic cells (DCs) function and T cell response, and reduces Natural Killer (NK) cells levels (Elli et al., 2019; McLornan, Khan, & Harrison, 2015). Consequently, ruxolitinib may lead to increased risk of opportunistic infection and reactivation of latent infections (Elli et al., 2019).

Pharmacokinetics/Pharmacodynamics and Drug Interactions

Ruxolitinib has a good oral bioavailability, and is rapidly absorbed and metabolized in the liver, primarily via CYP3A4 (Chen et al., 2014; Mascarenhas & Hoffman, 2012). Although renal excretion contributes only minimally to ruxolitinib clearance, it is the primary elimination route for ruxolitinib metabolites (Chen et al., 2014). Therefore, in patients with any hepatic impairment or with moderate or severe renal impairment, a reduction in the starting dose of ruxolitinib is recommended (Chen et al., 2014). The recommended starting dose is based on platelet count, and is then titrated based on safety and efficacy. The maximum recommended dose of ruxolitinib is 25 mg twice daily (Mascarenhas & Hoffman, 2012). Ruxolitinib dose should be reduced by approximately 50% when it is administered with strong CYP3A4 inhibitors or dual inhibitors of CYP2C9 and CYP3A4 enzymes (e.g., ketoconazole, fluconazole) (Umehara et al., 2019).

Ruxolitinib in Myelofibrosis

Ruxolitinib has demonstrated clinical benefit in patients with intermediate-2 and high-risk myelofibrosis in a phase I/II trial (study INCB18424-251) and in two phase III randomized clinical trials (COMFORT-I and COMFORT-II). In these studies, ruxolitinib was well-tolerated and demonstrated early and sustained clinical benefits in terms of reductions in spleen size and improvements in myelofibrosis-related symptoms (Verstovsek et al., 2012). In the initial phase I/II study, results were equivalent irrespective of JAK2 mutational status or subtype of MF (i.e., primary or post-PV MF or post-ET MF) (Harrison & Vannucchi, 2012; Verstovsek et al., 2010). A marked depression in the increased expression of proinflammatory cytokines was seen with ruxolitinib treatment; additionally, there was only a modest decrease in mutant JAK2 allele burden despite significant clinical benefit (Harrison & Vannucchi, 2012; Mascarenhas & Hoffman, 2012). Taken together, these data suggest that the efficacy of the drug may be mainly due to inhibition of JAK1 signaling and subsequent reduction in inflammatory cytokines, as well as aberrant JAK2 signaling, rather than being imputed to a decrease in *JAK* mutant allele burden (Harrison & Vannucchi, 2012; Mascarenhas & Hoffman, 2012). Although the follow-up was limited to 2 years and the study did not include a comparator arm, there was a trend to improvement in survival and a suggestion of a reduction in rate of transformation to acute leukemia in comparison with historical controls (Mascarenhas & Hoffman, 2012; Verstovsek et al., 2011). In the phase III, randomized, double-blind COMFORT-I (Controlled Myelofibrosis study with oral JAK Inhibitor

Therapy -I) trial ruxolitinib was compared with placebo in patients with intermediate-2 or high-risk MF and a baseline platelet count $\geq 100 \times 10^9$/L (Harrison & Vannucchi, 2012; Mascarenhas & Hoffman, 2012; Verstovsek et al., 2011). The primary endpoint was a reduction in spleen volume of at least 35% by magnetic resonance imaging (MRI) or computed tomography (CT), which was observed in 41.9% of patients with ruxolitinib versus 0.7% with placebo at week 24 ($p < 0.0001$) (Harrison & Vannucchi, 2012; Mascarenhas & Hoffman, 2012). This study also evaluated the improvement in disease-related symptoms (secondary endpoint): at week 24, 45.9% of the ruxolitinib-treated patients experienced a ≥50% improvement in constitutional symptoms, as compared with 5.3% in the placebo group ($p < 0.0001$) (Harrision et al., 2011; Mascarenhas & Hoffman, 2012). COMFORT-I showed no difference in clinical effect between JAK2 V617F positive or negative patients (Greenfield et al., 2018). Additionally, drug therapy was uniformly ineffective at reversing histopathological abnormalities in the peripheral blood or marrow, eliminating marker cytogenetic abnormalities, or significantly reducing the JAK2 V617F allele burden (Mascarenhas & Hoffman, 2012). In COMFORT-II (BAT) (Harrision et al., 2011; Mascarenhas & Hoffman, 2012) the proportion of patients with spleen volume reduction of at least 35% evaluated by MRI or CT at week 48 (primary endpoint) was 28.5% with ruxolitinib versus 0% with BAT ($p < 0.0001$) (Harrison & Vannucchi, 2012). The proportion of patients with spleen volume reduction of at least 35% evaluated by MRI or CT at week 24 (key secondary endpoint, and equivalent to the primary endpoint of COMFORT-I) was 31.9% with ruxolitinib versus 0% with BAT ($p < 0.0001$) (Harrison & Vannucchi, 2012). A combined analysis of the COMFORT-I and COMFORT-II studies demonstrated a 30% risk reduction of death and a significant survival advantage in those originally randomized to ruxolitinib in comparison to those crossing over (Greenfield et al., 2018). However, due to the short follow-up and the high rate of early cross-over from BAT or placebo to ruxolitinib, the COMFORT trials may be underpowered to provide a precise estimation of the effect of treatment on survival (Cervantes & Pereira, 2017; Greenfield et al., 2018).

Ruxolitinib in Polycythemia Vera

Ruxolitinib was shown to have a clinical benefit in patients with PV in a phase II study (Kiladjian et al., 2020). On the basis of the emerging efficacy and safety evidence from this study, the phase III RESPONSE trial was designed to compare the long-term efficacy and safety of ruxolitinib versus standard therapy in patients with PV who had an inadequate response to or had unacceptable side effects from HU (Kiladjian et al., 2020; Vannucchi et al., 2015). The starting dosage of ruxolitinib was 10 mg twice daily, which could be adjusted based on safety and efficacy to a minimum of 5 mg once daily and a maximum of 25 mg twice daily (McKeage, 2015). The primary endpoint (hematocrit control and at least a 35% reduction in spleen volume from baseline at week 32) was achieved in 21% of the patients in the ruxolitinib group versus 1% of those in the standard-therapy group ($p<0.001$) (Vannucchi et al., 2015). A complete hematological response was also achieved by significantly more patients in the ruxolitinib arm (McKeage, 2015; Vannucchi et al., 2015). Additionally, 49% versus 5% of the patients, respectively, had at least a 50% reduction in the total symptom score at week 32 (Vannucchi et al., 2015). The results of the 5-year analysis showed that the primary response, complete hematological remission, and overall clinicohematological response were maintained with long-term ruxolitinib therapy; in addition, modest reductions in JAK2 V617F allele burden and improvements in quality of life parameters were observed with longer-term ruxolitinib use (Kiladjian et al., 2020).

Toxicity and Safety

Reversible myelosuppression frequently occurs during treatment with ruxolitinib because of the drug's inhibitory effect on the JAK/STAT pathway (McKeage, 2015). In COMFORT-I study grade 3 or 4 anemia occurred in 34.2% and 11.0% of patients treated with ruxolitinib; and significant thrombocytopenia (grade 3 or 4) was seen in 8.0% and 3.9%, respectively (Harrison & Vannucchi, 2012). In the RESPONSE trial, low-grade anemia, thrombocytopenia and lymphopenia were the most frequent hematological adverse events (McKeage, 2015). Treatment-related anemia and thrombocytopenia are generally managed using dose interruptions and/or reductions, with drug discontinuation rarely required (Harrison & Vannucchi, 2012; McKeage, 2015). Treatment with ruxolitinib is associated with an increased risk of opportunistic and viral infections, due to its immunosuppressive activity (Lussana et al., 2018). Prior to initiation of therapy with ruxolitinib and other JAK inhibitors, screening for latent tuberculosis (TB) is highly recommended (Elli et al., 2019; Sant'Antonio et al., 2019). Prompt antiviral prophylaxis should be considered in hematological patients with a high risk of hepatitis B virus reactivation (Elli et al., 2019). Similarly, hepatitis C virus carriers must be identified and treated according to viral load (Elli et al., 2019). Antiviral prophylaxis with acyclovir should also be considered, as ruxolitinib-treated patients have a statistically significant increased risk of herpes zoster infection compared to controls (Sant'Antonio et al., 2019). Also, active surveillance of second solid neoplasia (in particular non-melanoma skin cancer) should always be performed during therapy with ruxolitinib (Elli et al., 2019). The use of ruxolitinib may increase total cholesterol, low-density lipoprotein cholesterol, triglycerides and transaminases (Harrison et al., 2012). Another potential limitation of ruxolitinib is the possible occurrence of a "withdrawal syndrome" during ruxolitinib treatment discontinuation, characterized by acute relapse of disease symptoms, accelerated splenomegaly, worsening of cytopenias, and occasional hemodynamic decompensation; therefore, treatment discontinuation must be done under close supervision and preferably in a tapering schedule (Tefferi & Pardanani, 2011).

Ruxolitinib-Based Combinations

The combination of ruxolitinib with other agents has been evaluated in numerous studies, namely with immunomodulators (lenalidomide), activin receptor type IIA ligand trap (sotatercept), hypomethylating agents (azacitidine and decitabine), BCL-2 inhibitors (navitoclax) and Bromodomain and Extraterminal Domain (BET) inhibitor (CPI-0610) (Bewersdorf et al., 2019; Bose & Verstovsek, 2017; Mascarenhas et al., 2019; Mullally et al., 2020).

While the clinical trial of ruxolitinib in combination with lenalidomide had terminated early due to lack of therapeutic benefit and significant side effects, pomalidomide with or without prednisone has been successfully tested to treat cytopenias in patients with MF (Bewersdorf et al., 2019). A study of the combination of ruxolitinib and thalidomide in patients with MF has recently begun enrolling patients (Bose & Verstovsek, 2017). The combination of ruxolitinib with sotatercept, a first-class activin receptor type IIA ligand trap, that inhibits the transforming growth factor (TGF)-β signaling pathway, has proven to be effective to improve MPN-associated MF and anemia (Bose & Verstovsek, 2017; Mullally et al., 2020). While azacitidine and decitabine have limited single-agent activity in MF, their combination with ruxolitinib might be especially effective in patients with myelodysplastic syndrome (MDS)/MPN-overlap, especially in the setting of high-risk features such as elevated bone marrow blast percentage (Bose & Verstovsek, 2017; Mullally et al., 2020). Navitoclax, a BCL-2 inhibitor has been tested in combination with ruxolitinib in a recent phase II trial in patients with MF; however, all patients had treatment-emergent AEs, with 77% experiencing grade ≥3 (Mullally et al., 2020). The combination of ruxolutinib with CPI-0610, a selective and potent small molecule Bromodomain and Extraterminal Domain (BET) inhibitor, that regulates key oncogenic pathways, including NF-κB and TGFβ signaling (important drivers of pro-inflammatory cytokine expression and bone marrow fibrosis, respectively) show, in a preliminary data of the phase II study MANIFEST, that CPI-0610 alone or in combination with ruxolitinib is generally well-tolerated and provides clinical benefits in MF patients with inadequate responses or who are refractory to ruxolitinib (Mascarenhas et al., 2019). Other agents that seem promising as potential partners for ruxolitinib include heat shock protein 90 (HSP90) inhibitors (PU-H71), cyclin-dependent kinases 4 and 6 inhibitors (ribociclib), nuclear export inhibitor (selinexor) and histone deacetylase (HDAC) inhibitors (Bose & Verstovsek, 2017; Mullally et al., 2020).

Other Potential Indications of Ruxolitinib

The MAJIC trial was a randomized phase II trial that compared ruxolitinib versus BAT in ET patients resistant or intolerant to HU (Harrison et al. 2017a). The study found no significant differences between the two arms, suggesting that ruxolitinib is not superior to current second-line treatments for ET (Harrison et al. 2017a).

Ruxolitinib is also being evaluated outside of MPN, and studies are ongoing or have been completed in relapsed/refractory solid tumors, androgen-independent metastatic prostate cancer, pancreatic cancer, and multiple myeloma and lymphoma (Mascarenhas & Hoffman, 2012). The activity of ruxolitinib as a single agent in post-MPN acute leukemia is poor (Harrison & Vannucchi, 2012). A synergism between ruxolitinib and decitabine in post-MPN acute myeloid leukemia (AML) has been demonstrated in preclinical studies (Bose et al., 2020). A synergism between ruxolitinib and dexamethasone in pre-clinical acute lymphoblastic leukemia (ALL) models has also been demonstrated (Verbeke et al., 2019).

Fedratinib

Fedratinib is a JAK2-selective kinase inhibitor recently approved by the FDA for the treatment of adult patients with intermediate-2 or high-risk MF, becoming the second approved JAK2 inhibitor in MF (Mullally et al., 2020). Being an agent selective for JAK2 could be advantageous because JAK1, JAK3, and TYK2 are critical for proper immune function, and agents with activity against these other Janus kinases, including ruxolitinib, have been shown to have immunosuppressive activity (Mullally et al., 2020). Fedratinib has been shown to have rapid absorption after oral administration (Bewersdorf et al., 2019). Dose adjustments based on renal function are recommended in patients with a CrCl <30 ml/min (Bewersdorf et al., 2019). In the phase I trial, evaluating fedratinib in MF, although the maximum tolerated dose (680 mg/day) was the most efficacious dose, it was also associated with the highest incidence of adverse events [AEs] (dose-limiting toxicity hyperamylasemia); therefore, a lower starting dose (400–500 mg) was used in phase II and III trials to provide an optimal risk/benefit balance (Bewersdorf et al., 2019; Mullally et al., 2020). The single-arm, phase II trial JAKARTA-2 evaluated fedratinib at 400 mg once daily in 97 patients with intermediate-1, intermediate-2, or high-risk PMF, post-PV MF, or post-ET

MF who were either resistant to or intolerant of ruxolitinib (Harrison et al. 2017b). As one of the major criticisms of the JAKARTA-2 trial was the definition of ruxolitinib resistance and intolerance, a recently published update using more stringent definitions as inclusion criteria has been presented; relapsed/refractory disease was defined as at least 3 months of prior treatment with ruxolitinib with an initial response, while ruxolitinib intolerance was defined as the development of red blood cell (RBC) transfusion requirements or grade ≥3 cytopenias after at least 28 days of previous ruxolitinib treatment (Bewersdorf et al., 2019). The investigators concluded that approximately one-third of JAKARTA-2 ruxolitinib resistant or intolerant patients had spleen volume responses during fedratinib therapy, regardless of prior ruxolitinib outcomes (Harrison et al. 2019).

A multi-center, randomized, phase III clinical trial (JAKARTA) evaluated the efficacy and safety of fedratinib therapy in patients with primary or secondary MF; fedratinib was shown to significantly reduce splenomegaly and symptom burden in patients with MF (Pardanani et al., 2105). The suspicion that the drug might cause Wernicke's Encephalopathy (based on 8 reported potential cases) led to suspension of the JAKARTA trials in 2013 (Mullally et al., 2020). However, after further analysis, only one of those cases was confirmed to be Wernicke's Encephalopathy and the FDA lifted the hold on fedratinib development in August 2017 (Bewersdorf et al., 2019). Despite this conflicting evidence, fedratinib is approved by FDA at a dose of 400 mg for the treatment of myelofibrosis, but encephalopathy remains a rare, but serious concern and is a listed black box warning (Bewersdorf et al., 2019). Since thrombocytopenia can be a dose-limiting AE to treatment with ruxolitinib, evaluating fedratinib as an alternative in patients with baseline thrombocytopenia is of significant clinical interest (Bewersdorf et al., 2019). Patients with myelofibrosis who presented with low baseline platelet counts achieved spleen responses and reduced symptom burden with fedratinib, whether used as first-line or salvage therapy after ruxolitinib failure (Harrison et al., 2019b).

JAK Inhibitors in the Pipeline

Momelotinib is a selective and orally-bioavailable JAK1/JAK2/ activin A receptor type 1 (ACVR1) inhibitor that has, in addition to the improvement in spleen volume and symptoms, also improved MF-associated anemia as proven in phase III trials (SIMPLIFY-1 and -2) (Mullally et al., 2020). Based on the favorable effect on anemia, momelotinib is currently being tested against danazol in the randomized, double-blind phase III trial, MOMENTUM (Bewersdorf et al., 2019).

Pacritinib is a novel JAK2/FLT3/IRAK1 inhibitor, which in addition to improvements in spleen volume and MF symptoms has less treatment-related myelosuppression than ruxolitinib and the ability to be dosed fully in patients irrespective of thrombocytopenia (Mullally et al., 2020; Tremblay & Mascarenhas, 2018). Safety and efficacy supporting its use were evaluated in 2 large phase III trials (PERSIST 1 and 2), with another phase III study ongoing (Mullally et al., 2020). Similar to fedratinib, its development was briefly placed on hold in February 2016, after reports of heart failure and intracranial hemorrhage in the PERSIST trials; however, after an additional review of those cases, the development hold on pacritinib was lifted (Bewersdorf et al., 2019).

Gandotinib (LY2784544) is a selective and potent inhibitor of JAK2V617F (Recio, 2018). A phase II study is currently underway to evaluate its efficacy in patients with MPNs, including those who have demonstrated an intolerance, failure of primary response, or have demonstrated disease progression while on ruxolitinib (Berdeja et al., 2018).

NS-018 is a JAK2/SRC inhibitor currently being tested in a phase I/II trial in patients with MF (Bose & Verstovsek, 2017). In vitro, this agent is 4.3-fold more selective for JAK2V617F than wild-type JAK2, which translated to reduction of leukocytosis and splenomegaly, improvement in BM fibrosis, and prolonged survival in a mouse model of MF without a decrease in circulating RBCs or platelet counts (Bose & Verstovsek, 2017).

Spleen Tyrosine Kinase (SYK) Inhibitors

Spleen tyrosine kinase (SYK) is a cytosolic non-receptor protein tyrosine kinase (NPTK) that belongs to the Src family of non-receptor type PTKs, mainly expressed in hematopoietic cells like B-cells, monocytes, macrophages, mast cells, and neutrophils (Liu, 2017). This protein contains two N-terminal SH2 domains and one C-terminal tyrosine kinase domain (Geahlen, 2014). SYK activation results from the interaction between SH2 domains with multiple receptors that contain ITAM (immunoreceptor tyrosine-based activation motifs) motifs, present, for example, in B-cell receptors, Fc receptors, adhesion receptors among others. After this activation, SYK phosphorylates multiple substrates leading to activation of downstream pathways essential in tumorigenesis, like PI3K/AKT, MAPK, and NF-kB (Mócsai, Ruland & Tybulewicz, 2010). This knowledge leads to the development of SYK inhibitors (Norman 2014; Thoma, et al. 2015).

However, the role of SYK in cancer is controversial and very dependent on tissue type (Geahlen 2014). In some neoplasias, this kinase has been described as a tumor suppressor (breast cancer, melanoma, pancreatic ductal adenocarcinoma) (Bailet, et al. 2009; Coopman & Mueller 2006; Layton, et al. 2009), while in cancer with origin on hematopoietic and epithelial tissues, SYK was described as oncogenic (Efremov & Laurenti 2011; Geahlen 2014). It plays a critical role in B-cell antigen receptor (BCR) signaling pathway and controls multiple physiological functions in B lymphocytes (Feng 2017; Liu 2017). SYK is also a key component in signal transduction from other immune receptors like Fc receptors and adhesion receptors. SYK along with other BCR signaling molecules, Bruton tyrosine kinase (BTK), PI3K delta (PI3Kδ), and tumor necrosis factor (TNF) superfamily receptors was also found to be involved in signal transduction independent from the BCR (Liu 2017). In animal models, Syk was found to be a critical point in B-cell antibody responses, differentiation into germinal center or plasma cells and memory B-cells (Liu 2017). Syk`s role in the regulation of cellular responses to extracellular antigens and antigen-immunoglobulin complexes is of particular importance to the initiation of inflammatory responses (Geahlen 2014). It has been demonstrated that constitutive activation of

SYK and the BCR pathway is essential for cell proliferation and survival in multiple B-cell malignancies (Sharman 2015). It was also recognized as a promoter of cell survival in numerous other cancer cell types, like retinoblastoma, breast, ovarian and pancreatic cancers (Geahlen 2014; Sappal 2018).As a consequence, SYK was recognized to be a potential target for the treatment of various cancers, namely hematologic neoplasms, autoimmune disorders, and other inflammatory states (Geahlen 2014; Liu 2017). Several oral Syk inhibitors (Syki) have been developed and accessed in clinical trials in lymphoid and myeloid malignancies, as well in solid tumors (Liu 2017; Sappal 2018). In addition to cancer, SYK inhibitors have been explored in autoimmune and inflammatory disorders. In fact, at the present, the only Syk inhibitor approved by the US Food and Drug Administration is fostamatinib (R788) and its active metabolite R406, in the autoimmune disorder, Chronic Immune Thrombocytopenia (Roskoski 2020), with an insufficient response to at least one prior line of therapy (Connel 2019). Besides fostamatinib, other inhibitors are currently in clinical trials to access their therapeutic potential, as Entospletinib (GS-9973), Cerdulatinib, HMPL-523 and TAK-659. (Liu 2017).

Characteristics and Clinical Experience with SYK Inhibitors

Fostamatinib, Entospletinib, Cerdulatinib and TAK-659, are some of the several oral Syk inhibitors that are being assessed in clinical trials (Liu & Mamorska-Dyga, 2017).

Fostamatinib (R788) is an oral SYK inhibitor, acting as a competitive inhibitor for the ATP binding site, that is rapidly metabolized in vivo to R406, a metabolite that inhibits signal transduction of Fc-activating receptors and B-cell receptor (Liu & Mamorska-Dyga, 2017). Fostamatinib has potent anti-inflammatory effects, demonstrating its activity, primarily, in rheumatoid arthritis and immune thrombocytopenia (Liu & Mamorska-Dyga, 2017). This drug presents antiproliferative and pro-apoptotic activity in B-cell lymphoma, chronic lymphocytic leukemia (CLL), and Waldenstrom macroglobulinemia (WMG) in preclinical studies with an *in vitro* IC_{50} of 41 nM (Buchner, *et al.* 2010; Kuiatse, *et al.* 2015; Young, *et al.*

2009). Additionally to SYK, Fostamatinib also presents effects on FLT3, aurora A kinase, and RET (McAdoo & Tam 2011).

Data suggested that chemotaxis and retention of Chronic Lymphocytic Leukemia (CLL) cells within lymphoid tissues depend on signaling through SYK, and that in vitro inhibition of SYK induces apoptosis of a number of lymphoma cell lines (Sharman 2015; Cheson, 2010), led to the assessment of SYK inhibitors, namely fostamatinib, in clinical trials. In a phase I/II study, in patients with refractory B-cell lymphomas, the highest overall response rate (ORR) was observed in CLL/Small Lymphocytic Lymphoma (SLL) patients (55%) and in diffuse large B-cell lymphoma (DLBCL) patients (22%). The dose limiting toxicity (DLT) was diarrhea, neutropenia, and thrombocytopenia. Median progression-free survival (PFS) was 4.2 months. This trial established the phase II dose at 200 mg twice daily (Friedberg et al., 2010). Fostamatinib was studied in patients with relapsed or refractory (R/R) DLBCL in a phase II, two-arm, randomized, double-blinded trial at either 100 mg twice a day (BID) or 200 mg BID. The efficacy at these doses and schedule were poor. The ORR was 3% across both arms and clinical benefit (stable disease or better) was achieved in 13% of all patients. Fostamatinib was generally well tolerated, being diarrhea, nausea, and fatigue the most common treatment-related adverse events (AEs) (Finn et al., 2016). The safety profile in these patients was similar to those described in other clinical trials with Fostamatinib in rheumatoid arthritis (Weinblatt, *et al.* 2008). Off-target effects on VEGFR and other tyrosine kinases were thought to be responsible for the most common AEs, namely hypertension (Rolf et al., 2015; Skinner et al., 2014). This SYK inhibitor is currently involved in clinical trials to access the therapeutic potential in ovarian cancer (NCT03246074), in renal transplant rejection (NCT03991780), among others.

Entospletinib (GS-9973) is a second-generation oral SYK inhibitor that in comparison to fostamatinib revealed an increased selectivity for Janus kinase 2 (JAK-2), c-KIT, FMS-like tyrosine kinase 3 (FLT 3), RET, and VEGFR2 (Currie et al., 2014). Preclinical studies showed attractive results in monotherapy and combination with other drugs (Burke, *et al.* 2014; Liu & Mamorska-Dyga 2017) Entospletinib was evaluated in a multicenter, phase II study, that enrolled R/R CLL and non-Hodgkin lymphoma (NHL) patients. Entospletinib was administered 800 mg twice a day. The ORR was 61% with no complete responses (CR). The median PFS for CLL was 13.8 months. The rate of serious adverse events (SAEs) was 29%. The most common AEs were dyspnea, pneumonia, febrile neutropenia, and pyrexia. The study showed that entospletinib had clinical activity in patients with R/R CLL (Sharman et al., 2015a). In an updated report of a cohort of 69 patients with indolent NHL (41 follicular lymphoma (FL), 11 lymphoplasmacytic lymphoma (LPL), 17 marginal zone lymphoma (MZL)), of the multicenter phase II study mentioned above (Sharman et al. 2015b), the ORR was 13.0%, with 7 PR, and one CR. The median PFS was 5.5 months. Entospletinib was generally well tolerated. The most common AEs were fatigue and GI toxicities, like nausea, diarrhea and vomiting. The most frequent laboratory abnormalities were elevation of ALT /AST and bilirubin, as well as anemia and neutropenia. Entospletinib was also evaluated in a phase II trial in R/R mantle cell lymphoma (MCL) patients, demonstrating a modest activity with an ORR of 15% and a median PFS of 5.6 months (Sharman et al., 2016). In a phase II study in patients with R/R DLBCL, entospletinib monotherapy had limited activity, with 74% of the patients experiencing a grade ≥ 3 AEs (Burke et al., 2018).

PI3Kδ inhibitors and BTK inhibitors have impacted the management of CLL and NHL. Nevertheless, the emergence of resistance to these therapies led to the investigation and development of other treatment strategies. Entospletinib was a potential therapeutic option due to the inhibition of SYK, located upstream of both BTK and PI3Kδ in the B-cell receptor (BCR) signaling pathway. Entospletinib mi monotherapy was evaluated in a multicenter, phase II study (NCT01799889) in patients with R/R CLL, who had received a prior therapy with a BCR inhibitor. Patients were treated with entospletinib 400 mg BID. The ORR was 32.7% and the median PFS was 5.6 months. The most common AEs were fatigue, diarrhea, and anemia (Awan et al., 2019). Also, the combination of entospletinib and idelalisib, a PI3Kδ inhibitor, was evaluated in an attempt to enhance the efficacy and reduce resistance in patients with R/R CLL and NHL. However, the study was terminated early because of treatment-emergent pneumonitis in 18% of patients (Barr et al., 2016).

Constitutive activation of SYK in acute myeloid leukemia (AML) has been reported. Targeted inhibition of SYK induced differentiation in vitro, demonstrating anti-leukemia activity in AML mouse models. SYK promotes leukemogenesis by directly phosphorylating the FLT3 receptor, modulating its activation and possibly promoting its role in leukemogenesis (Walker et al., 2016b; Walker et al., 2018). In AML, entospletinib 400 mg twice daily was evaluated in monotherapy and in combination with chemotherapy in a phase Ib/II study (NCT02343939). The aim was to evaluate the efficacy of entospletinib in untreated AML patients in monotherapy, followed by entospletinib plus standard 7+3 induction chemotherapy regimen (cytarabine 100 mg/m2/d, days 1-7 plus daunorubicin 60 mg/m2/d, days 1-3). Interestingly, the combination of entospletinib plus 7+3 induction demonstrated high remission rates in specific molecular subgroups. The presence of NPM1, FLT3-ITD mutations, and KMT2A gene rearrangements were associated with higher CR rates than historical controls (Walker et al, 2018). Entospletinib efficacy was also evaluated in patients with AML and acute lymphoblastic leukemia (ALL) specifically with t(v;11q23.3) KMT2A/MLL gene rearrangements, concluding that KMT2A rearranged AL is sensitive to entospletinib (Walker et al, 2018). In AML preclinical models, RAS pathway activation, through RAS, PTPN11, and potentially CBL mutations, or upregulation of expression of these target genes, renders resistance to SYK inhibitors. This was also observed in AML patients treated with the entospletinib with early relapse. Some preclinical data suggest that combining SYK with MEK inhibitors has the potential to prevent the emergence of resistance to SYK inhibition and even shows upfront efficacy (Cremer et al., 2019).

Increased activity of SYK in ALL cells may play a role in leukemia cell survival and proliferation. Deregulated SYK activity allows growth factor-independent proliferation and transformation of bone marrow-derived pre-B cells in mice. Inhibition of SYK has been shown to attenuate the growth of B-ALL *in vitro* and *in vivo* in mouse models (Minden et al., 2015). In pre-clinical models, entospletinib and vincristine had a synergistic anti-leukemia effect, which led to a phase Ib trial (NCT02404220) evaluating the combination of estospletinib with vincristine and dexamethasone for the treatment of relapsed or refractory adult Pre-B-ALL (Minden et al., 2015). However, due to the low response rate observed, the sponsor decided not to proceed with Phase II (dose-expansion) and the cohort was subsequently closed with no participant enrolled. Preclinical studies showed attractive results in monotherapy and combination with other drugs (Burke*, et al.* 2014; Liu & Mamorska-Dyga 2017)

HMPL-523 is an oral selective SYK inhibitor that is currently on clinical trials in lymphoma patients (NCT02857998 and NCT 03779113), but few details are available (Yang*, et al.* 2016). Preliminary results showed that this TKI is well tolerated as a single agent in Chinese patients with R/R B-cell lymphoma, and 600 mg once daily was determined as the dose to move for phase II of the trial (Fowler*, et al.* 2019; Zhu*, et al.* 2018).

Some of SYK inhibitors under study and with promising results are not exclusive of SYK targeting another kinase with potency, as the case of Cerdulatinib and TAK-659. Cerdulatinib is a dual SYK and JAK inhibitor that shows a wide range of antitumor activity in preclinical studies (Liu & Mamorska-Dyga 2017; Ma*, et al.* 2015). This TKI presented *in vitro* an IC_{50} of 32 nM for SYK and between 0.5 to 12 nM for JAK kinases (Guo*, et al.* 2017). Present under clinical trial (NCT01994382) in a phase I/II dose-escalation study in CLL and NHL. The few results show the highest response on follicular lymphoma and CLL. The most common adverse effects reported were fatigue, diarrhea, and anemia. So far, the dose of 35mg twice daily was the dose selected to pursue phase II of the trial (Coffey*, et al.* 2018; Hamlin*, et al.* 2019).

TAK-659, an oral dual SYK and FLT3 inhibitor, has been investigated in hematological malignancies and in solid tumors, due to the inhibition of the pro-survival, proliferative, chemoresistant, and activation effects promoted by the microenvironment (Liu & Mamorska-Dyga, 2017). This TKI presented in investigational studies the ability to inhibit pro-survival and proliferative effects in tumor models, and also presented a synergistic effect when combined with other drugs, as BCR inhibitor (Purroy*, et al.* 2017) In phase I study (NCT02000934) in patients with advanced solid tumors or lymphoma, TAK-659 showed an acceptable safety profile, and signs of clinical activity in DLBCL and FL. However, no solid tumor patient achieved an objective response (Kaplan et al., 2016). In a phase Ib/II study in adult patients with R/R AML, TAK-659 demonstrated an acceptable safety profile, as well as preliminary antitumor activity (Pratz et al., 2017). In safety evaluation, the maximal dose tolerated was 100 mg daily, and the most common adverse effects were fatigue, elevated AST, anemia, and diarrhea (Gordon, et al. 2020). The efficacy was variable according to patients' neoplasias, with 46% of ORR in DLBCL, but no response was observed in solid tumors (Gordon, et al. 2020; Petrich, *et al.* 2015). Due to this dual targeting, TAK-659 has also been tested in R/R AML (NCT02323113) (Kaplan, et al. 2016). The preliminary results showing that this TKI presented an acceptable PK profile and is moving to phase II stage. TAK-659 is involved in six ongoing clinical trials, where this TKI has been tested in monotherapy and combination with other chemotherapeutic agents (Vincristine, Paclitaxel, Venetoclax) in solid and hematological malignancies.

No Syk inhibitors are currently approved for therapeutic use in cancer therapy. Modest clinical results have dampened the enthusiasm in this new group of small molecule inhibitors targeting BCR-mediated signaling pathways in some malignancies. The second-generation compound, entospletinib, showed interesting results in clinical trials against CLL and in specific molecular subgroups of AML, suggesting that SYK inhibition is a possible therapeutic strategy in some hematological malignancies, however, further studies are warranted. The ongoing trials where SYK inhibitors are combined with other drugs may increase the therapeutic potential of these inhibitors. However, a more extensive follow-up is needed to make a robust analysis of clinical trial results.

ALK Inhibitors

Anaplastic lymphoma kinase (ALK) is a proven molecular target in several tumors that have ALK rearrangements, namely non-small cell lung cancer (NSCLC). ALK was discovered in 1994 when a chromosomal rearrangement t(2;5), leading to a nucleophosmin (*NPM1)-ALK* fusion gene, was found in anaplastic large-cell lymphoma (ALCL; Morris et al., 1994). Until now, more than 20 different *ALK* fusion partner genes have been reported (Lin et al., 2017). The spectrum of chimeric ALK proteins and their frequency varies along tumor types. The frequency of ALK rearrangements in ALCL is about 55% in adult patients and is present in almost all pediatric patients. In inflammatory myofibroblastic tumor these rearrangements occur in up to 50% of cases, in NSCLC the frequency of ALK rearrangements range from 3 to 7%, and in diffuse large B cell lymphoma, colorectal cancer, and renal cell carcinoma is inferior to 1%. ALK rearrangements have been detected in other cancers, including breast, esophageal, and ovarian cancers, and renal medullary carcinoma (Lin et al., 2017). ALK fusion proteins interact with multiple downstream pathways, such as mitogen-activated protein kinase (MAPK), signal transducer and activator of transcription 3 (STAT3) and phosphoinositide 3-kinase (PI3K)-AKT, which are involved in the processes of cellular proliferation, invasion, metastasis and resistance to apoptosis (Spagnuolo, Maione &Gridelli, 2018; Zhang et al., 2016). The discovery of the first ALK fusion-positive (ALK+) NSCLC (EML4-ALK, TPF-ALK) took place in 2007 (Rikova et al., 2007; Soda et al., 2007). In the following years, deep sequencing methods made possible for the identification of more than 90 fusion partners in ALK+ NSCLC in the beginning of 2020 (Ou, Zhu & Nagasaka, 2020). For each partner, several variants can be found depending on the position where the two genes fusion has occurred, which may influence tumor's response and patient prognosis (Christopoulos et al., 2018). EML4-ALK is still the major variant in ALK+ NSCLC (accounting for approximately 95% of all ALK fusion variants) (Ross et al., 2017). *ALK* rearrangements typically occur in younger patients who have never smoked or have a history of light smoking and that have adenocarcinoma histotype (Shaw et al., 2009). These rearrangements are typically mutually exclusive with EGFR and KRAS mutations (Takahashi et al., 2010). The presence of rearrangements or mutations in the ALK gene had given in this NSCLC subgroup of patients a major therapeutic advantage as it turns cancer cells sensitive to tyrosine kinase inhibitors and allows these drugs to bind to receptor tyrosine kinases, inhibiting downstream signaling pathways (Schrank et al., 2018).

Currently, five ALK inhibitors have been approved by FDA for treatment of ALK-positive NSCLC, crizotinib (2011), ceritinib (2014), alectinib (2015), brigatinib (2017), and lorlatinib (2018) (Roskoski, 2020). Approved ALK inhibitors bind to the abnormal ALK protein, specifically to its ATP pocket, blocking its access to energy and inhibiting its action. Crizotinib, the first approved oral ALK inhibitor, was developed initially as a c-MET inhibitor, but it also targets ALK, ROS1, and MET (Nwizu et al., 2011). The compound binds the ATP pocket of these kinases. The FDA granted accelerated approval to crizotinib based on promising data from phase I trial (PROFILE 10019), which reported 72% 6-months progress-free survival (PFS) and 57% overall response rate (ORR), and from phase II (PROFILE 100513) trial that demonstrated similar encouraging results of 53% and a median progression-free survival of 8.5 months in often heavily pretreated ALK-positive patients (Khan et al., 2019; Kim et al., 2012; Kwak et al., 2010). The subsequent phase 3 trials (PROFILE 1007 and 1014) reported comparative results of crizotinib to the single agent chemotherapy (premetexed or docetaxel and pemetrexed plus platinum chemotherapy) in previously treated NSCLC patients with significantly superior in median PFS and ORR (Shaw et al., 2013; Solomon et al., 2014). Crizotinib is in general well tolerated mostly with mild treatment-related adverse events that include vision disorder, nausea, diarrhea, vomiting of grade 1 and 2, elevated transaminases and neutropenia of grade 3 or 4 (Sharma et al., 2018). Although first-line ALK-targeted therapy often yields remarkable responses, the efficacy of crizotinib decreases after the onset of acquired resistance mechanisms, mainly secondary mutations in the *ALK* gene and activation of bypass tracks (Ferrara et al., 2020; Lin et al., 2017). Disease progression will involve multiple sites and distinct patterns of progression have been identified, including isolated CNS progression and extracranial oligoprogression (Rothenstein & Chooback, 2018). Most patients who progress under crizotinib, even those with undetectable resistance mutation in *ALK* gene, still respond to treatment with a next-generation ALK inhibitor. Therefore, the best therapeutic option is a second-generation ALK inhibitor (Rothenstein & Chooback, 2018). Ceritinib, alectinib, and brigatinib – the second-generation ALK TKIs – were investigated and demonstrated outstanding activity in both crizotinib-naïve and resistant ALK-rearranged NSCLC, with superior penetration of the blood-brain barrier and response rate on brain metastases (Ferrara et al., 2020). Ceritinib, a highly selective ATP competitive second generation ALK inhibitor, was investigated in ASCEND-4 and ASCEND-5 in ALK rearranged NSCLC patients. This inhibitor is 20 times more potent than crizotinib, being also active against many *ALK* mutations that confer resistance to crizotinib (e.g., C1156Y, F1174C, G1202R, and the gatekeeper mutation L1196M) (Ferrara et al., 2020). In ASCEND-4 trial the efficacy of ceritinib was analyzed in treatment-naïve patients versus pemetrexed-based platinum doublet therapy. The results of this trial show in patients treated with ceritinib a 72.5% ORR and 16.6 months median PFS in comparison with 26.7% and 11.1 months (Soria et al., 2017). Moreover, ASCEND-5 trial showed that even with prior ALK TKI therapy, patients treated with ceritinib had 45% ORR and 5.4 months PFS (Shaw et al., 2017).

Most of the adverse events related to ceritinib treatment were of grade 1 or 2 diarrhea, nausea, and vomiting, and increased alanine and aspartate aminotransferases of grade 3 or 4 (Sharma et al., 2018). The comparison of alectinib to crizotinib was analyzed in ALEX trial treatment-naïve ALK rearranged patients showed 34.8 months versus 10.9 months of median PFS, 82.9% versus 75.5% of ORR, and a similar 12-month OS of 84.3% and 82.5%, respectively (Camidge et al., 2019).

Alectinib showed some adverse events and the most common side effects were constipation, fatigue, myalgia and peripheral edema. In some patients grade 3 or higher AEs were observed (increased blood creatine phosphokinase and neutropenia) (Sharma et al., 2018). The ALTA study analyzed the efficacy of brigatinib in ALK-positive NSCLC patients pre-treated with crizotinib or chemotherapy. This trail showed 53% ORR, 15.6 months of median PFS, and 12-month OS of 80%.

The subsequent ALTA-1L phase 3 study showed significant results in favor of brigatinib versus crizotinib (ORR=71%, 12-month PFS=67%, and 12-month survival without intracranial disease progression=67%) (Kim et al., 2017; Camidge et al., 2018). The most frequent adverse events related to brigatinib included diarrhea, increased creatine kinase level, nausea, cough, and hypertension (Kim et al., 2017; Camidge et al., 2018).

The last ALK inhibitor to be approved was lorlatinib, a third-generation ALK inhibitor. This drug showed significant benefit in ALK rearranged patients regardless of treatment history (Giustini et al., 2020). Lorlatinib showed a 90% ORR with 66.7% intracranial response in the treatment-naïve cohort, 69.5% ORR with 87% intracranial response in patients previously treated with crizotinib, and 47% ORR with 63% intracranial response in patients treated with one or more TKIs (1 to 3), indicating benefit in heavily pretreated patients (Solomon et al., 2018).

In order to overcome the inevitable drug resistance and to enhance inhibitory activity against ALK, new ALK inhibitors have emerged. The most important new ALK inhibitors are entrectinib and ensartinib.

Entrectinib is a potent inhibitor of NTRK, ROS1, and ALK fusions. In a phase I basket study involving treatment-naïve patients, it demonstrated significant responses in NTRK-, ROS1-, and ALK-positive patients (Drilon et al., 2017). Ensartinib is 10-fold more potent than crizotinib at inhibiting the growth of ALK-positive lung cancer cell lines and showed activity in crizotinib-naïve patients, crizotinib-resistant patients, and patients with brain metastases with potential to overcome resistance to crizotinib with good CNS penetration (Lovly et al., 2011; Reckamp et al., 2016). Several clinical trials analyzing the efficacy of ALK inhibitors to treat other cancers are also ongoing. Some examples of these clinical trials include: crizotinib to treat bladder cancer (NTC02612194) and non-Hodgkin's lymphoma (NTC02693535), brigatinib to treat lymphoma patients (NTC01449461), lorlatinib to treat pediatric neuroblastoma (NTC03107988), alectinib to treat cancer patients with ALK or RET-positive tumors (NTC03194893), and ceritinib to treat tumors with ALK or RET-aberrations (NTC02465528 and NTC02186821).

Serine-Threonine Kinase Inhibitors

Braf Inhibitors

The *BRAF* gene is located on chromosome 7 (7q34) and encodes for a serine-threonine protein kinase (B-RAF) which is moved to the cell membrane on stimulation by growth factors (Davis et al., 2002; Dhomen & Marais, 2007). The wild-type *BRAF* gene causes downstream activation of the Mitogen-activated protein kinase (MAPK) signaling pathway, which is usually initiated by activation of a membrane tyrosine kinase receptor (Figure 1). This signal, through RAS activation, promotes BRAF activation, which in turn phosphorylates MEK and ERK sequentially, regulating growth, proliferation, apoptosis and differentiation of human cells (Caronia, Phay & Shah, 2011).

Activating BRAF mutations lead to the constitutive BRAF protein dimerization and to the subsequent activation of the RAF-MEK-ERK signaling cascade, inducing uncontrolled cell proliferation, apoptosis inhibition and cancer growth. The BRAF-V600E mutation was the first BRAF mutation described in 2002. Besides this mutation is the most common one, although more than 40 *BRAF* gene mutations have already been identified. It has been associated with several solid tumors, including melanoma (50-60%), thyroid carcinoma (30-50%), colorectal cancer (10%) and non-small cell lung cancer (NSCLC, 3%) (Bernicker, Allen & Cagle 2019; Ducreux et al., 2019; Yan et al., 2019). The identification of BRAF mutations in different tumor types has permitted the development of a new class of antineoplastic agents, ATP-competitive RAF inhibitors, of which Vemurafenib and Dabrafenib are the most extensively studied.

High constitutive activity of MAPK pathway has been shown in a majority of melanomas, in colorectal and in Lung cancer, making these diseases especially prone to oncogene-targeted therapy.

BRAF INHIBITORS IN MELANOMA

Vemurafenib

A multicenter phase 1 dose escalation trial using PLX4032 (Vemurafenib), administered orally, reported in 2010 a high rate of complete (CR) or partial tumor regressions (PR) in the 32 patients treated for metastatic melanoma with BRAF-V600E mutation (Flaherty et al., 2010). These favorable results elicited BRIM-2 (NCT00949702), a pivotal phase II trial aiming at patients who had received at least one previous line of therapy for metastatic melanoma. At median time of follow-up of 7 months, best overall response rate (ORR) was 52.3% (95% CI: 43–61%; 2.3% CR, 50% PR), with median duration of response of 6.8 months (95% CI: 5.6-NR) and median progression free survival (PFS) of 6.2 months (95% CI: 5.6–6.8%) (Ribas et al., 2011).

BRIM-3 (NCT01006980), a phase 3 randomized clinical trial comparing vemurafenib with dacarbazine, reported improved rates of overall survival (OS) and PFS in patients with previously untreated melanoma with the BRAF-V600E mutation treated with vemurafenib. Response rates were 48% for vemurafenib versus 5% for dacarbazine. Main side effects were arthralgia, rash, fatigue, alopecia, keratoacanthoma or squamous-cell carcinoma, photosensitivity, nausea, and diarrhea, with 38% of patients requiring dose reduction because of toxicity (Chapman et al., 2011).

Based on these reports, in August 17, 2011, the FDA approved vemurafenib for V600E BRAF mutation positive unresectable or metastatic melanoma.

Dabrafenib

Dabrafenib (by GlaxoSmithKline) is also a BRAF inhibitor used for patients with metastatic or unresectable V600E-BRAF mutated melanoma patients. FDA approval occurs in May 2013 resulted from the publication of an open-label phase 3 trial which reported significantly improved median

PFS with dabrafenib compared with dacarbazine (5.1 versus 2.7 months, HR 0.30, 95% CI 0.18-0.51; p<0.0001) (Hauschild et al., 2012).

BRAF INHIBITORS IN COLORECTAL CANCER

Ten-to-fifteen percent of colorectal cancers present mutated BRAF, which is a sign of a poorer prognosis. It is also associated to reduced response to anti-EGFR therapy in KRAS wild-type colorectal cancer. BRAF-V600E is the most common mutation seen in BRAF in colorectal cancer, but response to BRAF-inhibitors in this cancer is limited. The mechanism responsible for the lack of responsiveness in colorectal cancer is probably related to the reactivation of MAPK pathway by EGFR. EGFR expression is not as frequent in melanoma, which could explain its apparently unimportant role in melanoma.

Ongoing clinical trials are dwelling on the use of double or triple combination of EGFR targeted agents with BRAF inhibitors, apparently with some benefit in terms of response rate (Sanz-Garcia et al, 2017).

BRAF INHIBITORS IN LUNG CANCER

BRAF mutations have been reported in 3% of lung adenocarcinomas, making BRAF-mutations a potential target in this subset of patients (Ali et al., 2015; Cardarella et al., 2013; Marchetti et al., 2011).

A multiple non-melanoma, histology-independent phase 2 "basket" trial of vemurafenib in BRAF-V600 mutation–positive nonmelanoma cancers reported a response rate of 42% in the NSCLC cohort (Hyman et al., 2015).

The phase II multicenter non-randomized NCT01336634 trial enrolled previously treated and untreated patients with stage IV metastatic BRAF-V600E NSCLC. Patients received dabrafenib and overall response was achieved in 33% [95% CI 23–45] (Planchard et al., 2016a). Based on the interim analysis of this study, presented at ASCO 2013, (Planchard et al.,

2013) Dabrafenib was granted a "breakthrough therapy" designation by the FDA for BRAF mutation positive Adenocarcinoma in January 2014.

Another phase II, non-randomized, open-label study NCT01336634 investigated dabrafenib administered without and in combination with trametinib (MEK-inhibitor) in stage IV BRAF-mutant advanced NSCLC patients who failed at least one previous line of chemotherapy. Dabrafenib plus trametinib showed early antitumor activity in this subset of patients, with an ORR of 63.2% [95% CI 49.3-75.6] (Planchard et al., 2016b).

The ESMO guidelines, updated 18 September 2019, recommend the use of dabrafenib combined with trametinib for patients with stage IV NSCLC with BRAF V600 mutation should be exposed in first or second line to BRAF/MEK inhibition using dabrafenib/trametinib [III, A; ESMO-MBCS v1.1 score: 2] (Planchard et al., 2018; Planchard et al., 2019).

AKT Inhibitors

AKT, or protein kinase B (PKB), is a serine threonine kinase that plays a major role in PI3K/AKT/mTOR pathway (Figure 1). This signaling pathway contributes to the regulation of fundamental mechanisms such as survival, proliferation, glucose metabolism, protein synthesis, genome stability, inhibition of apoptosis, neovascularization, and differentiation (Jiang et al., 2020; Kaboli et al., 2020; Shariati & Meric-Bernstam, 2019). AKT has three isoforms – AKT1 or PKBα, AKT2 or PKBβ, and AKT3 or PKBγ (Keane et al., 2014). The activity of AKT, the regulation of multiple downstream effects of PI3K/AKT/mTOR, is modulated by several upstream signaling proteins and by important negative regulators such as PTEN, PP2A, and PHLPP (Brown & Banerji, 2017; Kaboli et al., 2020). The PI3K/AKT/mTOR pathway is one of the most frequently disrupted signaling pathways in cancers being present in up to 40% of all tumor types (Brown & Banerji, 2017). AKT activation is mainly triggered by the binding of ligands to cell membrane receptors, such as IGF-1, PDGF, cytokines, hormones, and mitogens (Shariati & Meric-Bernstam, 2019). The frequency of genetic alteration of AKT genes is relatively uncommon, ranging from

0.1% in non-Hodgkin lymphoma (NHL) to 2.5% in prostate and bladder cancer (Jiang et al., 2020). However, amplification of AKT1 gene occurs in 20% of neuroendocrine prostate cancers, 10% of pancreatic cancers, and 2-3% of breast and serous ovarian cancers, while AKT2 amplifications are found in 16% of pancreatic and uterine cancers, 13% of breast cancers, and 5-10% of ovarian, lung, and bladder cancers (Brown & Banerji, 2017). AKT3 amplifications have been observed mainly in breast cancers (Brown & Banerji, 2017). Nevertheless, AKT activation can arise as a result of overexpression of upstream proteins such as PTEN, PHLPP, PP2A, and INPP4B, or mutations in *PIK3CA* and *PTEN* genes (Brown & Banerji, 2017; Jiang et al., 2020; Shariati & Meric-Bernstam, 2019).

Several AKT inhibitors are now in preclinical and clinical evaluation. These inhibitors act in different aspects of AKT biology and activation: pleckstrin homology (PH) domain, ATP-binding site and phosphorylation status, and conformation of the protein and cellular location (Keane et al., 2014). However, the majority of AKT inhibitors fall into two classes – the allosteric inhibitors of PH domain, that prevent localization of AKT to the plasma membrane and block AKT phosphorylation and activation, and the ATP-competitive inhibitors, that lock AKT in PH-out domain inactive state (Brown & Banerji, 2017). Most AKT inhibitors in clinical evaluation inhibit AKT1, AKT2, and AKT3, being therefore pan-AKT inhibitors (Song et al., 2019). ATP-competitive inhibitors bind to the active site of AKT blocking ATP binding (Shariati & Meric-Bernstam, 2019). However, these inhibitors are non-selective against AKT isozymes, and poorly selective against closely related kinases since the catalytic domain is very similar (Nitulescu, 2016). The ATP-competitive inhibitors include afuresertib (GSK2110183), ipatasertib (GDC-0068), capivasertib (AZD5363), uprosertib (GSK2141795), and GSK690693. These inhibitors have been in phase I and phase II clinical trials for monotherapy and combination therapy with several indications. Besides the limited selectivity of ATP-competitive inhibitors these drugs also showed dose-limiting side effects during treatment and therefore a lack of efficacy due to dose reduction (Landel et al., 2020).

Afuresertib is an orally pan-AKT kinase inhibitor that is ATP-competitive. This drug show promising antitumor activity against hematologic malignancies as single-agent, including multiple myeloma, with a favorable safety profile (Spencer et al., 2014). The most frequent treatment-related adverse events were nausea (35.6%), diarrhea (32.9%), and dyspepsia (24.7%) (Spencer et al., 2014). This study also showed clinical activity against non-Hodgkin lymphoma, Langerhan's cell histiocytosis, and Hodgkin disease. Some clinical trials also study the effectivity of afuresertib in combination with chemotherapy and targeted therapies such as ofatumumab in relapsed or refractory chronic lymphocytic leukemia patients (NCT01532700) and with trametinib in solid tumors (NTC01476137).

Ipatasertib in a first phase I study (NCT01090960) demonstrated a robust and safe targeting of AKT in patients with solid tumors with good tolerability (Saura et al., 2017). Two phase II trials are studying the effectiveness of ipatasertib in association with oxaliplatin, 5-fluorouracil, and leucovorin in advanced or metastatic gastric cancer (NTC01896531) and in association with paclitaxel in breast cancer (NTC02301988).

The allosteric inhibitors already in clinical trials include perifosine, miransertib (ARQ092), MK2206, triciribine, KRX-0401, and ARQ751. These inhibitors offer greater specificity, reduced side-effects, and lower toxicity compared to ATP-competitive inhibitors (Landel et al., 2020). However, these non-competitive inhibitors do not have activity against mutated AKT forms like AKTE17K (Keane et al., 2014).

The first AKT inhibitors to enter clinical development was the perifosine (D-21266 or KRX-0401; Aeterna Zentaris), an oral allosteric alkyl-phospholipid AKT inhibitor that prevents AKT translocation to the plasma membrane blocking AKT activation by disrupting the interaction between AKT and the phospholipids (Brown & Banerji, 2017; Song et al., 2019). The initial clinical trials showed that doses of oral perifosine are limited by gastro-intestinal toxicity and several studies have tested different schedules in order to achieve administration of biologically active doses without intolerable toxicity (Brown & Banerji, 2017; Crul et al., 2002; Figg et al., 2014; Unger et al., 2010; Van Ummersen et al., 2004). This AKT inhibitor showed clinical activity in glioblastoma multiforme, well tolerated, being the gastrointestinal toxicities the most common side effect, although none resulted in treatment discontinuation (Kaley et al., 2019). Additional phase I clinical trials confirmed that perifosine in monotherapy was safe and well-tolerated in children with high-risk neuroblastoma (Kushner et al., 2017). In a phase I clinical study (NCT00019656) perifosine combined with sorafenib showed promising activity against Hodgkin lymphoma (Guidetti et al., 2014). Several clinical trials analyzed the effectivity of therapeutic combination of perifosine with chemotherapy/radiotherapy and targeted therapy in several hematological and solid tumors. The most relevant are the association with capecitabine in patients with metastatic colorectal cancer (NCT00398879), docetaxel (NTC00431054) in patients with epithelial ovarian cancer, temsirolimus in patients with recurrent/refractory pediatric solid tumors (NCT01049841), imatinib (NTC00455559) in GIST patients, sorafenib in lymphoproliferative diseases, and bortezomib and dexamethasone in multiple myeloma (NTC00401011, NTC01002248), among others. Although this allosteric inhibitor has been studied in several trials and was the only one AKT inhibitor to reach a Phase III clinical trial, it has not been found to be superior to other first- or second-line treatments. Overall, perifosine was shown in several clinical trials to have significant activity either as a single agent or in combination therapy (Jiang et al., 2020; Song et al., 2019).

MK-2206 is one of the most clinically advanced allosteric inhibitor that acts predominantly in AKT1/2 with low effect against AKT3 (Brown & Banerji, 2017). This drug exhibited potent antiproliferative activity against various cancer cell types harboring PI3KCA mutations, PTEN loss, upstream RTK gene amplification or overactivation, and mutation of AKT itself (Song et al., 2019). The effectivity of MK2206 for patients with non-small cell lung cancer in combination with other targeted therapies has been analyzed in clinical trials. For example, a phase I study analyzed the association of MK2206 with gefitinib (NTC01147211) and a phase II study analyzed the combination with erlotinib (NTC 01294306). Other clinical trials studied the effectivity of MK2206 in monotherapy in patients with breast cancer (NTC01277757, NTC01319539), colorectal cancer

(NTC01802320, NTC01186705), liver cancer (NTC01239355), and hematological neoplasias (acute myeloid leukemia: NTC01253447; lymphoma: NTC01258998, NTC01466868, NTC01481129). MK2206 has been also studied in clinical trials combined with several chemotherapy drugs, such as paclitaxel and docetaxel, and targeted therapy agents like lapatinib, selumetinib, gefitinb, erlotinib, everolimus, dinaciclib, bicalutamide, among others. For example, the efficacy of MK2206 in combination with bendamustine and rituximab in relapsed or refractory chronic lymphocytic leukemia showed a promising overall response of 92% and a median PFS and treatment-free survival of 16 and 24 months, respectively (Larsen et al., 2017). These results suggest that MK2206 combined with chemo-immunotherapy might be a promising therapeutic option to treat cancer.

MEK/ERK Inhibitors

MEK kinase is an important component of the MAPK signaling cascade, mainly because, its two isoforms MEK1 and MEK2, are the only specific activators of ERK1 and ERK2 and they are also the only known catalytic substrates of RAF kinases. Unlike RAS mutations, MEK mutations appear only in a small percentage of all cancers (~1%) being mainly described in melanomas and colorectal cancer patients (Murugan et al., 2009; Nikolaev et al., 2011). Because the low prevalence of these mutations, MEK inhibition was not considered a potential treatment approach. However, the development of selective inhibitors against the active form of MEK already proved to be effective. Also, the rapid incidence of resistance to BRAF inhibitors prompted the investigation of other MAPK pathway inhibitors. The selectivity of MEK inhibitors results from the fact that they do not compete with ATP binding, unlike other kinase inhibitors, which make them highly specific towards their targets. Crystal structure studies showed that MEK inhibitors bind to an allosteric pocket adjacent to the ATP-binding site, without overlapping with, locking MEK in a conformation that avoids interactions with ERK activation loops (Ohren et al., 2004). One of the first

MEK inhibitors to enter clinical trials was CI-1040, a small-molecule with dual-specificity for MEK1/2. The first results obtained in several advanced malignancies were very promising, however progressive studies demonstrated its lack of efficacy pending further investigation (Lorusso et al., 2005). Since then, several molecules have been studied and currently four MEK inhibitors have been approved by FDA and EMA, namely trametinib, cobitini, binitinib and selumetinib.

Trametinib (Mekinist; GSK1120212) is an orally available, potent small MEK1 and MEK2 inhibitor, approved for the treatment of BRAF-mutated melanomas and non-small cell lung cancer (NSCLC). Besides blocking MEK activity, trametinib also inhibits MEK activation through RAF, producing a prolonged ERK inhibition (Gilmartin et al., 2011; Yamaguchi et al., 2011). The first preclinical data demonstrated that cell lines harboring either BRAF mutations or activating mutations in NRAS and KRAS were more sensitive to trametinib (Gilmartin et al., 2011). Similar results were observed further in BRAF-mutant xenografts where trametinib showed to inhibit tumor growth (Gilmartin et al., 2011). Based on this data, a phase I dose-escalation trial enrolling 206 patients with different advanced solid tumors was initiated. The authors were able to show that trametinib was well tolerated and that the most common adverse events were rash and diarrhea and recommended a daily dose of 2mg of trametinib for further studies (NCT00687622) (Infante et al., 2012). Several phase II/III clinical trials were initiated with trametinib alone or in combination with other drugs. The most important is the METRIC trial (NCT01245062), where 322 melanoma patients with V600E or V600K BRAF mutations were randomly assigned to received either oral trametinib or intravenous chemotherapy. Trametinib improved rates of progression-free (4.8 vs. 1.5 months, respectively) and overall survival (81% vs. 67%, respectively) comparing to chemotherapy group (NCT01072175) (Flaherty et al., 2012). A 5-years follow-up evaluation of these patients demonstrated that no new or unexcepted adverse effects appear after long-term use of trametinib and some patients even experienced long-term survival benefit (NCT01245062) (Robert et al., 2019a). The safety of trametinib administered in combination with dabrafenib (a BRAF inhibitor) was also evaluated in patients with previously untreated, unresectable or metastatic, BRAF V600 mutation-positive melanoma in two clinical trials, the COMBI-d (NCT01584648) and COMBI-v (NCT01597908) trials. Both studies demonstrated a clinical benefit for the combination treatment with significant improvement in overall survival when compared with dabrafenib (Long et al., 2015) and with vemurafenib, both in monotherapy (Robert et al., 2015). The most commonly occurring adverse reactions were pyrexia, nausea, rash, chills, diarrhea, vomiting, hypertension, and peripheral edema (Long et al., 2015; Robert et al., 2015). Nonetheless, one third of these patients were showed to have long-term benefit after 5-years follow up (Robert et al., 2019b). A more recent study evaluated the same drug combination as adjuvant treatment in stage III melanoma with BRAF V600 mutations (COMBI-AD trial; NCT01682083), showing that this combination therapy leads to an estimated 3-year rate of relapse-free survival of 58%, significantly lower than the 39% observed in the placebo group (Long et al., 2017). The latest trametinib approval indicated its combination with dabrafenib to treat patients with non-small lung cancer patients with BRAF V600E mutations. An overall response rate higher than 60%, with a median PFS longer than 9 months were observed in patients receiving this drug combination comparing to the dabrafenib group (27% ORR and 5.5 months median PFS) (NCT01336634) (Planchard et al., 2017).

Cobimetinib (Cotellic; GDC-0973), a structural analogue of CI-1040, is an orally bioavailable, highly selective inhibitor of the MEK1 and MEK2 (Rice et al., 2012). Cobimetinib is currently approved by FDA and EMA in combination with vemurafenib (a BRAF inhibitor) for the treatment of unresectable or metastatic melanoma with BRAF V600E or V600K mutation. The recommended dose of administration is 60mg once daily for 21 days followed by a 7-day break in combination with 960mg twice daily of vemurafenib (NCT01271803) (Ribas et al., 2014). To prove the hypothesis that cobimetinib and vemurafenib combination improve clinical outcomes in melanoma patients, a randomized phase III study (coBRIM; NCT01689519) was performed (Ascierto et al., 2016). Patients receiving the combination schedule had a clear advantage in terms of response rate (70% vs. 50%), overall survival (22.3 vs. 17.4 months) and progression-free survival (11.0 vs. 8.8 months). The combination presented an acceptable and manageable safety profile. Adverse events were more common in the combination arm and included serous retinopathy, decreased left ventricular ejection fraction and increased creatine phosphokinase, however they were generally manageable (Ascierto et al., 2016). This study ultimately leads to the approval of this drug schedule for this specific melanoma patient subpopulation.

Binimetinib (Mektovi; MEK162) is an orally available, MEK1 and MEK2 inhibitor. A phase I study determined the maximum tolerated dose of binimetinib as single agent of 60 mg twice daily, however due to ocular toxicities the recommended dose for further studies was 45 mg two times a day (NCT00959127) (Bendell et al., 2017). Then, the NEMO trial (NCT01763164) showed that binimetinib improved the median progression-free survival compared with dacarbazine (2.8 and 1.5, respectively) and also presents a well tolerability in patients with NRAS-mutant melanoma (Dummer et al., 2017). The approval of binimetinib was based on a two-part phase III trial (COLOMBUS; NCT01909453) of encorafenib plus binimetinib versus encorafenib plus vemurafenib in monotherapy in patients with unresectable or metastatic BRAF V600-mutant melanoma. First, authors observed that the combination consisting of 450 mg of encorafenib once daily plus 45 mg of binimetinib twice daily improved median progression-free survival (7.3 vs. 14.9) and median overall survival (16.9 vs. 33.6 months) when compared to vemurafenib in monotherapy (Dummer et al., 2018a; Dummer et al., 2018b). Recently an update on this clinical trial demonstrated a long term benefit in these melanoma patients (Ascierto et al., 2020).

Selumetinib is the most recently approved MEK1 and MEK2 inhibitor (KOSELUGO; AZD6244, ARRY-142886). This MEK inhibitor was approved by FDA for the treatment of pediatric patients with neurofibromatosis type 1 and symptomatic, inoperable plexiform neurofibromas and is under regulatory review by EMA. This approval was a result of a phase II SPRINT trial (NCT01362803) that enrolled 50 children with neurofibromatosis type 1 treated with selumetinib 25 mg/m2 twice daily in 28-day cycles on in continuous schedule. In the first trial report, authors demonstrated that selumetinib induced a durable tumor shrinkage and confirmed partial responses in approximately 70% of the patients (Dombi et al., 2016). These responses were also accompanied by clinically meaningful benefit, observed for example in life quality improvement through the interference in pain control (Gross et al., 2020). Most common adverse events were vomiting, nausea, rash, abdominal pain, diarrhea, among others (Dombi et al., 2016; Gross et al., 2020). Other clinical trials are ongoing using selumetinib, most of them testing a combination therapy with other drugs, for the treatment of gliomas, neurofibromatosis type 1 and 2 and advanced/recurrent solid tumors.

Several other MEK inhibitors are currently under development and just entered early stages of clinical trials. These inhibitors include mirdametinib (PD-0325901), FCN-159, CS3006, HL-085 and JSI-1187. All these compounds, along with the previously described ones, continue to be evaluated in a very wide range of tumors, but their real clinical potential seems to be in their combination with other drugs. Particularly, the combination of MEK inhibitors with immune checkpoint inhibitors is a highly investigated treatment option. For example, a few clinical trials are currently evaluating the potential of atezolizumab in combination with cobimetinib for the treatment of soft tissue sarcoma (NCT04216953), non-small cell lung cancer (NCT03600701) and other advanced or refractory rare tumors (NCT03108131). Other combinations with BRAF inhibitors, autophagy inhibitors and CDK inhibitors are also under study.

The inhibition of ERK, the downstream kinase of the MAPK pathway, has gained an increased interest over the past few years, not only because it would reverse the abnormally activated pathway due to all the upstream mutations, but also because it would possibly overcome the acquired resistance induced by the upstream inhibitors. Several ERK inhibitors are currently under pre-clinical and clinical evaluation for the treatment of different malignancies, but none has been approved by FDA or EMA.

Ulixertinib (BVD-523) is a novel first-class small molecule, highly selective, targeting ERK1 and ERK2 by ATP-competition. This compound showed good preclinical efficacy, particularly in cell lines with activating mutations in the MAPK signaling pathway (Germann et al., 2017). The same research group also verified that ulixertinib not only inhibited ERK1 and ERK2 activity, but also increased ERK phosphorylation by a negative feedback loop (Germann et al., 2017). The first-in-human trial with ulixertinib (NCT01781429) enrolled patients with BRAF-, NRAS- and MEK-mutated solid tumors and reported that partial responses were observed in 17% of patients. This drug show to be well tolerable, and its toxicity was manageable, being the more common treatment-related adverse events rash, fatigue, and gastrointestinal disturbances, such as nausea, vomiting, and diarrhea (Sullivan et al., 2018). Clinical evaluation of ulixertinib is currently still ongoing. One clinical trial is studying ulixertinib in a combination schedule with hydroxychloroquine in advanced MAPK-mutated gastrointestinal adenocarcinoma patients (NCT04145297) and, another study, with palbociclib in patients with advanced pancreatic and other solid tumors (NCT03454035). A recent large-scale basket trial (MATCH trial) is evaluating the clinical potential of ulixertinib in patients with advanced solid tumors, Non-Hodgkin lymphoma, or histiocytic disorders with MAPK mutations (NCT03698994), but no results were yet reported.

LY3214996 is a potent and selective ATP-competitive inhibitor of ERK1 and ERK2, that is under clinical evaluation after the demonstration of its antitumor activity in *in vitro* and *in vivo* cancer models with ERK pathway mutations (BRAF, KRAS, NRAS, MEK and NF1) (Bhagwat et al., 2020). Ongoing trials with LY3214996 are evaluating its potential in several advanced/metastatic tumors (NCT02857270) and acute myeloid leukemia (NCT04081259), in combination with abemaciclib, in recurrent glioblastoma patients (NCT04391595) and in combination with hydroxychloroquine, in patients with advanced pancreatic cancer (NCT04386057).

Other ERK inhibitor in clinical evaluation is MK-8353, a highly potent and selective ATP-competitive ERK1/2 inhibitor, with good oral bioavailability. This inhibitor demonstrated an antitumor activity in several BRAF/KRAS tumor models. Unlike the previously ERK inhibitors described, MK-8353 inhibits ERK kinase activity and prevents the phosphorylation of ERK by MEK (Boga et al., 2018). Two combination schedules with MK-8353 are under clinical investigation, one with selumetinib (NCT03745989) and other with pembrolizumab (NCT02972034), in patients with advanced/metastatic solid tumors. Three other ERK inhibitors are under early stages of clinical evaluation, LTT 462, ASN007 and KO-947, however information regarding their development is not available.

CDK Inhibitors

Cancer is characterized by uncontrolled proliferation resulting from aberrant activity of various cell cycle proteins. Cyclin-dependent kinases (CDKs) are proteins that directly regulate cell cycle progression. The knowledge of the relevance of CDKs and checkpoint kinases in inducing cell-cycle arrest and apoptosis in neoplastic cells lead to the development of small molecule inhibitors targeting these kinases. Certain cancers, as hormone receptor-positive breast cancer, have a higher probability to have disturbances in CDK4/6 (Otto & Sicinski, 2017).

Breast cancer (BC) represents one of the leading causes of cancer worldwide and a main cause of death by cancer. In recent years, intrinsic gene expression profiling has permitted BC classification into major subtypes, characterized by specific biological properties, distinct morphologies and clinical implications, which translate into different prognosis (Dai et al., 2015). The most commonly diagnosed subset of BC patients is estrogen receptor (ER)- and/or progesterone receptor (PR)-positive. Endocrine therapy is a highly effective treatment for this group of patients, in the adjuvant and metastatic settings (Maximov, Lee & Jordan, 2013). Nevertheless, some patients will develop metastatic disease (MBC), usually related to endocrine therapy resistance, and new therapeutic approaches are needed (Chlebowski, 2013). The relevance of CDK in cancer leads to the development of CDK inhibitors as palbociclib, Abemaciclib and ribociclib (Figure 2).

Palbociclib

Palbociclib, the first CDK4/6 inhibitor to be approved for BC treatment, is a small selective inhibitor of CDK4/6, orally administered (Fry et al., 2004). Early trials on this drug showed its efficacy in BC ER+/HER2−. Myelosuppression turned out to be the main dose-limiting toxicity (DLT) in the phase I palbociclib trial (Flaherty et al., 2012; Schwartz et al., 2011). The PALOMA-1/TRIO-18 trial, an open-label randomized phase II clinical trial, focused on the safety and efficacy of palbociclib plus letrozole versus letrozole alone as first line treatment of postmenopausal women with previously untreated BC ER+/HER2−. Median progression-free survival (PFS) was greatly increased in the combination arm (20.2 months vs. 10.2 months). Grade 3-4 neutropenia was reported in 54% of patients in the palbociclib plus letrozole group versus 1% of patients in the letrozole group (Finn et al., 2015). Based on these results, the FDA granted accelerated approval of palbociclib (IBRANCE, Pfizer Inc.) in 2015, for the treatment of postmenopausal women with BC ER+/HER2− in combination with letrozole (Beaver et al.,2015). Phase III PALOMA-2 (NCT01740427), a randomized multicenter double-blind clinical trial, confirmed the clinical benefit and safety of palbociclib plus letrozole, translating into significantly longer PFS of 24.8 months in the combination arm versus 14.5 months in the letrozole group. As expected, the main side effect was myelotoxicity (Finn et al., 2016). Lastly, phase III PALOMA-3 trial (NCT01942135), compared palbociclib plus fulvestrant (an ER antagonist and downregulator) with placebo plus fulvestrant, for pre- and postmenopausal patients with MBC ER+/HER2- that had progressed on previous endocrine therapy. Median PFS was 9.5 months (95% CI 9.2-11.0) in the fulvestrant plus palbociclib arm and 4.6 months (3.5-5.6) in the fulvestrant plus placebo group (hazard ratio 0.46, 95% CI 0.36-0.59, $p<0{\cdot}0001$). Grade 3-4 adverse events occurred in 73% in palbociclib group (vs. 22% in the placebo group), and neutropenia remained the most common grade 3-4 adverse event (Cristofanilli et al., 2016). Based on these results, FDA approved palbociclib (Ibrance®, Pfizer) in combination with fulvestrant on February 2016, for the treatment of women advanced or metastatic breast cancer (MBC) hormone receptor (HR)-positive and HER2-negative, with disease progression following endocrine therapy (Faslodex, AstraZeneca) (Walker et al., 2016a). Ongoing studies are focusing on the use of Palbociclib in early BC patients ER+/HER2−, in the adjuvant and neoadjuvant setting, including the randomized phase III study PENELOPE-B (NCT01864746) and PALLAS (NCT02513394).

Ribociclib

In a similar manner to Palbociclib, Ribociclib blocks BC cell lines Rb-positive by inhibition of Rb phosphorylation (Barroso-Sousa, Shapiro & Tolaney, 2016). The phase I Ribociclib study NCT01237236, indicated that the most common DLTs were neutropenia and thrombocytopenia (Infante et al., 2016). In the MONALEESA-1 phase II trial (NCT01919229), letrozole with or without ribociclib was administered to postmenopausal women with early BC ER+/HER2− prior to surgery, being well tolerated in the combination arm (Curigliano et al., 2016). Phase III MONALEESA-2 (NCT01958021) trial focused on first-line treatment for postmenopausal BC patients HR+/HER2− who had not received previous systemic therapy for advanced disease; patients received either ribociclib plus letrozole or placebo plus letrozole. Results showed that the combination treatment of ribociclib and letrozole was associated with a significantly better PFS (25.3 months vs 16 months) (Hortobagyi et al., 2016). Based on these results, on March 2017, FDA approved ribociclib (KISQALI®; Novartis Pharmaceuticals Corp.), in combination with an aromatase inhibitor as initial endocrine-based therapy for the treatment of postmenopausal women with BC/MBC HR+/HER2- (Shah et al., 2018). MONALEESA-3 (NCT02422615), a randomized double-blind phase III trial, also focused on the evaluation on the efficacy of ribociclib or placebo with fulvestrant on postmenopausal women with HR+/HER2− ABC patients, but who received no or only one line of previous endocrine treatment. Results showed a median PFS significantly better with the combination of ribociclib with fulvestrant (20.5 months versus 12.8 months) (Slamon et al., 2018).

Consequently, the FDA would approve this treatment association in HR+/HER2− MBC/ABC patients as first-line or second-line therapy in July 2018. MONALEESA-7 (NCT02278120) phase III trial explored a different subset of patients, the premenopausal patients with BC HR+/HER2− receiving either oral tamoxifen or a non-steroidal aromatase inhibitor (letrozole or anastrozole, both oral, daily) and goserelin, with or without ribociclib. Results showed that Ribociclib plus endocrine therapy significantly improved the PFS, with a median of 23.8 months versus 13.0 months (Tripathy et al., 2018). Ongoing trials are exploring the association of ribociclib with other agents such as everolimus (TRINITI-1 trial, NCT01857193) or erdafitinib (NCT03238196).

Abemaciclib

Abemaciclib is another oral CDK4/6 inhibitor and, consequently, an inhibitor of RB phosphorylation arresting cell-cycle on G1 phase, with the resultant reduction of cell proliferation. Abemaciclib can cross the blood-brain barrier at lower doses and persist on target for a longer period higher than palbociclib, making this drug more appealing for patients with brain metastases (Tolaney et al., 2017). MONARCH-1 (NCT02102490), a single-arm phase II study, evaluated the safety and efficacy of abemaciclib in monotherapy for heavily treated HR+/HER2− MBC/BC patients (brain metastases were excluded). Abemaciclib was administered until disease progression, resulting in a clinical benefit rate of 42.4% and a median PFS of 6.0 months (Dickler et al., 2017). Based on these results, the FDA approved abemaciclib in monotherapy on September 2017, for women and men with BC or MBC HR-positive, HER2-negative, under disease progression following endocrine therapy and prior chemotherapy in the metastatic setting. MONARCH 2 (NCT02107703), the subsequent randomized double-blind placebo-controlled phase III clinical trial, studied HR+/HER2− ABC patients with disease progression following endocrine therapy who had not received chemotherapy in the metastatic setting. Patients were randomized to receive either abemaciclib or placebo orally with fulvestrant. Results showed that abemaciclib with fulvestrant significantly improved median PFS, compared with fulvestrant alone (16.4 versus 9.3 months) (Sledge et al., 2017). Based on these results, on September 2017, FDA also approved abemaciclib (Vernezio®, Eli Lilly and Company) in combination with fulvestrant, as second-line therapy for women with HR-positive, HER2-negative advanced or metastatic breast cancer with disease progression following endocrine therapy. MONARCH 3 (NCT02246621) are another randomized (2:1) double-blinded, placebo-controlled, multicenter clinical trial, aimed to HR+/HER2− MBC patients who did not receive prior treatment, as first-line. Patients were randomized to receive abemaciclib plus anastrozole/letrozole versus placebo plus anastrozole/letrozole. Association with abemaciclib presented a median PFS advantage compared to the placebo arm (28.2 versus 14.8 months), (Johnston et al., 2019) leading to FDA approval in combination with aromatase inhibitors in this subset of patients as first-line therapy, in February 2018.

PHOSPHATIDYLINOSITOL 3-KINASE INHIBITORS

Phosphatidylinositol-3-kinase (PI3K)/AKT/mammalian target of rapamycin (mTOR) signaling is one of the most important intracellular pathways, which modulates cellular processes, including cell growth, proliferation and migration (Curigliano & Shah, 2019; Yang et al., 2019). This pathway is frequently activated in several solid tumors and hematological malignancies, making PI3K an attractive therapeutic target (Curigliano & Shah, 2019). PI3Ks are a family of lipid kinases that phosphorylate inositol lipids at the 3′-position of the inositol ring, generating PI-3-phosphate (PI(3)P1), PI-3,4-bisphosphate (PI(3,4)P2) and PI-3,4,5-trisphosphate (PI(3,4,5)P3); PIP3 facilitates the plasma membrane recruitment of pleckstrin homology (PH)-domain containing proteins such as the serine/threonine kinase AKT (Curigliano & Shah, 2019; Rodgers et al., 2017). Activated AKT phosphorylates a diverse spectrum of protein targets. PI3K-dependent AKT signaling is inhibited by phosphatase and tensin homologue (PTEN), which hydrolyses PIP3 (Rodgers et al., 2017).

In mammals, the PI3K family is divided into three different classes (I, II, and III) based on their coding genes, structure and substrate preference; class I PI3K is further subdivided into IA (activated by receptor tyrosine kinases) and IB (activated by G protein–coupled receptors) (Greenwell, Ip & Cohen, 2017; Wang, Ding & Meng, 2015). Class IA PI3Ks (PI3Kα, PI3Kβ and PI3Kδ) are heterodimers of one p110 (α, β or δ) catalytic subunit and one p85 regulatory subunit; class IB includes PI3Kγ, which is also a heterodimer enzyme containing the catalytic subunit p110γ and one regulatory subunit p101 or p84 (Wang, Ding & Meng, 2015). PI3Kα and PI3Kβ are ubiquitously expressed in all cells and tissues, while the δ and γ isoforms are preferentially expressed on leukocytes; PI3Kγ expression has also been described in several cells of the cardiovascular system and in platelets (Carnevale & Lembo, 2012; Greenwell, Ip & Cohen, 2017; Wang, Ding & Meng, 2015). PI3Kδ signaling has an essential role in many aspects of B-cell development and activation, particularly the p110δ. This has led to the development of highly p110δ-specific inhibitors for treatment of B-cell malignancies (Curigliano & Shah, 2019). In addition, PI3Kδ plays an important role in T-regulatory lymphocytes (Tregs) function, as well as in the differentiation of peripheral T-helper cells into the Th1 and Th2 lineages (Curigliano & Shah, 2019; Rodgers et al., 2017). The inactivation of p110δ in Tregs unleashes CD8+ cytotoxic T cells and induces tumor regression; thus, p110δ inhibitors can break tumor-induced immune tolerance (Ali et al., 2014). However, the activation of immune response resulting from the inhibition of PI3Kδ, has important clinical implications with regard to the toxicity associated with PI3Kδ-selective inhibitors (e.g., autoimmune toxicity) (Curigliano & Shah, 2019; Rodgers et al., 2017). PI3K inhibitors are subdivided into dual PI3K/mTOR inhibitors, pan-PI3K inhibitors and isoform-specific inhibitors (Wang, Ding & Meng, 2015). The PI3Kδ inhibitors are discussed below.

Idelalisib

Mechanisms of Action and Pharmacokinetics

Idelalisib (GS-1101, CAL-101) is an orally bioavailable, selective PI3Kδ inhibitor that competes with adenosine-5'-triphosphate (ATP) for binding to the catalytic subunit p110δ (Ramanathan et al., 2016). PI3Kδ is a downstream signal transducer for several receptors including B-cell receptor (BCR), CD40 receptor, chemokine receptors CXCR4 and CXCR5, IL-6 receptor, and integrins. Thus, by inhibiting PI3Kδ-mediated signaling, idelalisib inhibits B-cell proliferation, survival, motility, and homing to and maintenance of the tumor microenvironment in B-cell malignancies (Ramanathan et al., 2016; Wang, Ding & Meng, 2015). Idelalisib was the first PI3K inhibitor approved by the US Food and Drug Administration (FDA) for use in combination with rituximab for the treatment of relapsed or refractory (R/R) chronic lymphocytic leukemia (CLL), as well as for the treatment of R/R small lymphocytic lymphoma (SLL) and follicular lymphoma (FL) previously treated with two or more prior systemic therapies (Yang et al., 2019). Idelalisib has also demonstrated efficacy in CLL with adverse prognostic factors, including del(17p) and/or TP53 mutation (Ramanathan et al., 2016). *In vitro* studies demonstrated that Idelalisib have high potency against PI3Kδ, and substantially lower for PI3Kα, PI3Kβ, and PI3Kγ (Castillo, Furman & Winer, 2012; Ramanathan et al., 2016). The approved dose of Idelalisib is 150 mg twice daily, but dose reduction to 100 mg twice daily is allowed under specific toxicities (Ramanathan et al., 2016).

Idelalisib is primarily metabolized in the liver by aldehyde oxidase (AO) to its major circulating plasma metabolite, GS-563117. Other metabolic pathways involved to a lesser extent include oxidation by cytochrome P450 (CYP) 3A and glucuronidation by uridine 5'-diphospho-glucuronosyltransferase (UGT) 1A4. GS-563117 is inactive against PI3Kδ (Ramanathan et al., 2016; Wang, Ding & Meng, 2015). Both idelalisib and its metabolite are highly protein-bound (94% and 99%, respectively). Excretion is mostly hepatobiliary (Madanat et al., 2016). The presence of baseline hepatic impairment increases idelalisib exposure but do not require dose modification; however, careful monitoring for toxicity is recommended and its dose modified, as appropriate. The minor changes observed in idelalisib (and its metabolite) exposure in subjects with severe renal impairment were not considered to be clinically meaningful; therefore, dose adjustment in renal impairment is not necessary (Curigliano & Shah, 2019; Cuneo et al., 2019; Ramanathan et al., 2016).

Drug Interactions

Idelalisib may be affected by CYP3A inducers and inhibitors. Idelalisib and GS-563117 exposure has been shown to be substantially decreased by strong CYP3A4 and P-glycoprotein (P-gp) inducers (e.g., rifampicin); therefore, their co-administration should be avoided (Curigliano & Shah, 2019). The increase in idelalisib exposure caused by potent CYP3A inhibition (e.g., ketoconazole) is not considered to be of clinical relevance (Ramanathan et al., 2016). It is recommended that patients taking concomitant CYP3A inhibitors should be monitored for idelalisib toxicity signs and its dose modified as appropriate (Curigliano & Shah, 2019). Exposure to concomitant medications metabolized via CYP3A (e.g., midazolam) is expected to increase upon coadministration with idelalisib; these findings were consistent with the mechanism-based inhibition of CYP3A by GS-563117 (Ramanathan et al., 2016). Therefore, the use of CYP3A4-metabolized drugs should be avoided or closely monitored (Cuneo et al., 2019). Clinical studies have not revealed any significant effect of idelalisib on pharmacokinetics of digoxin, a P-gp substrate (Curigliano & Shah, 2019; Jin et al., 2015).

Idelalisib in Chronic Lymphocytic Leukemia

The first phase I trial evaluating the clinical efficacy of idelalisib in monotherapy in 54 relapsed or refractory CLL (R/R) heavily pre-treated patients, of which 80% had bulky lymphadenopathy, 70% had treatment-refractory disease, 91% had unmutated *IGHV*, and 24% del(17p) and/or TP53 mutations. Despite de adverse characteristics, the study show an overall response rate (ORR) of 72%, a median progression free survival (PFS) of 15.8 months and a 3-year overall survival (OS) of 75%; unlike standard chemoimmunotherapy, notable responses were seen even in patients with high-risk disease (Brown et al., 2014; Madanat et al., 2016; Nair & Cheson, 2016). Due to promising clinical activity and acceptable safety profile observed in phase I studies, the combination of idelalisib with rituximab (R) was further evaluated in a multicenter randomized phase III trial (Furman et al., 2014, Nair & Cheson, 2016). Patients were eligible if they had disease progression within 24 months of their last treatment and were unfit to receive cytotoxic therapy (Nair & Cheson, 2016). The trial was terminated early due to a significantly longer median PFS in the idelalisib-R group compared with placebo-R group (not reached versus 5.5 months, $p < 0.0001$) (Furman et al., 2014; Jin et al., 2015). The tendency for improved PFS in the idelalisib-R group was also observed in patients with poor prognostic features (del(17p) and/or TP53 mutation, or unmutated IGHV) . Based on these data, idelalisib-R was approved by the US FDA for R/R CLL in July 2014 (Nair & Cheson, 2016).

The idelalisib-R combination was also evaluated as front-line therapy in 64 patients over 65 years old in a phase II study. The ORR was 97%, with a complete response rate (CR) of 19%. In patients with del(17p)/TP53 mutations the ORR was 100% and 97% in those with unmutated IGHV. Progression-free survival was 83% at 36 months. (Madanat et al., 2016; Nair & Cheson, 2016; O'Brien et al., 2015). Combination of idelalisib with ofatumumab (Ofa), a second-generation, fully humanized IgG anti-CD20 monoclonal antibody was evaluated in a phase III randomized trial (Jones et al., 2015; Nair & Cheson, 2016). The study included patients with R/R CLL, with a median age of 68 years (61–7), and a median previous therapies of 3 (2–4). The median PFS was longer in the idelalisib-Ofa group versus Ofa-alone group (16.3 months versus 8 months, $p < 0.0001$); however, no difference was observed in median OS (Jones et al., 2015; Nair & Cheson, 2016). The combination of idelalisib with bendamustine and rituximab (BR) was assessed in a multicenter, double-blind, placebo-controlled phase III trial, in R/R CLL. Most patients had high-risk disease, namely del(17p), mutated TP53 and unmutated IGHV, and most had previously received a fludarabine-containing regimen. Patients randomized to the idelalisib arm achieved higher ORRs (70%) vs the placebo arm (45%). At a median follow-up of 14 months, median PFS was superior in the idelalisib-BR arm vs. placebo-BR arm (20.8 vs. 11.1 months; $p<0.0001$). These results were consistent across subgroups of patients with high-risk features. This combination could represent a new treatment option for the management of R/R disease (Madanat et al., 2016; Zelenetz et al., 2017).

Idelalisib in Indolent B-Cell Lymphoma

The efficacy of idelalisib in monotherapy was first reported in a phase I study of patients with previously treated indolent B-cell lymphoma (FL, SLL, marginal-zone lymphoma and lymphoplasmacytic lymphoma) (Flinn et al., 2014). Based on these encouraging results, a phase II trial of idelalisib in monotherapy was conducted in 125 heavily pre-treated patients with relapsed indolent non-Hodgkin lymphoma; the median duration of response was 12.5 months, and the median PFS duration was 11 months (Barrientos, 2016; Gopal et al., 2014; Madanat et al., 2016). Based on these data, the US FDA granted idelalisib accelerated approval for treatment of patients with relapsed FL and SLL who had received at least 2 prior systemic therapies (de Vos et al., 2016). A post hoc subgroup analysis of this phase II trial, published in 2017, identified 72 (58%) patients with Follicular Lymphoma (FL), with baseline characteristics consistent with a high-risk population. It was shown an ORR of 55.6% (CR of 13.9%) and that idelalisib was effective across evaluated patient categories, regardless of the number of prior therapies, refractoriness to previous regimens, bulky disease, and age. Median PFS was 11.0 months overall, however median PFS in patients with CR was 30.6 months. At 24 months, OS was estimated to be 69.8%, and all patients achieving a CR had survived. Discontinuation of idelalisib due to adverse events occurred in 18 patients. Despite this, the investigators conclude that given the unmet need in high-risk patients with R/R FL, the overall benefit of idelalisib in such patients outweighs these safety concerns (Salles et al., 2017).

Safety and Adverse Events

The use of idelalisib is associated with a unique side effects profile, due to the selective inhibition of the PI3Kδ isoform (Nair & Cheson, 2016). In phase I-II trials, 9–20% of the patients discontinued treatment because of adverse events (AEs); a phase III trial in R/R CLL reported treatment discontinuation because of AEs in 8% of the patients (de Weerdt et al., 2017). Immune-mediated disorders and infections are the leading causes of treatment interruption (Cuneo et al., 2019). Several upfront trials were terminated due to the observation of increased risk of death related to infection for patients randomized to combinations containing idelalisib. The majority of deaths was due to bacterial sepsis, sometimes associated with neutropenia, and pneumocystis jiroveci pneumonia (PJP) and cytomegalovirus (CMV) infections were also seen. This experience was communicated to healthcare professionals via an US FDA alert, and a black box warning for fatal hepatoxicity, severe diarrhea or colitis, pneumonitis, serious infections and intestinal perforation is now included in the idelalisib product insert (Zirlik & Veelken, 2018). Diarrhea is one of the most common drug-related adverse reactions that can eventually lead to idelalisib dose reduction and/or discontinuation (Cuneo et al., 2019). Although a definitive underlying mechanism for idelalisib-associated diarrhea is unknown, it is thought that the immune dysregulation associated with PI3K inhibition results in inhibition of regulatory T cells and consequent damage by CD8+ cytotoxic T cells (Cuneo et al., 2019; de Weerdt et al., 2017). Characteristic histologic features include lymphocytic colitis in combination with characteristic epithelial cell apoptosis and neutrophilic cryptitis (de Weerdt et al., 2017). Diarrhea can occur at any time after initiation of idelalisib: diarrhea that occurs within the first 8 weeks of idelalisib use is usually grade 1–2, tends to be self-limiting and usually responds to common antidiarrheal agents; late-onset diarrhea is generally grade ≥3 (median time to onset of 7.1 months) and responds poorly to antidiarrheal or empiric antimicrobial therapy (Coutré et al., 2015; de Weerdt et al., 2017). Accompanying symptoms (e.g., cramps, blood, mucus) are uncommon (Coutré et al., 2015; de Weerdt et al., 2017). In atypical cases or in cases unresponsive to treatment, colonoscopy is advised (Coutré et al., 2015; Cuneo et al., 2019). Self-limiting, uncomplicated diarrhea (grade 1 or grade 2) can usually be managed with antidiarrheal therapy (e.g., loperamide) and diet modification, without discontinuation of idelalisib. In patients with grade ≥3 diarrhea, or grade 2 diarrhea that is unresolved after 24–48 h, it is advisable to interrupt idelalisib treatment; after exclusion infectious causes, initiation of budesonide or steroid therapy, oral or intravenously, is recommended (Coutré et al., 2015; Cuneo et al., 2019). The duration of steroid therapy should be based on individual clinical response; Interruption of idelalisib and concurrent initiation of oral budesonide in 23 patients with grade 3 diarrhea led to resolution in all cases after a mean of 12 days (Coutré et al., 2015; de Weerdt et al., 2017). In patients who have interrupted idelalisib, rechallenge with a reduced dose (e.g., 100 mg twice daily) may be attempted after resolution of diarrhea (Cuneo et al., 2019).

An elevation of alanine transaminase (ALT) and aspartate transaminase (AST) blood levels of any grade frequently occurs (35%-50%) during treatment with idelalisib, usually during the first 3 months, and is more prevalent in younger (<65 years), previously untreated patients (Cuneo et al., 2019; de Weerdt et al., 2017). Proposed mechanism for liver injury is an adaptive immune response elicited by the on-target inhibition of PI3Kδ in regulatory T cells (Cuneo et al., 2019). In grades 1 and 2 transaminitis, idelalisib can be continued with careful weekly monitoring (Cuneo et al., 2019). In grade 3 transaminitis (elevations in ALT and/or AST > 5 and < 20 x the upper limit of normal (ULN), idelalisib should be temporarily discontinued; most transaminase elevations are reversible with drug interruption (Cuneo et al., 2019; de Weerdt et al., 2017). In the absence of other causes, transaminitis > 5 x ULN, persisting without a significant decline after 7 days from the drug withdrawal, a steroid-based treatment may be given (Cuneo et al., 2019). Idelalisib may be reassumed at a lower dose of 100 mg twice daily when transaminase levels have returned to normal; in most patients, there is no recurrence of ALT and AST elevation after reinitiating idelalisib at a lower dose (de Weerdt et al., 2017). The presence of transaminase elevation 20 times over the UNL (grade 4) should prompt permanent discontinuation of idelalisib (Cuneo et al., 2019).

Across clinical trials, pneumonitis occurred in 3% of idelalisib-treated patients, with some fatal cases (Coutré et al., 2015). Bronchoalveolar lavage shows an increase of lymphocytes and lung biopsy shows changes consistent with hypersensitivity pneumonitis (Coutré et al., 2015; Cuneo et al., 2019).

Any patient who presents with acute/subacute onset pulmonary signs/symptoms, such as cough, dyspnea, fever and hypoxia, should be evaluated for pneumonitis (Coutré et al., 2015; Cuneo et al., 2019). Bilateral interstitial infiltrates are usually found on chest X-ray, and high-resolution computed tomography shows various abnormalities, including ground-glass opacities, consolidation and pleural effusion (Cuneo et al., 2019; de Weerdt et al., 2017). In the absence of clear infectious etiology or lack of clinical response to empiric antibiotic treatment, idelalisib should be discontinued; high-dose steroids may also be used (Cuneo et al., 2019; de Weerdt et al., 2017). In patients with a diagnosis of interstitial pneumonitis, idelalisib should not be resumed (Cuneo et al., 2019). Pneumocystis jiroveci pneumonia (PJP) has been reported in a small number of patients on idelalisib treatment; as most of these cases occurred in patients not receiving PJP prophylaxis, trimethoprim-sulfametoxazole is indicated as prophylactic regimen for PJP during treatment with idelalisib and up to 2 to 6 months after discontinuation (de Weerdt et al., 2017). Before commencing idelalisib, all patients should have cytomegalovirus (CMV) status assessed. In seropositive patients, CMV viral load should be regularly monitored at least on a monthly basis (Cheah & Fowler, 2016; Cuneo et al., 2019). Asymptomatic patients with CMV viremia should be carefully monitored and preemptive ganciclovir or valganciclovir may be considered; for patients with evidence of viremia and clinical signs of infection, ganciclovir or valganciclovir should be initiated and idelalisib discontinued until the viremia has resolved (Cheah & Fowler, 2016). Screening for latent tuberculosis infection is recommended; if positive, suppressive anti-tuberculosis treatment is indicated (Cuneo et al., 2019). Vaccinations against *S. pneumoniae* and influenza are recommended to all patients (Cuneo et al., 2019).

Blood counts should be monitored at least every 2 weeks for the first 3 months of therapy (Coutré et al., 2015). Neutropenia is common during the first months of idelalisib treatment, with grade 3–4 occurring in 23–43%; neutropenia may be managed with growth factor support, whereas dose reduction is rarely necessary (de Weerdt et al., 2017). Grade 3 anemia has been reported in 3–11% of patients, and grade 3 thrombocytopenia in 17–

30% (de Weerdt et al., 2017). Any grade rash was reported in 10–22% of patients with relapsed/refractory disease treated with idelalisib, and the frequency may be higher in treatment-naïve patients (de Weerdt et al., 2017). Patients should be monitored for cutaneous reactions and treatment discontinued in the event of severe cases (Driscoll, 2016).

Copanlisib

Mechanisms of Action and Pharmacokinetics

Copanlisib (BAY 80-6946) is an intravenous pan–class I PI3K inhibitor with preferential inhibitory activity against the PI3K-α and PI3K-δ isoforms (Eltantawy et al., 2019). Beneficial off-target effects include upregulation of apoptotic pathways and the inhibition of CXCR12 mediated chemotaxis of malignant B-cells and NF-κB signaling in lymphoma cell lines (Mensah, Blaize & Bryan, 2018). Copanlisib was approved in September 2017 by the FDA for the treatment of patients with relapsed FL who have received at least two prior systemic therapies (Curigliano & Shah, 2019). The recommended dose is 60 mg infused over 1 hour on days 1, 8, and 15 of a 28-day cycle and continued until disease progression or unacceptable toxicity (Eltantawy et al., 2019). Copanlisib has a large volume of distribution and a terminal phase half-life of 39.1h at the maximum tolerated dose of 0.8 mg/kg (Gerisch et al., 2017); no accumulation was observed after once-weekly administration (Eltantawy et al., 2019). Copanlisib is principally metabolized by CYP3A (Curigliano & Shah, 2019). The M-1 metabolite is active and its pharmacological activity against PI3Kα and PI3Kδ is comparable with that of the parent compound (Curigliano & Shah, 2019). Approximately 50% of parent compound is excreted unchanged into urine and feces (Gerisch et al., 2017). In the setting of mild to moderate renal and hepatic impairment, dose adjustments are not warranted because these had no clinically significant effect on the pharmacokinetics of copanlisib (Eltantawy et al., 2019).

Drug Interactions

Copanlisib administration should be avoided in combination with strong CYP3A4 inducers or inhibitors, and a dose reduction to 45 mg is advised with concurrent use of strong CYP3A inhibitors (Curigliano & Shah, 2019; Eltantawy et al., 2019).

Clinical Studies and Efficacy

The multicenter, single-arm, phase II CHRONOS-1 study led to copanlisib's FDA approval. The results of this study were reported in 2 parts (Eltantawy et al., 2019). Part A evaluated the efficacy and safety of copanlisib in patients with RR indolent or aggressive lymphoma; the ORR was noted to be 43.7% and 27.1% in the indolent and aggressive groups, respectively; in the indolent cohort the median duration of response (DOR) was 12.8 months and a median PFS was 9.7 months (Driscoll, 2016; Eltantawy et al., 2019). Part B focused on evaluating exclusively the efficacy and safety of copanlisib in patients with RR indolent lymphoma. In the 2-year follow-up of the primary analysis, an ORR of 60.6% was achieved, the median DOR was 14.1 months and median PFS was greater than 1 year (Eltantawy et al., 2019; Gerisch et al., 2017).

There are three ongoing phase III studies designed to expand on the safety and efficacy of copanlisib: CHRONOS-2, a randomized study of copanlisib vs placebo in patients with rituximab-refractory indolent Non-Hodgkin's Lymphoma (iNHL); CHRONOS-3, intended to evaluate copanlisib in combination with rituximab in relapsed iNHL; and CHRONOS-4, a randomized trial of copanlisib in combination with standard chemoimmunotherapy in relapsed iNHL (Mensah, Blaize & Bryan, 2018).

Safety and Adverse Events

Although copanlisib is generally well-tolerated, it can be is associated with several potentially serious adverse effects (Cheson et al., 2019). Two of the most common toxicities not seen with other PI3K inhibitors include hyperglycemia and hypertension, which are likely related to targeting the PI3Kα isoform (Cheson et al., 2019). Other toxicities of copanlisib are similar to other drugs of the same pharmacologic class, such are diarrhea/colitis, pneumonitis, hepatotoxicity and infectious complications; nonetheless, copanlisib appears to have a more favorable safety profile than either idelalisib or duvelisib with regard to these toxicities (Cheson et al., 2019; Mensah, Blaize & Bryan, 2018).

PI3Kα is fundamental for most biological responses exerted by insulin; therefore, inhibition of PI3Kα transiently blocks skeletal muscle glucose uptake and enhances hepatic glucose production, creating a hyperglycemic state (Cheson et al., 2019). Not surprisingly, grade 3 or 4 hyperglycemia occurred in 41% of 317 patients treated with copanlisib monotherapy, with serious hyperglycemic events in 2.8% of patients (Curigliano & Shah, 2019). In the majority of the patients, blood glucose levels typically peaked 5–8 h post-infusion and subsequently decline to baseline levels; however, in some patients, blood glucose levels remain elevated 1 day after copanlisib infusion (Curigliano & Shah, 2019). FDA recommends to withhold copanlisib in patients with a preinfusion fasting plasma glucose of ≥160 mg/dL or a random glucose of ≥200 mg/dL until the fasting glucose is ≤160 mg/dL or the random glucose is ≤200 mg/dL; for those patients with a postdose blood glucose ≥500 mg/dL, on first occurrence, copanlisib should be withheld until the fasting glucose is ≤160 mg/dL or the random blood glucose is ≤200 mg/dL; dose reductions from 60 mg to 45 mg and then to 30 mg are based on subsequent hyperglycemia occurrences (Eltantawy et al., 2019). If the hyperglycemia becomes difficult to manage, copanlisib should be discontinued (Cheson et al., 2019). Patients with diabetes mellitus should only be treated with copanlisib following adequate glucose control and should be monitored closely (Curigliano & Shah, 2019).

In the CHRONOS-1 trial, 29.6% of patients developed hypertension, almost all grade 3 with no grade 4 (Cheson et al., 2019). Hypertension associated with copanlisib peaks 2 hours postinfusion and typically resolves within 24 hours (Eltantawy et al., 2019). Optimal blood pressure control and monitoring prior to and during infusion is required (Mensah, Blaize & Bryan, 2018). For patients with a predose blood pressure of ≥150/90 mmHg, it is recommended to hold copanlisib until 2 consecutive evaluations under150/90 mmHg are obtained, measured at least 15 minutes apart; for patients with a postdose blood pressure ≥150/90 mmHg despite initiation or optimization of antihypertensive therapy, copanlisib can be reduced from 60 to 45 mg, or from 45 to 30 mg (Eltantawy et al., 2019).

Noninfectious pneumonitis is an uncommon event with copanlisib, occurring in approximately 5% of treated patients, with 1.9% of patients experiencing grade 3 events. Those patients were successfully managed by suppression the drug and administration of steroids (Cheson et al., 2019). In the CHRONOS-1 trial, copanlisib was associated with relatively low rates of lung infections. Given the infrequency of pneumonia, routine prophylaxis is not recommended (Eltantawy et al., 2019).

Copanlisib seems to be associated with a lower incidence of colitis than idelalisib (grade 3 diarrhea was reported in 5% of 168 patients treated with copanlisib monotherapy, with no cases of grade 4 toxicity), possibly owing to its intermittent and parenteral dose schedule (Cheson et al., 2019). In patients with grade 3 diarrhea, copanlisib should be withheld until diarrhea resolves to grade 1 or better; it then can be restarted at 45 mg; if diarrhea of grade 3 or worse recurs, copanlisib should be discontinued (Cheson et al., 2019). In the CHRONOS-1 study, there was no significant clinical treatment-induced liver injury; therefore, there is no mandate for frequent liver enzyme monitoring (Cheson et al., 2019).

Bone marrow suppression was not uncommon in patients treated with copanlisib. Approximately 25% of patients may experience grade 3 or 4 neutropenia (Mensah, Blaize & Bryan, 2018). Grade 3 anemia was reported in 4% of 168 patients treated with copanlisib monotherapy, and grade 3 thrombocytopenia in 7% (Cheson et al., 2019).

Duvelisib

Mechanisms of Action and Pharmacokinetics

Duvelisib (IPI-145) is an oral first-class, dual PI3K inhibitor (PI3Kδ and PI3Kγ) (Frustaci et al., 2019; Rodrigues, Sagrillo & Fraga, 2019). In 2018, duvelisib was approved by the US FDA for the treatment of adult patients with relapsed or refractory CLL/ SLL after at least two prior therapies; in addition, duvelisib received accelerated approval for adult patients with relapsed or refractory FL after at least two prior systemic therapies (Rodrigues, Sagrillo & Fraga, 2019). Maximum tolerated dose was determined to be 75 mg twice daily, with 25 mg twice daily selected for further evaluation in phase II and III studies (Flinn et al., 2018a). Duvelisib is rapidly absorbed, with a maximum concentration after 1–3 h (Rodrigues, Sagrillo & Fraga, 2019). It is widely distributed to peripheral tissues (as indicated by a large volume of distribution) and has an elimination half-life of 2.7 to 7.5 hours. Most of the compound is hepatically transformed into its inactive major metabolite, IPI-656, before enteric elimination (Flinn et al., 2018a).

Drug Interactions

Duvelisib is primarily metabolized by cytochrome P450 CYP3A4; therefore, concomitant use with a strong inhibitor of CYP3A4 can increase the risk of toxic effects (Rodrigues, Sagrillo & Fraga, 2019).

Clinical Studies and Efficacy

The 2 pivotal clinical trials with duvelisib were DUO and DYNAMO. In the phase III DUO study in R/R CLL/SLL, patients were randomized to duvelisib or ofatumumab. The ORR was 73.8% with duvelisib versus 45.3% with ofatumumab, and, after a median follow-up of 22.4 months, the study reached its primary end point by duvelisib significantly improving PFS in all patients compared to ofatumumab (median PFS: 13.3 vs. 9.9 months; $P < .0001$), including those with high-risk features like del(17p) and/or TP53 mutations (Flinn et al., 2018b; Frustaci et al., 2019). DYNAMO was a single-arm phase 2 clinical trial that assessed the efficacy and safety of duvelisib in monotherapy in patients with relapsed iNHL refractory to rituximab and to either chemotherapy or radioimmunotherapy. The study enrolled 129 patients, with a median age of 65 years (30-90) and heavily pre-treated, with a median of 3 prior lines. The ORR was 47%, median DOR was 10 months and median PFS was 9.5 months (Flinn et al., 2019).

Safety and Adverse Events

Consistent with previous observations with idelalisib, transaminase elevations and diarrhea resulted the most frequent non-hematologic adverse events and the most common non-hematological grade ≥3 side effect (Frustaci et al., 2019). Transaminase elevations were observed early in treatment, and most patients were managed with dose modifications, with few patients requiring treatment discontinuation (Flinn et al., 2018a). Severe diarrhea/colitis appeared 6–9 months after starting duvelisib, differently from the more common grade 1–2 intestinal toxicity appearing earlier (Frustaci et al., 2019). Neutropenia was the most frequent hematologic side effect across clinical studies (Frustaci et al., 2019). Infections of all grades were also common, including a few cases of PJP and CMV infection (Flinn et al., 2018a).

Other PI3KΔ Inhibitors in the Pipeline

Umbralisib (TGR-1202)

Umbralisib is a next-generation, oral, dual inhibitor of PI3Kδ and casein kinase-1ε (CK-1ε), in development for treatment of patients with previously treated marginal zone lymphoma (MZL) and FL (Burris et al., 2018). In a phase I study, the safety profile of umbralisib was distinct from the other PI3Kδ inhibitors, with lower rates of immune-mediated toxicities such as colitis (Burris et al., 2018; Davids et al. 2019). Preclinical data suggest that CK-1ε inhibition may lead to augmentation of regulatory T-cell activity, which could hypothetically lead to immunosuppression and thereby lower the risk of immune-mediated toxicities (Davids et al. 2019). Umbralisib is also being investigated in combination with other drugs, such as umbralisib plus ibrutinib (in patients with R/R CLL and mantle cell lymphoma) and the umbralisib, ublituximab and venetoclax triple combination (in patients with R/R CLL) (Davids et al. 2019; Yang et al., 2019).

Parsaclisib (IBI-376)

Parsaclisib is a next-generation, potent, and highly selective PI3Kδ inhibitor being evaluated in R/R B-cell NHL, either alone or in combination with a Janus kinase 1 inhibitor (itacitinib) or chemotherapy (rituximab, ifosfamide, carboplatin, and etoposide). Parsaclisib demonstrated a differentiated safety profile relative to first-generation PI3Kδ inhibitors (e.g., idelalisib and duvelisib), most notably by the near absence of grade ≥2 transaminitis. Diarrhea/colitis and rash were two of the most frequent toxicities observed with parsaclisib (Forero-Torres et al., 2019).

Tenalisib (RP6530)

Tenalisib is a novel, next generation, highly specific, dual equipotent PI3K δ/γ inhibitor. It shows acceptable safety and encouraging clinical activity in R/R T-cell lymphoma (Oki et al., 2018).

Buparlisib

Buparlisib is a novel pan-PI3K inhibitor that has been developed to inhibit all class I PI3K isoforms. It is currently in clinical development for various cancers, including primary and secondary brain tumors. Buparlisib has an excellent brain penetration that is unaffected by efflux transporters at the blood-brain barrier with excellent oral bioavailability and intracranial target engagement (de Gooijer et al., 2018).

ACP-319 (Previously AMG-319)

ACP-319 is a novel selective PI3Kδ inhibitor with early pre-clinical and clinical anti-tumor activity in CLL and lymphoma. ACP-319 has been evaluated in combination with acalabrutinib (a second-generation inhibitor of Bruton tyrosine kinase) in patients with R/R B-cell malignancies (Spriano ate al., 2019).

Acalisib (GS-9820)

Acalisib is a second generation PI3Kδ inhibitor. Based on the drug's similar efficacy and toxicity profile to idelalisib, no further clinical development was planned (Lampson & Brown, 2017).

Pictilisib (GDC-0941)

Pictilisib is a potent, pan-PI3K inhibitor that inhibits all four isoforms of class I PI3K (Lampson & Brown, 2017). It was investigated for the treatment of several solid tumors, including breast cancer. In two phase II trials, efficacy of pictilisib was limited by the higher incidence of adverse events and dose reductions/discontinuations; as a result, further development of pictilisib by the sponsor is not planned (Schöffski et al., 2018).

KA-2237

KA-2237 is a dual inhibitor of the class I β and δ isoforms of the 110 kDa catalytic subunit of PI3K that has shown strong activity in mantle cell lymphoma (MCL); therefore, KA-2237 may be a potential candidate for MCL therapy, especially in the ibrutinib-resistant cases (Huang et al., 2016).

Pilaralisib (SAR245408)

Pilaralisib is a pan-PI3K inhibitor. It has shown clinical activity in solid tumors and B-cell malignancies, with an acceptable safety profile (Brown et al., 2015).

AZD8186

AZD8186 is reported to have good biochemical potency against the PI3K β and δ isoforms. It has been shown to inhibit the growth of PTEN-deficient breast and prostate tumors alone and in combination with docetaxel (Hancox et al., 2015).

Other Kinases Inhibitors

AK Inhibitors

The aurora kinases (AURK) are a family of highly conserved serine/threonine kinases comprising three mammalian isoforms, the aurora kinase A (AURKA), aurora kinase B (AURKB) and aurora kinase C (AURKC). These kinases are responsible for the regulation of key processes of cell division, namely mitotic entry, spindle assembly and cytokinesis (Carmena, Ruchaud & Earnshaw 2009; Wang, Jiang & Zhang, 2014). Due to their essential role in cell cycle, AURK deregulations were already associated with several types of cancer. AURKA and AURKAB were found of be overexpressed and/or amplified in several solid tumors, including gastric, pancreatic, ovarian and cervical cancers (Ding et al., 2020; Fard et al., 2019; Gritsko et al., 2003; Li et al., 2003; Twu et al., 2009), and also in hematological malignancies, including chronic myeloid leukemia, acute myeloid leukemia and T-cell lymphomas (Kanagal-Shamanna et al., 2013; Lucena-Araujo et al., 2011; Marsola et al., 2018). Moreover, the expression AURKs were showed to predict patient prognosis in various cancers, such as breast, colorectal, nasopharyngeal, gastric, bladder and endometrial carcinomas (Aradottir et al., 2014; Burgess et al., 2019; Koh et al., 2017; Liu et al., 2012; Umene et al., 2015; Wang et al., 2011). Furthermore, AURKA also interacts with cancer promoting signaling pathways, namely WNT, RAS-MAPK and MYC among others, favoring proliferation, survival and therapeutic resistance (D'Assoro, Haddad & Galanis, 2016; den Hollander et al., 2010; Jacobsen et al., 2018). Despite its overexpression in some tumor cells, AURKC is the less characterized aurora kinase and its role in tumorigenesis is not clearly elucidated (Khan et al., 2011; Tsou et al., 2011). Given the previously described role of AURK in cancer, the development of small-molecule inhibitors targeting these specific kinases might become an important therapeutic strategy for cancer treatment.

Several aurora kinase inhibitors (AURKi) have been developed and clinically evaluated throughout the last decade, although none have been approved so far by US FDA or EMA for clinical practice. The most promising AURKi is alisertib (MLN8237), an orally available of second generation, highly selective and ATP-competitive reversible AURKA inhibitor. However, it also inhibits AURKB at higher concentrations (Manfredi et al., 2017). Alisertib binds to the ATP-binding site in AURKA and AURKB and inhibits the autophosphorylation at Thr288 (Fancelli et al., 2006). Studies evaluating alisertib showed that it induced cell cycle arrest, apoptosis, autophagy, polyploidy and mitotic catastrophe in vitro, and induced tumor regression in vivo (Qi et al., 2019; Tan et al., 2020; Wang et al., 2015; Yang et al., 2020; Yuan et al., 2015). Given its proven preclinical activity alisertib has been evaluated for safety and efficacy in several clinical phase I and II trials. These showed that alisertib had favorable pharmacokinetics and good safety profiles, with manageable toxicity, in advanced solid tumors and hematological malignancies (Barr et al., 2015; Cervantes et al., 2012; Dees et al., 2012; Melinchar et al., 2015). Given the upregulation of AURKA in aggressive lymphomas and the supporting efficacy in vitro, alisertib was evaluated in a phase II trial in 48 patients with relapsed or refractory diffuse large B-cell lymphoma (DLBCL), mantle-cell lymphoma (MCL), transformed follicular lymphoma, Burkitt's lymphoma, and peripheral T-cell lymphoma (PTCL), in the dose of 50 mg twice a day for 7 consecutive days, in a 21 days cycle. The overall response rate (ORR) was 27%. The most common grade 3–4 adverse events reported were neutropenia in over half of the patients, anemia and thrombocytopenia in a third of the patients and a few with stomatitis, febrile neutropenia and fatigue (Friedberg et al., 2013). Due to the reported efficacy and tolerability of alisertib, a multi-center, randomized phase III study (LUMIERE trial; NCT01482962) was conducted in patients with relapsed/refractory PTCL.

Two hundred and seventy-one patients were assigned to either the alisertib or the comparator arm, and results showed an ORR of 33% for alisertib and 45% for the comparator arm with median PFS of 115 days and 104 days, respectively. Most common adverse events were anemia and neutropenia. In this trial, alisertib demonstrated efficacy in PTCL patients, however it did not show significant benefit over the comparator arm (O'Connor et al., 2018). More recently, pharmacological efficacy of alisertib has been evaluated in combination protocols, involving other target therapies. A phase I study in lymphoid malignancies, mainly including diffuse large B-cell lymphoma, classical Hodgkin lymphoma and follicular lymphoma patients, evaluated alisertib in combination with vorinostat, a histone deacetylase inhibitor. This trial demonstrated some clinical activity and an acceptable safety profile for the combination schedule (Siddiqui et al., 2019). Another study showed clinical evidence of antitumor activity with manageable safety when treating patients with advanced solid tumors with a combination schedule of alisertib plus a VEGFR inhibitor (Shah et al., 2019). The most frequent grade 3-4 drug-related adverse event was neutropenia; however, fatigue, nausea, alopecia and gastrointestinal disorders were also reported (Cervantes et al., 2012; Dees et al., 2012; Melinchar et al., 2015).

Currently, other AURKis are in clinical evaluation, these include barasertib and chiauranib. Barasertib (AZD1152) is a compound that needs serum conversion to a more active ATP-competitive molecule, barasertib-hQPA, which selectively inhibits AURKB over AURKA and AURKC (Mortlock et al., 2007). The binding of barasertib-hQPA to AURKB inhibits H3 histone phosphorylation leading to cytokinesis defects of tumor cell division, endoreplication and induction of apoptosis (Wilkinson et al., 2007; Yang et al., 2007). Barasertib also showed antitumor activity against AML cell lines harboring internal tandem duplications within the FLT3 tyrosine kinase receptor (Grundy et al., 2010). This preclinical analysis has translated the evaluation of barasetib to clinical evaluation showing a good absorption and tolerable toxicity, both in solid tumors (Boss et al., 2011; Schwatrz et al., 2013) and hematological malignancies (Collins et al., 2015; Denis et al., 2012; Lownberg et al., 2011). The most commonly reported adverse events for barasertib treatment was neutropenia, followed by nausea, stomatitis and fatigue (Collins et al., 2015; Lownberg et al., 2011; Schwatrz et al., 2013). Currently, an active phase I/II clinical trial is evaluating safety, tolerability, pharmacokinetics and efficacy of nanoparticles with barasertib in monotherapy or combination in acute myeloid leukemia patients, however no results have been reported so far (NCT03217838).

Chiauranib (CS2164) is a novel orally available multi-kinase inhibitor that blocks simultaneously AURKB, angiogenesis kinases (VEGFR2, VEGFR1, VEGFR3, PDGFRα and c-KIT), and the chronic inflammation-related kinase CSF-1R, targeting three important pathways in tumorigenesis (Zhou et al., 2017). Besides its activity against angiogenesis-related kinases and CSF-1R, chiauranib directly bounds to AURKB inducing G2/M cell cycle arrest at cellular level. This inhibition results in decreased H3 phosphorylation, confirming AURKB inhibition (Zhou et al., 2017). Preclinical evaluation of chiauranib demonstrated its antitumor activity in acute myeloid leukemia models (Deng et al., 2019), in hepatocellular carcinoma both *in vitro* and *in vivo* (Zhou et al., 2016), and in non-Hodgkin's lymphomas through inhibition of proliferation and induction of apoptosis (Deng et al., 2018). The first reported clinical trial with chiauranib was conducted in patients with advanced solid tumors demonstrating a potential antitumor activity with acceptable safety (NTC02122809) (Sun et al., 2019). Clinical trials evaluating chiauranib in ovarian cancer, hepatocellular carcinoma, small cell lung cancer and non-Hodgkin lymphoma are currently ongoing.

Several other AURKi have been studied throughout the last years, these include pan-AURK inhibitors, such as Danusertib (PHA-739358), Tozasertib (VX-680) and AMG-900, or AURKB inhibitors like ENMD-2076. Despite their evaluations in a few clinical trials, no significant results have been reported so far and no ongoing trials are evaluating them. Despite some disappointing clinical results with AURAK inhibitors, there is still much preclinical research being applied to these specific kinases, some focused on the improvement of the already known molecules and other focused on the development of new and more effective AURK inhibitors, such as AKI604, a recently reported AURKA inhibitors (Long et al., 2018) that already proved efficacy in *in vitro* models (Wang et al., 2020).

PLK Inhibitors

Polo-like kinases (PlKs) are a conserved family of serine/threonine kinases that regulates several essential steps during cell cycle progression and mitosis. PlKs have a highly conserved catalytic kinase domain in the N-terminal (Ser/Thr kinase), responsible for ATP binding and enzyme activity and, in the C- terminal, one or two regulatory Polo-box domain (PBD), which are crucial for subcellular localization and binding of specific phosphopeptides. There are five PlKs that have been identified: PlK1, PlK2, PlK3, PlK4 and PlK5. The later, unlike the others, lacks the kinase domain being a PBD-containing protein (Archambault & Glover, 2009; Barr, Silljé & Nigg, 2004; de Cácer et al., 2011; de Cácer, Manning & Malumbres, 2011; Eckerdt, Yuan & Strebhardt, 2005; Liu, 2015; Lowery, Lim & Yaffe, 2005; Pellegrino et al., 2010; Yu, Liu & Li, 2012;). Despite having a ubiquitous distribution in human tissues, PlKs have a differential distribution in different tissues/organs as well as different functions. Classically, PlKs have been identified as important regulatory molecules for cell cycle progression, cell proliferation and differentiation. Later it was found that their expression is altered in several human cancers therefore having an associated prognostic value and, in that way, PlKs can be consider as potential targets for cancer treatment (Archambault & Glover, 2009; Barr, Silljé & Nigg, 2004; Fu & Wen, 2017; Liu, 2015; Winkles & Alberts, 2005). PLK1 is the most studied and known PlKs member and considering its role in cell division and its overexpression in several human cancers, PlK1 play a role in oncogenesis. While others are attributed a role of tumor suppressor, although in some cases they can also contribute to the development of cancer (de Cácer, Manning & Malumbres, 2011; Gatz et al., 2019; Kawakami et al., 2018; van de Weerdt & Medema, 2006; Weiβ & Efferth, 2012; Weichert et al., 2004). Recognizing the role that PlKs have in the progression of the cell cycle, either as a positive or negative regulator, have stimulated the interest of PlKs in cancer. This knowledge had motivated the development of molecules that, interfering with the N-terminal in the kinase domain or PBD domain in the C-terminal, that can be used for cancer therapy, and the list of these small compounds has been growing (de Cácer, Manning & Malumbres, 2011; Lens, Voest & Medema, 2010; Timme et al., 2020).

Volasertib (BI6727), is a small-molecule ATP-competitive kinase inhibitor that belongs to a class of dihydropteridinone, that seems to selectively inhibits PLK1 enzymatic activity in an irreversible way. It induces G2/M arrest followed by apoptosis in a variety of tumor cells, but in normal cells the effect in cell cycle is reversible without apoptosis, which may be valuable, as it can improve the efficacy and decrease side effects and drug related toxicity (Hao & Kota, 2015; Rudolph et al., 2009). The effect of volasertib on pediatric cancer cell lines was investigated in two separate studies using various cell lines (Abbou et al., 2016; Gorlick et al., 2014). All cell lines in these studies proved to be sensitive to volasertib, although with variable response, showing rhabdomyosarcoma cells a specific sensitivity (Gatz et al., 2019). These results may open new perspectives of treatments and benefit young patients with rhabdomyosarcoma and probably other cancers (Gatz et al., 2019; Goroshchuk et al., 2019). Preclinical and phase I and phase II trials have been carried out to study the effects of volasertib as a single agent or in combination with other agents, for several cancers such as acute myeloid leukemia (AML) (NCT02003573), non-small cell lung cancer (NCT00824408), advanced solid tumors in Japanese patients (NCT01348347), ovarian cancer patients resistant or refractory to platinum-based cytotoxic therapy (NCT01121406), glioblastoma, high-risk myelodysplastic syndrome (MDS) or chronic myelomonocytic leukemia patients that are not candidates for hematopoietic stem cell transplant (NCT01957644) (Dong et al., 2018; Nguyen et al., 2017; Pujade-Lauraine et al., 2016; van den Bossche et al., 2019). Currently, volasertib is being evaluated for safety and efficacy in a Phase III (NCT01721876) clinical trial, for the treatment of patients aged 65 or older with previously untreated AML, who are ineligible for intensive remission induction therapy. In this phase III clinical trial, volasertib is being tested in combination with low-dose Cytarabine (POLO-AML-2). In a different phase II trial

(NCT00804856) but also in patients with AML, it is being evaluated the safety, pharmacokinetics, maximum tolerated dose, and efficacy of intravenous volasertib, as a single agent (monotherapy) or in combination with subcutaneous cytarabine. In another phase I trial (NCT01772563), that is in progress, the objective is to evaluate the potential of drug to drug interaction of intravenously administered volasertib in association with a P-gap and CYP3A4 inhibitor (Itraconazole p.o.) in patients suffering of various solid tumors. In addition, the FDA gave Orphan Drug Status to volasertib for the treatment of acute myeloid leukemia (AML).

Rigosertib (ON 01910.Na) is a small molecule, non-ATP-competitive multikinase inhibitor that inhibits the RAS, PI3K and PLK1 signaling pathways (Chapman et al., 2012; Gumireddy et al., 2005; Navada & Silverman, 2016). The therapeutic potential of Rigosertib has been subject of multiple studies and clinical trials in several solid and hematological tumors, some of which have already been concluded, such as the ONTIME study, in refractory myelodysplastic syndrome patients with excess blasts (NCT01241500; Garcia-Manero et al., 2016). Patients with head and neck squamous cell carcinoma (HNSCC), non-small cell lung squamous cell carcinoma (SCC), skin SCC, cervical SCC, penile SCC, anal SCC or esophageal SCC, where enrolled in a phase II clinical trial (NCT01807546) to evaluate the safety and efficacy of oral rigosertib. Relapsed or metastatic SCC, that were previously treated with platinum-based chemotherapy and/or chemo-radiation therapy were also included. In patients with advanced untreated metastatic pancreatic cancer a phase III, multicenter, randomized, controlled study was done to compare the effect of gemcitabine alone vs. rigosertib plus gemcitabine (NCT01360853). After the ONTIME study, the INSPIRE phase III clinical trial, for patients with the same clinical conditions (MDS intractable with hypomethylating drugs), shown some promising results that motivate the continuation of this clinical research line (NCT02562443) (Garcia-Manero et al., 2016; Xu et al., 2014). Although initially the results did not show an advantage, namely in terms of overall survival, it was later found that patients with primary resistant disease treated with hypomethylating drugs and high-risk patients benefited from treatment with Rigosertib (Jonasova et al., 2019; Nazha et al., 2017). This drug is also under study in different solid tumors. A phase I/IIa clinical trial is ongoing to study Rigosertib plus Nivolumab in stage IV lung adenocarcinoma patients with KRAS mutation who progressed on first-line treatment (NCT04263090). The therapeutic potential of Rigosertib is also being under study in patients with recessive Dystrophic Epidermolysis bullosa (RDEB) with locally advanced Squamous Cell Carcinoma (SCC). This pilot trial aims to know how Rigosertib can selectively target RDEB cancer cells while leaving normal cells unaffected (Santini, 2019).

Onvansertib (NMS-1286937/PCM-075) is an oral, third generation, PLK1 inhibitor. Preclinical studies have demonstrated that Onvansertib has a synergistic effect with several anticancer drugs, namely irinotecan, FLT3 and HDAC inhibitors and taxanes, among others. The promising results will contribute to improve clinical efficacy of treatments in different malignancies such as acute myeloid leukemia (AML), metastatic castration-resistant prostate cancer (mCRPC), KRAS-mutated colorectal cancer, triple-negative breast cancer (TNBC), among others (Affatato, et al. 2020; Giordano et al., 2019; Lenz et al., 2020; Wang et al., 2020). Currently, there are some ongoing clinical trials to test onvansertib both in hematological and solid malignancies. In a phase II trial in adult patients with mCRPC, who have signs of early progressive disease, Onvansertib is being tested in combination with abiraterone and prednisone (NCT03414034). For patients with metastatic colorectal cancer with a KRAS mutation, onvansertib is in an ongoing phase 1b/2 study in combination with FOLFIRI and Bevacizumab for a second line treatment (NCT03829410). In adult patients with relapsed or refractory AML, a Phase 1b/2 clinical trial is underway to test Onvansertib in combination with low dose of cytarabine or decitabine (NCT03303339; Green & Konig, 2020; Zeidan et al., 2019). Onvansertib has an FDA Orphan Drug Designation, as well as a European indication for treatment of patients with AML (Eckerdt, Yaun & Strebhardt, 2005). It had been demonstrated that onvansertib inhibits tumor growth in patients with acute myeloid leukemia who are resistant to venetoclax. These results suggest that onvansertib may be a new frontline therapeutic option for AML patients venetoclax-resistant (Zeidan et al., 2019).

Poloxin is the first small-molecule inhibitor of PLK1, that specifically targets the polo-box domain (PBD) in the C-terminal. Poloxin induces Plk1 mislocalization, chromosome congression defects, mitotic arrest, and apoptosis in HeLa cells. Experimental studies have shown that Poloxin inhibits growth and triggers apoptosis of HeLa cell lines as well as in several human cancer cell lines from metastatic breast cancer, triple-negative breast cancer, colon adenocarcinoma grade 3-4, lung adenocarcinoma, prostate cancer and Pharynx cancer, in a dose-dependent manner. However, a similar effect was observed in normal human cell lines. This fact suggests that PLK1 is essential for cellular proliferation, regardless of whether or not they are normal. Since studies have shown this lack of specificity, its interest and therapeutic potential have been questioned, namely in cancer, unless a molecule PLK1- PBD specific can be developed. So far, there are no studies in the clinical or even preclinical phase. Despite the inconclusive results, it is expected that Poloxin may emerge and move on to preclinical and clinical studies and come to be a new therapeutic possibility in cancer (Archambault & Normandin, 2017; Reindl et al., 2008; Rubner, Schubert & Berg, 2019; Sanhaji et al., 2012; Yuan et al., 2011).

CONCLUSION

Cancer treatment is one of the biggest challenges in contemporary Medicine. Cancer patients with advanced stages of disease or in relapse, special those showing some sort of resistance to conventional treatments, deserve new targeted therapeutic strategies to overcome this situation.

Current knowledge in genomics and tumor biology, identify a large proportion of actionable kinases, relevant in cancer development and progression and many that can be druggable. So far, more than 28 oncology drugs targeting kinases have been approved and are on clinical practice; a considerable number of others are ongoing various stages of clinical evaluation.

Kinase inhibitors represent a new and promising approach to cancer therapy, with demonstrated beneficial clinical effects. In the future, scientific advances may, eventually, allow the combination of mutagenesis screens, through next generation sequencing and proteomic techniques, with the computational modeling of compound interactions with all possible mutant variants of a targeted kinase. This may allow the development of well-tolerated and more efficacious kinase inhibitors and improving the therapeutic approach of patients with cancer.

REFERENCES

Aalipour, A., & Advani, R. H. (2014). Bruton's tyrosine kinase inhibitors and their clinical potential in the treatment of B-cell malignancies: focus on ibrutinib. *Therapeutic Advances in Hematology*, 5(4), 121–133.

Abbou, S., Lanvers-Kaminsky, C., Daudigeos-Dubus, E., Dret, L. L. E., Laplace-Builhe, C., Molenaar, J., Vassal, G., Geoerger, B., & within the ITCC Biology and Preclinical Evaluation Committee. (2016). Polo-like kinase inhibitor Volasertib exhibits antitumor activity and synergy with Vincristine in pediatric malignancies. *Anticancer Research*, 36 (2): 599-609.

Ackermann, C. J., Stock, G., Tay, R., Dawod, M., Gomes, F., & Califano, R. (2019). Targeted Therapy For RET-Rearranged Non-Small Cell Lung Cancer: Clinical Development And Future Directions. *OncoTargets and Therapy*, 12, 7857–7864.

Adjei, A. A., & Hidalgo, M. (2005). Intracellular signal transduction pathway proteins as targets for cancer therapy. *Journal of Clinical Oncology: Official Journal of the American Society of Clinical Oncology*, 23(23), 5386–5403.

Advani, R. H., Buggy, J. J., Sharman, J. P., Smith, S. M., Boyd, T. E., Grant, B., Kolibaba, K. S., Furman, R. R., Rodriguez, S., Chang, B. Y., Sukbuntherng, J., Izumi, R., Hamdy, A., Hedrick, E., & Fowler, N. H. (2013). Bruton tyrosine kinase inhibitor ibrutinib (PCI-32765) has significant activity in patients with relapsed/refractory B-cell malignancies. *Journal of Clinical Oncology: Official Journal of the American Society of Clinical Oncology*, 31(1), 88–94.

Affatato, R., Carrassa, L., Chilà, R., Lupi, M., Restelli, V., and Damia, G. (2020). Identification of PLK1 as a new therapeutic target in mucinous ovarian carcinoma. *Cancers (Basel)*, 12 (3): 672.

Aguilera, D. G., & Tsimberidou, A. M. (2009). Dasatinib in chronic myeloid leukemia: a review. *Therapeutics and Clinical Risk Management*, 5 (2): 281-289.

Ali S, Wang K., Johnson A., Suh J., Heilmann A., Lipson D., Yelensky, R., Chmielecki, J., Elvin, J., Konduri, K., Subbiah, V., Stephens, P., Ross, J., Miller V. (2015). Comprehensive genomic profiling characterizes the cpectrum of non-V600E activating BRAF alterations Including BRAF fusions in lung cancer. *European Journal of Cancer*, 51:S597.

Ali, K., Soond, D. R., Pineiro, R., Hagemann, T., Pearce, W., Lim, E. L., Bouabe, H., Scudamore, C. L., Hancox, T., Maecker, H., Friedman, L., Turner, M., Okkenhaug, K., & Vanhaesebroeck, B. (2014). Inactivation of PI(3)K p110δ breaks regulatory T-cell-mediated immune tolerance to cancer. *Nature*, 510(7505), 407–411.

Alves, R., Fonseca, A. R., Gonçalves, A. C., Ferreira-Teixeira, M., Lima, J., Abrantes, A. M., Alves, V., Rodrigues-Santos, P., Jorge, L., Matoso, E., Carreira, I. M., Botelho, M. F., & Sarmento-Ribeiro, A. B. (2015). Drug transporters play a key role in the complex process of Imatinib resistance in vitro. *Leukemia research*, 39(3), 355–360.

Andorsky, D. J., Kolibaba, K. S., Assouline, S., Forero-Torres, A., Jones, V., Klein, L. M., Patel-Donnelly, D., Smith, M., Ye, W., Shi, W., Yasenchak, C. A., and Sharman, J. P. (2019). An open-label phase 2 trial of entospletinib in indolent non-Hodgkin lymphoma and mantle cell lymphoma. *British Journal of Haematology*, 184 (2): 215-222.

Aparicio, T., Ghiringhelli, F., Boige, V., Le Malicot, K., Taieb, J., Bouché, O., Phelip, J. M., François, E., Borel, C., Faroux, R., Dahan, L., Jacquot, S., Genet, D., Khemissa, F., Suc, E., Desseigne, F., Texereau, P., Lepage, C., Bennouna, J., & PRODIGE 9 Investigators (2018). Bevacizumab Maintenance versus No Maintenance During Chemotherapy-Free Intervals in Metastatic Colorectal Cancer: A Randomized Phase III Trial (PRODIGE 9). *Journal of clinical oncology: official journal of the American Society of Clinical Oncology*, 36(7), 674–681.

Aradottir, M., Reynisdottir, S. T., Stefansson, O. A., Jonasson, J. G., Sverrisdottir, A., Tryggvadottir, L., Eyfjord, J. E., & Bodvarsdottir, S. K. (2014). Aurora A is a prognostic marker for breast cancer arising in BRCA2 mutation carriers. *The Journal of Pathology. Clinical research*, 1(1), 33–40.

Archambault, V., & Glover, D. M. (2009). Polo-like kinases: conservation and divergence in their functions and regulation. *Nature reviews. Molecular cell biology*, 10(4), 265–275.

Archambault, V., & Normandin, K. (2017). Several inhibitors of the Plk1 Polo-Box Domain turn out to be non-specific protein alkylators. *Cell Cycle*, 16 (12): 1220-1224.

Argyropoulos, K. V., & Palomba, M. L. (2018). First-Generation and Second-Generation Bruton Tyrosine Kinase Inhibitors in Waldenström Macroglobulinemia. *Hematology/Oncology Clinics of North America*, 32(5): 853–864.

Arighi, E., Borrello, M. G., & Sariola, H. (2005). RET tyrosine kinase signaling in development and cancer. *Cytokine & Growth Factor Reviews*, 16(4-5), 441–467.

Asami, T., Kawahata, W., Kashimoto, S., & Sawa, M. (2018). Abstract B152: CB1763, a highly selective, novel non-covalent BTK inhibitor, targeting ibrutinib-resistant BTK C481S mutant. *Molecular Cancer Therapeutics*, 17(1 Supplement): B152.

Ascierto, P. A., Dummer, R., Gogas, H. J., Flaherty, K. T., Arance, A., Mandala, M., Liszkay, G., Garbe, C., Schadendorf, D., Krajsova, I., Gutzmer, R., de Groot, J. W. B., Loquai, C., Gollerkeri, A., Pickard, M. D., & Robert, C. (2020). Update on tolerability and overall survival in COLUMBUS: Landmark analysis of a randomised phase 3 trial of Encorafenib plus Binimetinib vs Vemurafenib or Encorafenib in patients with BRAF V600-mutant melanoma. *European Journal of Cancer*, 126: 33-44.

Ascierto, P. A., McArthur, G. A., Dréno, B., Atkinson, V., Liszkay, G., Giacomo, A. M. D., Mandalà, M., Demidov, L., Stroyakovskiy, D.,

Thomas, L., de la Cruz-Merino, L., Dutriaux, C., Garbe, C., Yan, Y., Wongchenko, M., Chang, I., Hsu, J. J., Koralek, D. O., Rooney, I., Ribas, A., and Larkin, J. (2016). Cobimetinib combined with Vemurafenib in advanced BRAF(V600)-mutant melanoma (coBRIM): Updated efficacy results from a randomised, double-blind, phase 3 trial. *Lancet Oncology*, 17 (9): 1248-1260.

Aw, A. & Brown, J. R. (2017) Current Status of Bruton's Tyrosine Kinase Inhibitor Development and Use in B-Cell Malignancies. *Drugs Aging*, 34: 509-527.

Awan, F. T., Thirman, M. J., Patel-Donnelly, D., Assouline, S., Rao, A. V., Ye, W., Hill, B., & Sharman, J. P. (2019). Entospletinib monotherapy in patients with relapsed or refractory chronic lymphocytic leukemia previously treated with B-cell receptor inhibitors: results of a phase 2 study. *Leukemia & lymphoma*, 60(8), 1972–1977.

Babon, J. J., Lucet, I. S., Murphy, J. M., Nicola, N. A., & Varghese, L. N. (2014). The molecular regulation of Janus kinase (JAK) activation. *The Biochemical Journal*, 462(1): 1–13.

Bacher, U., Haferlach, C., Kern, W., Haferlach, T., & Schnittger, S. (2008). Prognostic relevance of FLT3-TKD mutations in AML: the combination matters--an analysis of 3082 patients. *Blood*, 111(5), 2527–2537.

Bachow, S. H., and Lamanna, N. (2016). What appears safe is sometimes not: a reason for caution. *Blood*, 127 (20): 2367-2368.

Bailet, O., Fenouille, N., Abbe, P., Robert, G., Rocchi, S., Gonthier, N., Denoyelle, C., Ticchioni, M., Ortonne, J.-P., Ballotti, R., Deckert, M., and Tartare-Deckert, S. (2009). Spleen Tyrosine Kinase Functions as a Tumor Suppressor in Melanoma Cells by Inducing Senescence-like Growth Arrest. *Cancer Research*, 69 (7): 2748.

Bang, Y. J., Van Cutsem, E., Feyereislova, A., Chung, H. C., Shen, L., Sawaki, A., Lordick, F., Ohtsu, A., Omuro, Y., Satoh, T., Aprile, G., Kulikov, E., Hill, J., Lehle, M., Rüschoff, J., Kang, Y. K., & ToGA Trial Investigators (2010). Trastuzumab in combination with chemotherapy versus chemotherapy alone for treatment of HER2-positive advanced gastric or gastro-oesophageal junction cancer (ToGA): a phase 3, open-label, randomised controlled trial. *Lancet (London, England)*, 376(9742), 687–697.

Bardelli, A., & Siena, S. (2010). Molecular mechanisms of resistance to cetuximab and panitumumab in colorectal cancer. *Journal of Clinical Oncology: Official Journal of the American Society of Clinical Oncology*, 28(7), 1254–1261.

Barr, F. A., Sillјé, H. H., & Nigg, E. A. (2004). Polo-like kinases and the orchestration of cell division. *Nature reviews. Molecular Cell Biology*, 5(6), 429–440.

Barr, p. M., Li, H., Spier, C., Mahadevan, D., LeBlanc, M., Haq, M. U., Huber, B. D., Flowers, C. R., Wagner-Johnston, N. D., Horwitz, S. M., Fisher, R. I., Cheson, B. D., Smith, S. M., Kahl, B. S., Bartlett, N. L., & Friedberg, J. W. (2015). Phase II Intergroup Trial of Alisertib in Relapsed and Refractory Peripheral T-Cell Lymphoma and Transformed Mycosis Fungoides: SWOG 1108. *Journal of Clinical Oncology*, 33 (21): 2399-2404.

Barr, P. M., Saylors, G. B., Spurgeon, S. E., Cheson, B. D., Greenwald, D. R., O'Brien, S. M., Liem, A. K., Mclntyre, R. E., Joshi, A., Abella-Dominicis, E., Hawkins, M. J., Reddy, A., Di Paolo, J., Lee, H., He, J., Hu, J., Dreiling, L. K., & Friedberg, J. W. (2016). Phase 2 study of idelalisib and entospletinib: pneumonitis limits combination therapy in relapsed refractory CLL and NHL. *Blood*, 127(20), 2411–2415.

Barr, P. M., Saylors, G. B., Spurgeon, S. E., Cheson, B. D., Greenwald, D. R., O'Brien, S. M., Liem, A. K. D., McLntyre, R. E., Joshi, A., Abella-Dominicis, E., Hawkins, M. J., Reddy, A., Di Paolo, J., Lee, H., He, J., Hu, J., Dreiling, L. K., and Friedberg, J. W. (2016). Phase 2 study of idelalisib and entospletinib: pneumonitis limits combination therapy in relapsed refractory CLL and NHL. *Blood*, 127 (20): 2411-2415.

Barrientos J. C. (2016). Idelalisib for the treatment of indolent non-Hodgkin lymphoma: a review of its clinical potential. *OncoTargets and Therapy*, 9, 2945–2953.

Barroso-Sousa, R., Shapiro, G. I., & Tolaney, S. M. (2016). Clinical Development of the CDK4/6 Inhibitors Ribociclib and Abemaciclib in Breast Cancer. *Breast care (Basel, Switzerland)*, 11(3), 167–173.

Beaver, J. A., Amiri-Kordestani, L., Charlab, R., Chen, W., Palmby, T., Tilley, A., Zirkelbach, J. F., Yu, J., Liu, Q., Zhao, L., Crich, J., Chen, X. H., Hughes, M., Bloomquist, E., Tang, S., Sridhara, R., Kluetz, P. G., Kim, G., Ibrahim, A., Pazdur, R., … Cortazar, P. (2015). FDA Approval: Palbociclib for the Treatment of Postmenopausal Patients with Estrogen Receptor-Positive, HER2-Negative Metastatic Breast Cancer. *Clinical cancer research: An Official Journal of the American Association for Cancer Research*, 21(21), 4760–4766.

Ben Hassine, I., Gharbi, H., Soltani, I., Teber, M., Farrah, A., Ben Hadj Othman, H., Amouri, H., Bellaaj, H., lakhal, R. B., Romdhane, N. B., Abbes, S., & Menif, S. (2017). hOCT1 gene expression predict for optimal response to Imatinib in Tunisian patients with chronic myeloid leukemia. *Cancer Chemotherapy and Pharmacology*, 79 (4): 737-745.

Bendell, J. C., Javle, M., Bekaii-Saab, T. S., Finn, R. S., Wainberg, Z. A., Laheru, D. A., Weekes, C. D., Tan, B. R., Khan, G. N., Zalupski, M. M., Infante, J. R., Jones, S., Papadopoulos, K. P., Tolcher, A. W., Chavira, R. E., Christy-Bittel, J. L., Barrett, E., & Patnaik, A. (2017). A phase 1 dose-escalation and expansion study of Binimetinib (MEK162), a potent and selective oral MEK1/2 inhibitor. *British Journal of Cancer*, 116 (5): 575-583.

Berdeja, J., Palandri, F., Baer, M. R., Quick, D., Kiladjian, J. J., Martinelli, G., Verma, A., Hamid, O., Walgren, R., Pitou, C., Li, P. L., & Gerds, A. T. (2018). Phase 2 study of gandotinib (LY2784544) in patients with myeloproliferative neoplasms. *Leukemia Research*, 71, 82–88.

Bernicker, E. H., Allen, T. C., & Cagle, P. T. (2019). Update on emerging biomarkers in lung cancer. *Journal of Thoracic Disease*, 11(Suppl 1), S81–S88.

Bewersdorf, J. P., Jaszczur, S. M., Afifi, S., Zhao, J. C., & Zeidan, A. M. (2019). Beyond Ruxolitinib: Fedratinib and Other Emergent Treatment Options for Myelofibrosis. *Cancer Management and Research*, 11: 10777–10790.

Bhagwat, S. V., McMillen, W. T., Cai, S., Zhao, B., Whitesell, M., Shen, W., Kindler, L., Flack, R. S., Wu, W., Anderson, B., Zhai, Y., Yuan, X.-J., Pogue, M., Van Horn, R. D., Rao, X., McCann, D., Dropsey, A. J.,

Manro, J., Walgren, J., Yuen, E., Rodriguez, M. J., Plowman, G. D., Tiu, R. V., Joseph, S., & Peng, S.-B. (2020). ERK inhibitor LY3214996 targets ERK pathway-driven cancers: A therapeutic approach toward precision medicine. *Molecular and Cancer Therapeutics*, 19 (2): 325-336.

Bhattacharya, P., Shetakẹ, N. G., Pandey, B. N., & Kumar, A. (2018). Receptor tyrosine kinase signaling in cancer radiotherapy and its targeting for tumor radiosensitization. *International Journal of Radiation Biology*, 94(7), 628–644.

Bhullar, K. S., Lagarón, N. O., McGowan, E. M., Parmar, I., Jha, A., Hubbard, B. P., & Rupasinghe, H. (2018). Kinase-targeted cancer therapies: progress, challenges and future directions. *Molecular Cancer*, 17(1), 48.

Boga, S. B., Deng, Y., Zhu, L., Nan, Y., Cooper, A. B., Shipps, G. W., Jr, Doll, R., Shih, N. Y., Zhu, H., Sun, R., Wang, T., Paliwal, S., Tsui, H. C., Gao, X., Yao, X., Desai, J., Wang, J., Alhassan, A. B., Kelly, J., Patel, M., … Samatar, A. A. (2018). MK-8353: Discovery of an Orally Bioavailable Dual Mechanism ERK Inhibitor for Oncology. *ACS Medicinal Chemistry Letters*, 9(7), 761–767.

Bokemeyer, C., Bondarenko, I., Makhson, A., Hartmann, J. T., Aparicio, J., de Braud, F., Donea, S., Ludwig, H., Schuch, G., Stroh, C., Loos, A. H., Zubel, A., & Koralewski, P. (2009). Fluorouracil, leucovorin, and oxaliplatin with and without cetuximab in the first-line treatment of metastatic colorectal cancer. *Journal of clinical oncology: official journal of the American Society of Clinical Oncology*, 27(5), 663–671.

Bond, D. A. & Woyach, J. A. (2019). Targeting BTK in CLL: Beyond Ibrutinib. *Current Hematologic Malignancy Reports*, 14: 197-205.

Bonner, J. A., Harari, P. M., Giralt, J., Azarnia, N., Shin, D. M., Cohen, R. B., Jones, C. U., Sur, R., Raben, D., Jassem, J., Ove, R., Kies, M. S., Baselga, J., Youssoufian, H., Amellal, N., Rowinsky, E. K., & Ang, K. K. (2006). Radiotherapy plus cetuximab for squamous-cell carcinoma of the head and neck. *The New England Journal of Medicine*, 354(6), 567–578.

Bonner, J. A., Harari, P. M., Giralt, J., Cohen, R. B., Jones, C. U., Sur, R. K., Raben, D., Baselga, J., Spencer, S. A., Zhu, J., Youssoufian, H., Rowinsky, E. K., & Ang, K. K. (2010). Radiotherapy plus cetuximab for locoregionally advanced head and neck cancer: 5-year survival data from a phase 3 randomised trial, and relation between cetuximab-induced rash and survival. *The Lancet. Oncology*, 11(1), 21–28.

Bose, P., & Verstovsek, S. (2017). JAK2 inhibitors for myeloproliferative neoplasms: what is next?. *Blood*, 130(2): 115–125.

Bose, P., Verstovsek, S., Cortes, J. E., Tse, S., Gasior, Y., Jain, N., Jabbour, E. J., Estrov, Z., Alvarado, Y., DiNardo, C. D., Pemmaraju, N., Kornblau, S. M., Kadia, T. M., Daver, N. G., Naqvi, K., Short, N. J., Masarova, L., Villareal, J., Pierce, S. A., Nogueras-Gonzalez, G., … Ravandi, F. (2020). A phase 1/2 study of ruxolitinib and decitabine in patients with post-myeloproliferative neoplasm acute myeloid leukemia. *Leukemia*, 10.1038/s41375-020-0778-0.

Boss, D. S., Witteveen, P. O., van der Sar, J., Lolkema, M. P., Voest, E. E., Stockman, P. K., Ataman, O., Wilson, D., Das, S., & Schellens, J. H. (2011). Clinical evaluation of AZD1152, an i.v. inhibitor of Aurora B kinase, in patients with solid malignant tumors. *Annals of oncology : official journal of the European Society for Medical Oncology*, 22(2), 431–437.

Botrel, T., Clark, L., Paladini, L., & Clark, O. (2016). Efficacy and safety of bevacizumab plus chemotherapy compared to chemotherapy alone in previously untreated advanced or metastatic colorectal cancer: a systematic review and meta-analysis. *BMC cancer*, 16(1), 677.

Bousoik, E., & Aliabadi, H. M. (2018). "Do We Know Jack" About JAK? A Closer Look at JAK/STAT Signaling Pathway. *Frontiers in Oncology*, 8: 287.

Brauer, K., Werth, D., von Schwarzenberg, K., Bringmann, A., Kanz, L., Grünebach, F., & Brossart, P. (2006). BCR-ABL Activity Is Critical for the Immunogenicity of Chronic Myelogenous Leukemia Cells. *Blood*, 108(11): 2202.

Braun, T., Eide, C., & Druker, B. (2020). Response and Resistance to BCR-ABL1-Targeted Therapies. *Cancer Cell*, 37: 530-542.

Bray, F., Ferlay, J., Soerjomataram, I., Siegel, R. L., Torre, L. A., & Jemal, A. (2018). Global cancer statistics 2018: GLOBOCAN estimates of incidence and mortality worldwide for 36 cancers in 185 countries. *CA: A Cancer Journal for Clinicians*, 68(6), 394–424.

Broccoli, A., Casadei, B., Morigi, A., Sottotetti, F., Gotti, M., Spina, M., Volpetti, S., Ferrero, S., Spina, F., Pisani, F., Merli, M., Visco, C., Paolini, R., Zilioli, V. R., Baldini, L., Di Renzo, N., Tosi, P., Cascavilla, N., Molica, S., Ilariucci, F., … Zinzani, P. L. (2018). Italian real life experience with ibrutinib: results of a large observational study on 77 relapsed/refractory mantle cell lymphoma. *Oncotarget*, 9(34), 23443–23450.

Brown, J. R. (2018). How I treat CLL patients with ibrutinib. *Blood*, 131(4): 379-386.

Brown, J. R., Byrd, J. C., Coutre, S. E., Benson, D. M., Flinn, I. W., Wagner-Johnston, N. D., Spurgeon, S. E., Kahl, B. S., Bello, C., Webb, H. K., Johnson, D. M., Peterman, S., Li, D., Jahn, T. M., Lannutti, B. J., Ulrich, R. G., Yu, A. S., Miller, L. L., & Furman, R. R. (2014). Idelalisib, an inhibitor of phosphatidylinositol 3-kinase p110δ, for relapsed/refractory chronic lymphocytic leukemia. *Blood*, 123(22), 3390–3397.

Brown, J. R., Davids, M. S., Rodon, J., Abrisqueta, P., Kasar, S. N., Lager, J., Jiang, J., Egile, C., & Awan, F. T. (2015). Phase I Trial of the Pan-PI3K Inhibitor Pilaralisib (SAR245408/XL147) in Patients with Chronic Lymphocytic Leukemia (CLL) or Relapsed/Refractory Lymphoma. *Clinical cancer research: an official journal of the American Association for Cancer Research*, 21(14), 3160–3169.

Brown, J. R., Moslehi, J., O'Brien, S., Ghia, P., Hillmen, P., Cymbalista, F., Shanafelt, T. D., Fraser, G., Rule, S., Kipps, T. J., Coutre, S., Dilhuydy, M. S., Cramer, P., Tedeschi, A., Jaeger, U., Dreyling, M., Byrd, J. C., Howes, A., Todd, M., Vermeulen, J., … Burger, J. A. (2017). Characterization of atrial fibrillation adverse events reported in ibrutinib randomized controlled registration trials. *Haematologica*, 102(10), 1796–1805.

Brown, J. S., & Banerji, U. (2017). Maximising the potential of AKT inhibitors as anti-cancer treatments. *Pharmacology & therapeutics*, 172, 101–115.

Buchner, M., Baer, C., Prinz, G., Dierks, C., Burger, M., Zenz, T., Stilgenbauer, S., Jumaa, H., Veelken, H., and Zirlik, K. (2010). Spleen tyrosine kinase inhibition prevents chemokine- and integrin-mediated stromal protective effects in chronic lymphocytic leukemia. *Blood*, 115 (22): 4497-506.

Burger, J. A., & Wiestner, A. (2018). Targeting B cell receptor signalling in cancer: preclinical and clinical advances. *Nature reviews. Cancer*, 18(3), 148–167.

Burger, J. A., Barr, P. M., Robak, T., Owen, C., Ghia, P., Tedeschi, A., Bairey, O., Hillmen, P., Coutre, S. E., Devereux, S., Grosicki, S., McCarthy, H., Simpson, D., Offner, F., Moreno, C., Dai, S., Lal, I., Dean, J. P., & Kipps, T. J. (2020). Long-term efficacy and safety of first-line ibrutinib treatment for patients with CLL/SLL: 5 years of follow-up from the phase 3 RESONATE-2 study. *Leukemia*, 34(3), 787–798.

Burger, J. A., Keating, M. J., Wierda, W. G., Hartmann, E., Hoellenriegel, J., Rosin, N. Y., de Weerdt, I., Jeyakumar, G., Ferrajoli, A., Cardenas-Turanzas, M., Lerner, S., Jorgensen, J. L., Nogueras-González, G. M., Zacharian, G., Huang, X., Kantarjian, H., Garg, N., Rosenwald, A., & O'Brien, S. (2014). Safety and activity of ibrutinib plus rituximab for patients with high-risk chronic lymphocytic leukaemia: a single-arm, phase 2 study. *The Lancet. Oncology*, 15(10), 1090–1099.

Burger, J. A., Tedeschi, A., Barr, P. M., Robak, T., Owen, C., Ghia, P., Bairey, O., Hillmen, P., Bartlett, N. L., Li, J., Simpson, D., Grosicki, S., Devereux, S., McCarthy, H., Coutre, S., Quach, H., Gaidano, G., Maslyak, Z., Stevens, D. A., Janssens, A., … RESONATE-2 Investigators (2015). Ibrutinib as Initial Therapy for Patients with Chronic Lymphocytic Leukemia. *The New England Journal of Medicine*, 373(25), 2425–2437.

Burgess, E. F., Livasy, C., Trufan, S., Hartman, A., Guerreri, R., Naso, C., Clark, P. E., Grigg, C., Symanowski, J., & Raghavan, D. (2019). High aurora kinase expression identifies patients with muscle-invasive bladder cancer who have poor survival after neoadjuvant chemotherapy. *Urologic Oncology*, 37(12):900-906.

Burke, J. M., Shustov, A., Essell, J., Patel-Donnelly, D., Yang, J., Chen, R., Ye, W., Shi, W., Assouline, S., & Sharman, J. (2018). An Open-label, Phase II Trial of Entospletinib (GS-9973), a Selective Spleen Tyrosine Kinase Inhibitor, in Diffuse Large B-cell Lymphoma. *Clinical Lymphoma, Myeloma & Leukemia*, 18(8), e327–e331.

Burke, J. M., Shustov, A., Essell, J., Patel-Donnelly, D., Yang, J., Chen, R., Ye, W., Shi, W., Assouline, S., and Sharman, J. (2018). An Open-label, Phase II Trial of Entospletinib (GS-9973), a Selective Spleen Tyrosine Kinase Inhibitor, in Diffuse Large B-cell Lymphoma. *Clinical Lymphoma Myeloma and Leukemia*, 18 (8): e327-e331.

Burke, R. T., Meadows, S., Loriaux, M. M., Currie, K. S., Mitchell, S. A., Maciejewski, P., Clarke, A. S., Dipaolo, J. A., Druker, B. J., Lannutti, B. J., and Spurgeon, S. E. (2014). A potential therapeutic strategy for chronic lymphocytic leukemia by combining Idelalisib and GS-9973, a novel spleen tyrosine kinase (Syk) inhibitor. *Oncotarget*, 5 (4): 908-15.

Burris, H. A., Flinn, I. W., Patel, M. R., et al. (2018). Umbralisib, a novel PI3Kδ and casein kinase-1ε inhibitor, in relapsed or refractory chronic lymphocytic leukaemia and lymphoma: an open-label, phase 1, dose-escalation, first-in-human study. *The Lancet. Oncology*, 19(4): 486–496.

Burstein H. J. (2005). The distinctive nature of HER2-positive breast cancers. *The New England Journal of Medicine*, 353(16), 1652–1654.

Byrd, J. C., Brown, J. R., O'Brien, S., Barrientos, J. C., Kay, N. E., Reddy, N. M., Coutre, S., Tam, C. S., Mulligan, S. P., Jaeger, U., Devereux, S., Barr, P. M., Furman, R. R., Kipps, T. J., Cymbalista, F., Pocock, C., Thornton, P., Caligaris-Cappio, F., Robak, T., Delgado, J., … RESONATE Investigators (2014). Ibrutinib versus ofatumumab in previously treated chronic lymphoid leukemia. *The New England Journal of Medicine*, 371(3), 213–223.

Byrd, J. C., Furman, R. R., Coutre, S. E., Flinn, I. W., Burger, J. A., Blum, K. A., Grant, B., Sharman, J. P., Coleman, M., Wierda, W. G., Jones, J. A., Zhao, W., Heerema, N. A., Johnson, A. J., Sukbuntherng, J., Chang, B. Y., Clow, F., Hedrick, E., Buggy, J. J., James, D. F., … O'Brien, S.

(2013). Targeting BTK with ibrutinib in relapsed chronic lymphocytic leukemia. *The New England Journal of Medicine*, 369(1), 32–42.

Byrd, J. C., Harrington, B., O'Brien, S., Jones, J. A., Schuh, A., Devereux, S., Chaves, J., Wierda, W. G., Awan, F. T., Brown, J. R., Hillmen, P., Stephens, D. M., Ghia, P., Barrientos, J. C., Pagel, J. M., Woyach, J., Johnson, D., Huang, J., Wang, X., Kaptein, A., … Furman, R. R. (2016). Acalabrutinib (ACP-196) in Relapsed Chronic Lymphocytic Leukemia. *The New England Journal of Medicine*, 374(4), 323–332.

Byrd, J. C., Hillmen, P., O'Brien, S., Barrientos, J. C., Reddy, N. M., Coutre, S., Tam, C. S., Mulligan, S. P., Jaeger, U., Barr, P. M., Furman, R. R., Kipps, T. J., Thornton, P., Moreno, C., Montillo, M., Pagel, J. M., Burger, J. A., Woyach, J. A., Dai, S., Vezan, R., … Brown, J. R. (2019). Long-term follow-up of the RESONATE phase 3 trial of ibrutinib vs ofatumumab. *Blood*, 133(19), 2031–2042.

Caldemeyer, L., Dugan, M., Edwards, J., & Akard, L. (2016). Long-Term Side Effects of Tyrosine Kinase Inhibitors in Chronic Myeloid Leukemia. *Current Hematologic Malignancy Reports*, 11 (2): 71-79.

Cameron, D., Casey, M., Press, M., Lindquist, D., Pienkowski, T., Romieu, C. G., Chan, S., Jagiello-Gruszfeld, A., Kaufman, B., Crown, J., Chan, A., Campone, M., Viens, P., Davidson, N., Gorbounova, V., Raats, J. I., Skarlos, D., Newstat, B., Roychowdhury, D., Paoletti, P., … Geyer, C. E. (2008). A phase III randomized comparison of lapatinib plus capecitabine versus capecitabine alone in women with advanced breast cancer that has progressed on trastuzumab: updated efficacy and biomarker analyses. *Breast cancer research and treatment*, 112(3), 533–543.

Cameron, D., Piccart-Gebhart, M. J., Gelber, R. D., Procter, M., Goldhirsch, A., de Azambuja, E., Castro, G., Jr, Untch, M., Smith, I., Gianni, L., Baselga, J., Al-Sakaff, N., Lauer, S., McFadden, E., Leyland-Jones, B., Bell, R., Dowsett, M., Jackisch, C., & Herceptin Adjuvant (HERA) Trial Study Team (2017). 11 years' follow-up of trastuzumab after adjuvant chemotherapy in HER2-positive early breast cancer: final analysis of the HERceptin Adjuvant (HERA) trial. *Lancet (London, England)*, 389(10075), 1195–1205.

Camidge, D. R., Dziadziuszko, R., Peters, S., Mok, T., Noe, J., Nowicka, M., Gadgeel, S. M., Cheema, P., Pavlakis, N., de Marinis, F., Cho, B. C., Zhang, L., Moro-Sibilot, D., Liu, T., Bordogna, W., Balas, B., Müller, B., & Shaw, A. T. (2019). Updated Efficacy and Safety Data and Impact of the EML4-ALK Fusion Variant on the Efficacy of Alectinib in Untreated ALK-Positive Advanced Non-Small Cell Lung Cancer in the Global Phase III ALEX Study. *Journal of Thoracic Oncology: Official Publication of the International Association for the Study of Lung Cancer*, 14(7), 1233–1243.

Camidge, D. R., Kim, H. R., Ahn, M. J., Yang, J. C., Han, J. Y., Lee, J. S., Hochmair, M. J., Li, J. Y., Chang, G. C., Lee, K. H., Gridelli, C., Delmonte, A., Garcia Campelo, R., Kim, D. W., Bearz, A., Griesinger, F., Morabito, A., Felip, E., Califano, R., Ghosh, S., … Popat, S. (2018). Brigatinib versus Crizotinib in ALK-Positive Non-Small-Cell Lung Cancer. *The New England Journal of Medicine*, 379(21), 2027–2039.

Cardarella, S., Ogino, A., Nishino, M., Butaney, M., Shen, J., Lydon, C., Yeap, B. Y., Sholl, L. M., Johnson, B. E., & Jänne, P. A. (2013). Clinical, pathologic, and biologic features associated with BRAF mutations in non-small cell lung cancer. *Clinical cancer research: an official journal of the American Association for Cancer Research*, 19(16), 4532–4540.

Cardoso, F., Kyriakides, S., Ohno, S., Penault-Llorca, F., Poortmans, P., Rubio, I. T., Zackrisson, S., Senkus, E., & ESMO Guidelines Committee. Electronic address: clinicalguidelines@esmo.org (2019). Early breast cancer: ESMO Clinical Practice Guidelines for diagnosis, treatment and follow-up†. *Annals of oncology: official journal of the European Society for Medical Oncology*, 30(8), 1194–1220.

Cardoso, F., Senkus, E., Costa, A., Papadopoulos, E., Aapro, M., André, F., Harbeck, N., Aguilar Lopez, B., Barrios, C. H., Bergh, J., Biganzoli, L., Boers-Doets, C. B., Cardoso, M. J., Carey, L. A., Cortés, J., Curigliano, G., Diéras, V., El Saghir, N. S., Eniu, A., Fallowfield, L., … Winer, E. P. (2018). 4th ESO-ESMO International Consensus Guidelines for Advanced Breast Cancer (ABC 4)†. *Annals of oncology: official journal of the European Society for Medical Oncology*, 29(8), 1634–1657.

Carmena, M., Ruchaud, S., & Earnshaw, W. C. (2009). Making the Auroras glow: regulation of Aurora A and B kinase function by interacting proteins. *Current Opinion in Cell Biology*, 21(6), 796–805.

Carnevale, D., & Lembo, G. (2012). PI3Kγ in hypertension: a novel therapeutic target controlling vascular myogenic tone and target organ damage. *Cardiovascular Research*, 95(4): 403–408.

Caronia, L. M., Phay, J. E., & Shah, M. H. (2011). Role of BRAF in thyroid oncogenesis. *Clinical Cancer Research: an Official Journal of the American Association for Cancer Research*, 17(24), 7511–7517.

Castells, M., Thibault, B., Delord, J. P., & Couderc, B. (2012). Implication of tumor microenvironment in chemoresistance: tumor-associated stromal cells protect tumor cells from cell death. *International Journal of Molecular Sciences*, 13(8), 9545–9571.

Castillo, J. J., Furman, M., &Winer, E. S. (2012). CAL-101: a phosphatidylinositol-3-kinase p110-delta inhibitor for the treatment of lymphoid malignancies. *Expert Opinion on Investigational Drugs*, 21(1): 15–22.

Castillo, J. J., Treon, S. P., &Davids, M. S. (2016). Inhibition of the Bruton Tyrosine Kinase Pathway in B-Cell Lymphoproliferative Disorders. *Cancer Journal*, 22: 34–39.

Cervantes, A., Elez, E., Roda, D., Ecsedy, J., Macarulla, T., Venkatakrishnan, K., Roselló, S., Andreu, J., Jung, J., Sanchis-Garcia, J. M., Piera, A., Blasco, I., Maños, L., Pérez-Fidalgo, J. A., Fingert, H., Baselga, J., & Tabernero, J. (2012). Phase I pharmacokinetic/ pharmacodynamic study of MLN8237, an investigational, oral, selective aurora a kinase inhibitor, in patients with advanced solid tumors. *Clinical Cancer Research*, 18 (17): 4764-4774.

Cervantes, F., & Pereira, A. (2017). Does ruxolitinib prolong the survival of patients with myelofibrosis?. *Blood*, 129(7): 832–837.

Chanan-Khan, A., Cramer, P., Demirkan, F., Fraser, G., Silva, R. S., Grosicki, S., Pristupa, A., Janssens, A., Mayer, J., Bartlett, N. L., Dilhuydy, M. S., Pylypenko, H., Loscertales, J., Avigdor, A., Rule, S., Villa, D., Samoilova, O., Panagiotidis, P., Goy, A., Mato, A., … HELIOS investigators (2016). Ibrutinib combined with bendamustine and rituximab compared with placebo, bendamustine, and rituximab for previously treated chronic lymphocytic leukaemia or small lymphocytic lymphoma (HELIOS): a randomised, double-blind, phase 3 study. *The Lancet. Oncology*, 17(2), 200–211.

Chapman, C. M., Sun, X., Roschewski, M., Aue, G., Farooqui, M., Stennett, L., Gibellini, F., Arthur, D., Pérez-Galán, P. & Wiestner, A. (2012). ON 01910.Na is selectively cytotoxic for Chronic Lymphocytic Leukemia cells through a dual mechanism of action involving PI3K/AKT inhibition and induction of oxidative stress. *Clinical Cancer Research*, 18 (7): 1979-1991.

Chapman, P. B., Hauschild, A., Robert, C., Haanen, J. B., Ascierto, P., Larkin, J., Dummer, R., Garbe, C., Testori, A., Maio, M., Hogg, D., Lorigan, P., Lebbe, C., Jouary, T., Schadendorf, D., Ribas, A., O'Day, S. J., Sosman, J. A., Kirkwood, J. M., Eggermont, A. M., … BRIM-3 Study Group (2011). Improved survival with vemurafenib in melanoma with BRAF V600E mutation. *The New England Journal of Medicine*, 364(26), 2507–2516.

Chau, N. G., & Haddad, R. I. (2013). Vandetanib for the treatment of medullary thyroid cancer. *Clinical Cancer Research: an Official Journal of the American Association for Cancer Research*, 19(3), 524–529.

Cheah, C. Y., & Fowler, N. H. (2016). Idelalisib in the management of lymphoma. *Blood*, 128(3): 331–336.

Chen, X., Shi, J. G., Emm, T., Scherle, P. A., McGee, R. F., Lo, Y., Landman, R. R., Punwani, N. G., Williams, W. V., & Yeleswaram, S. (2014). Pharmacokinetics and pharmacodynamics of orally administered ruxolitinib (INCB018424 phosphate) in renal and hepatic impairment patients. *Clinical Pharmacology in Drug Development*, 3(1): 34–42.

Cheson, B. D. (2010). Syk [sic] of the same old chemotherapy? *Blood*, 115 (13): 2561–2562.

Cheson, B. D., O'Brien, S., Ewer, M. S., Goncalves, M. D., Farooki, A., Lenz, G., Yu, A., Fisher, R. I., Zinzani, P. L., & Dreyling, M. (2019). Optimal Management of Adverse Events from Copanlisib in the

Treatment of Patients with Non-Hodgkin Lymphomas. *Clinical Lymphoma, Myeloma & Leukemia*, 19(3), 135–141.

Chlebowski R. T. (2013). Changing concepts of hormone receptor-positive advanced breast cancer therapy. *Clinical Breast Cancer*, 13(3), 159–166.

Christopoulos, P., Endris, V., Bozorgmehr, F., Elsayed, M., Kirchner, M., Ristau, J., Buchhalter, I., Penzel, R., Herth, F. J., Heussel, C. P., Eichhorn, M., Muley, T., Meister, M., Fischer, J. R., Rieken, S., Warth, A., Bischoff, H., Schirmacher, P., Stenzinger, A., & Thomas, M. (2018). EML4-ALK fusion variant V3 is a high-risk feature conferring accelerated metastatic spread, early treatment failure and worse overall survival in ALK+ non-small cell lung cancer. *International Journal of Cancer*, 142(12), 2589–2598.

Cicenas, J., Zalyte, E., Bairoch, A., & Gaudet, P. (2018). Kinases and Cancer. *Cancers*, 10(3), 63.

Coffey, G. P., Feng, J., Betz, A., Pandey, A., Birrell, M., Leeds, J. M., Der, K., Kadri, S., Lu, P., Segal, J., Wang, Y. L., Michelson, G., Curnutte, J. T., and Conley, P. B. (2018). Cerdulatinib Pharmacodynamics and Relationships to Tumor Response Following Oral Dosing in Patients with Relapsed/Refractory B-cell Malignancies. *Clinical cancer research: an official journal of the American Association for Cancer Research*, 25(4), 1174–1184.

Cohen, M. H., Gootenberg, J., Keegan, P., & Pazdur, R. (2007). FDA drug approval summary: bevacizumab (Avastin) plus Carboplatin and Paclitaxel as first-line treatment of advanced/metastatic recurrent nonsquamous non-small cell lung cancer. *The oncologist*, 12(6), 713–718.

Cohen, M. H., Johnson, J. R., Chen, Y. F., Sridhara, R., & Pazdur, R. (2005). FDA drug approval summary: erlotinib (Tarceva) tablets. *The oncologist*, 10(7), 461–466.

Cohen, M. H., Williams, G. A., Sridhara, R., Chen, G., & Pazdur, R. (2003). FDA drug approval summary: gefitinib (ZD1839) (Iressa) tablets. *The oncologist*, 8(4), 303–306.

Cohen, M. H., Williams, G., Johnson, J. R., Duan, J., Gobburu, J., Rahman, A., Benson, K., Leighton, J., Kim, S. K., Wood, R., Rothmann, M., Chen, G., U, K. M., Staten, A. M., & Pazdur, R. (2002). Approval Summary for Imatinib Mesylate Capsules in the Treatment of Chronic Myelogenous Leukemia. *Clinical Cancer Research*, 8 (5): 935.

Collins, G. P., Eyre, T. A., Linton, K. M., Radford, J., Vallance, G. D., Soilleux, E., & Hatton, C. (2015). A Phase II trial of AZD1152 in relapsed/refractory diffuse large B-cell lymphoma. *British Journal of Haematology,* 170 (6): 886-890.

Connell, N. T., & Berliner, N. (2019). Fostamatinib for the treatment of chronic immune thrombocytopenia. *Blood*, 133 (19), 2027–2030.

Coopman, P. J., and Mueller, S. C. (2006). The Syk tyrosine kinase: A new negative regulator in tumor growth and progression. *Cancer Letters*, 241 (2): 159-173.

Cortes, J. E., Gambacorti-Passerini, C., Deininger, M. W., Mauro, M. J., Chuah, C., Kim, D.-W., Dyagil, I., Glushko, N., Milojkovic, D., le Coutre, P., Garcia-Gutierrez, V., Reilly, L., Jeynes-Ellis, A., Leip, E., Bardy-Bouxin, N., Hochhaus, A., & Brümmendorf, T. H. (2017). Bosutinib versus Imatinib for Newly Diagnosed Chronic Myeloid Leukemia: Results From the Randomized BFORE Trial. *Journal of Clinical Oncology*, 36 (3): 231-237.

Cortes, J. E., Kantarjian, H. M., Brümmendorf, T. H., Kim, D.-W., Turkina, A. G., Shen, Z.-X., Pasquini, R., Khoury, H. J., Arkin, S., Volkert, A., Besson, N., Abbas, R., Wang, J., Leip, E., & Gambacorti-Passerini, C. (2011). Safety and efficacy of bosutinib (SKI-606) in chronic phase Philadelphia chromosome–positive chronic myeloid leukemia patients with resistance or intolerance to Imatinib. *Blood*, 118 (17): 4567-4576.

Cortes, J. E., Kantarjian, H., Shah, N. P., Bixby, D., Mauro, M. J., Flinn, I., O'Hare, T., Hu, S., Narasimhan, N. I., Rivera, V. M., Clackson, T., Turner, C. D., Haluska, F. G., Druker, B. J., Deininger, M. W. N., & Talpaz, M. (2012). Ponatinib in Refractory Philadelphia Chromosome–Positive Leukemias. *New England Journal of Medicine*, 367 (22): 2075-2088.

Cortes, J. E., Khaled, S., Martinelli, G., Perl, A. E., Ganguly, S., Russell, N., Krämer, A., Dombret, H., Hogge, D., Jonas, B. A., Leung, A. Y., Mehta, P., Montesinos, P., Radsak, M., Sica, S., Arunachalam, M., Holmes, M., Kobayashi, K., Namuyinga, R., Ge, N., … Levis, M. J. (2019). Quizartinib versus salvage chemotherapy in relapsed or refractory FLT3-ITD acute myeloid leukaemia (QuANTUM-R): a multicentre, randomised, controlled, open-label, phase 3 trial. *The Lancet. Oncology*, 20(7), 984–997.

Cortes, J. E., Kim, D.-W., Nicolini, F. E., Saikia, T., Charbonnier, A., Apperley, J. F., Rathnam, K., Deininger, M. W., De Lavallade, H., Khattry, N., Whiteley, A., Mauro, M. J., Verhoef, G., Gambacorti-Passerini, C., Lucchesi, A., Apte, S., Nikki, G., Yao, S.-L., Kothekar, M., … Chimote, G. (2019). Phase 1 Trial of K0706, a Novel Oral BCR-ABL1 Tyrosine Kinase Inhibitor (TKI): In Patients with Chronic Myelogenous Leukemia (CML) and Phildelphia Positive Acute Lymphoblastic Leukemia (Ph+ ALL) Failing ≥ 3 Prior TKI Therapies: Initial Safety and Efficacy. *Blood*, 134 (Supplement_1): 4158-4158.

Cortes, J. E., Kim, D.-W., Pinilla-Ibarz, J., le Coutre, P., Paquette, R., Chuah, C., Nicolini, F. E., Apperley, J. F., Khoury, H. J., Talpaz, M., DiPersio, J., DeAngelo, D. J., Abruzzese, E., Rea, D., Baccarani, M., Müller, M. C., Gambacorti-Passerini, C., Wong, S., Lustgarten, S., … Kantarjian, H. (2013). A Phase 2 Trial of Ponatinib in Philadelphia Chromosome–Positive Leukemias. *New England Journal of Medicine*, 369 (19): 1783-1796.

Coutré, S. E., Barrientos, J. C., Brown, J. R., de Vos, S., Furman, R. R., Keating, M. J., Li, D., O'Brien, S. M., Pagel, J. M., Poleski, M. H., Sharman, J. P., Yao, N. S., & Zelenetz, A. D. (2015). Management of adverse events associated with idelalisib treatment: expert panel opinion. *Leukemia & Lymphoma*, 56(10), 2779–2786.

Cramer, P., V Tresckow, J., Robrecht, S., Bahlo, J., Fürstenau, M., Langerbeins, P., Pflug, N., Al-Sawaf, O., Heinz, W. J., Vehling-Kaiser, U., Dürig, J., Tausch, E., Hensel, M., Sasse, S., Fink, A. M., Fischer, K., Kreuzer, K. A., Böttcher, S., Ritgen, M., Kneba, M., … Hallek, M. (2020). Bendamustine, followed by ofatumumab and ibrutinib in chronic lymphocytic leukemia (CLL2-BIO): primary endpoint analysis of a multicentre, open-label phase-II trial. *Haematologica*, haematol.2019.223693. Advance online publication.

Cremer, A., Ellegast, J. M., Alexe, G., Frank, E. S., Ross, L., Chu, S. H., Pikman, Y., Robichaud, A., Goodale, A., Häupl, B., Mohr, S., Rao, A. V., Walker, A. R., Blachly, J. S., Piccioni, F., Armstrong, S. A., Byrd, J. C., Oellerich, T., & Stegmaier, K. (2020). Resistance Mechanisms to SYK Inhibition in Acute Myeloid Leukemia. *Cancer Discovery*, 10(2), 214–231.

Cristofanilli, M., Turner, N. C., Bondarenko, I., Ro, J., Im, S. A., Masuda, N., Colleoni, M., DeMichele, A., Loi, S., Verma, S., Iwata, H., Harbeck, N., Zhang, K., Theall, K. P., Jiang, Y., Bartlett, C. H., Koehler, M., & Slamon, D. (2016). Fulvestrant plus palbociclib versus fulvestrant plus placebo for treatment of hormone-receptor-positive, HER2-negative metastatic breast cancer that progressed on previous endocrine therapy (PALOMA-3): final analysis of the multicentre, double-blind, phase 3 randomised controlled trial. *The Lancet. Oncology*, 17(4), 425–439.

Crosby, M. E. (2007). Cell Cycle: Principles of Control. *The Yale Journal of Biology and Medicine*, 80(3), 141–142.

Crul, M., Rosing, H., de Klerk, G. J., Dubbelman, R., Traiser, M., Reichert, S., Knebel, N. G., Schellens, J. H., Beijnen, J. H., & ten Bokkel Huinink, W. W. (2002). Phase I and pharmacological study of daily oral administration of perifosine (D-21266) in patients with advanced solid tumours. *European journal of cancer (Oxford, England : 1990)*, 38(12), 1615–1621.

Cuellar, S., Vozniak, M., Rhodes, J., Forcello, N., & Olszta, D. (2018). BCR-ABL1 tyrosine kinase inhibitors for the treatment of chronic myeloid leukemia. *Journal of Oncology Pharmacy Practice*, 24 (6): 433-452.

Cuneo, A., Barosi, G., Danesi, R., Fagiuoli, S., Ghia, P., Marzano, A., Montillo, M., Poletti, V., Viale, P., & Zinzani, P. L. (2019). Management of adverse events associated with idelalisib treatment in chronic lymphocytic leukemia and follicular lymphoma: A multidisciplinary position paper. *Hematological Oncology*, 37(1): 3–14.

Curigliano, G., & Shah, R. R. (2019). Safety and Tolerability of Phosphatidylinositol-3-Kinase (PI3K) Inhibitors in Oncology. *Drug Safety*, 42(2): 247–262.

Curigliano, G., Gómez Pardo, P., Meric-Bernstam, F., Conte, P., Lolkema, M. P., Beck, J. T., Bardia, A., Martínez García, M., Penault-Llorca, F., Dhuria, S., Tang, Z., Solovieff, N., Miller, M., Di Tomaso, E., & Hurvitz, S. A. (2016). Ribociclib plus letrozole in early breast cancer: A presurgical, window-of-opportunity study. *Breast (Edinburgh, Scotland)*, 28, 191–198.

Currie, K. S., Kropf, J. E., Lee, T., Blomgren, P., Xu, J., Zhao, Z., Gallion, S., Whitney, J. A., Maclin, D., Lansdon, E. B., Maciejewski, P., Rossi, A. M., Rong, H., Macaluso, J., Barbosa, J., Di Paolo, J. A., & Mitchell, S. A. (2014). Discovery of GS-9973, a selective and orally efficacious inhibitor of spleen tyrosine kinase. *Journal of Medicinal Chemistry*, 57(9), 3856–3873.

Currie, K. S., Kropf, J. E., Lee, T., Blomgren, P., Xu, J., Zhao, Z., Gallion, S., Whitney, J. A., Maclin, D., Lansdon, E. B., Maciejewski, P., Rossi, A. M., Rong, H., Macaluso, J., Barbosa, J., Di Paolo, J. A., and Mitchell, S. A. (2014). Discovery of GS-9973, a Selective and Orally Efficacious Inhibitor of Spleen Tyrosine Kinase. *Journal of Medicinal Chemistry*, 57 (9): 3856-3873.

D'Assoro, A. B., Haddad, T., & Galanis, E. (2016). Aurora-A kinase as a promising therapeutic target in cancer. *Frontiers in Oncology*, 5: 295.

Dai, X., Li, T., Bai, Z., Yang, Y., Liu, X., Zhan, J., & Shi, B. (2015). Breast cancer intrinsic subtype classification, clinical use and future trends. *American Journal of Cancer Research*, 5(10), 2929–2943.

Dai, X., Li, T., Bai, Z., Yang, Y., Liu, X., Zhan, J., & Shi, B. (2015). Breast cancer intrinsic subtype classification, clinical use and future trends. *American journal of cancer research*, 5(10), 2929–2943.

Daver, N., Cortes, J., Ravandi, F., Patel, K. P., Burger, J. A., Konopleva, M., & Kantarjian, H. (2015). Secondary mutations as mediators of resistance to targeted therapy in leukemia. *Blood*, 125(21), 3236–3245.

Daver, N., Schlenk, R. F., Russell, N. H., & Levis, M. J. (2019). Targeting FLT3 mutations in AML: review of current knowledge and evidence. *Leukemia*, 33(2), 299–312.

Davids, M. S., Kim, H. T., Nicotra, A., Savell, A., Francoeur, K., Hellman, J. M., Bazemore, J., Miskin, H. P., Sportelli, P., Stampleman, L., Maegawa, R., Rueter, J., Boruchov, A. M., Arnason, J. E., Jacobson, C. A., Jacobsen, E. D., Fisher, D. C., Brown, J. R., & Blood Cancer Research Partnership of the Leukemia and Lymphoma Society (2019). Umbralisib in combination with ibrutinib in patients with relapsed or refractory chronic lymphocytic leukaemia or mantle cell lymphoma: a multicentre phase 1-1b study. *The Lancet. Haematology*, 6(1), e38–e47.

Davids, M. S., Kim, H. T., Nicotra, A., Savell, A., Francoeur, K., Hellman, J. M., Bazemore, J., Miskin, H. P., Sportelli, P., Stampleman, L., Maegawa, R., Rueter, J., Boruchov, A. M., Arnason, J. E., Jacobson, C. A., Jacobsen, E. D., Fisher, D. C., Brown, J. R., & Blood Cancer Research Partnership of the Leukemia and Lymphoma Society (2019). Umbralisib in combination with ibrutinib in patients with relapsed or refractory chronic lymphocytic leukaemia or mantle cell lymphoma: a multicentre phase 1-1b study. *The Lancet. Haematology*, 6(1), e38–e47.

Davies, H., Bignell, G. R., Cox, C., Stephens, P., Edkins, S., Clegg, S., Teague, J., Woffendin, H., Garnett, M. J., Bottomley, W., Davis, N., Dicks, E., Ewing, R., Floyd, Y., Gray, K., Hall, S., Hawes, R., Hughes, J., Kosmidou, V., Menzies, A., … Futreal, P. A. (2002). Mutations of the BRAF gene in human cancer. *Nature*, 417(6892), 949–954.

de Cárcer, G., Escobar, B., Higuero, A. M., García, L., Ansón, A., Pérez, G., Mollejo, M., Manning, G., Meléndez, B., Abad-Rodríguez, J., & Malumbres, M. (2011a). Plk5, a polo box domain-only protein with specific roles in neuron differentiation and glioblastoma suppression. *Molecular and Cellular Biology*, 31 (6): 1225-39.

de Cárcer, G., Manning, G., & Malumbres, M. (2011b). From Plk1 to Plk5: Functional evolution of Polo-like kinases. *Cell Cycle*, 10 (14): 2255-62.

de Gooijer, M. C., Zhang, P., Buil, L., Çitirikkaya, C. H., Thota, N., Beijnen, J. H., & van Tellingen, O. (2018). Buparlisib is a brain penetrable pan-PI3K inhibitor. *Scientific Reports*, 8(1), 10784.

de Graaff, E., Srinivas, S., Kilkenny, C., D'Agati, V., Mankoo, B. S., Costantini, F., & Pachnis, V. (2001). Differential activities of the RET tyrosine kinase receptor isoforms during mammalian embryogenesis. *Genes & Development*, 15(18), 2433–2444.

de Lima, L. T., Vivona, D., Bueno, C. T., Hirata, R. D. C., Hirata, M. H., Luchessi, A. D., de Castro, F. A., Chauffaille, M. d. L. F., Zanichelli, M. A., Chiattone, C. S., Hungria, V. T. M., & Guerra-Shinohara, E. M. (2014). Reduced ABCG2 and increased SLC22A1 mRNA expression are associated with imatinib response in chronic myeloid leukemia. *Medical Oncology*, 31 (3): 1-11.

de Vos, S., Wagner-Johnston, N. D., Coutre, S. E., Flinn, I. W., Schreeder, M. T., Fowler, N. H., Sharman, J. P., Boccia, R. V., Barrientos, J. C., Rai, K. R., Boyd, T. E., Furman, R. R., Kim, Y., Godfrey, W. R., & Leonard, J. P. (2016). Combinations of idelalisib with rituximab and/or bendamustine in patients with recurrent indolent non-Hodgkin lymphoma. *Blood Advances*, 1(2), 122–131.

de Weerdt, I., Koopmans, S. M., Kater, A. P., & van Gelder, M. (2017). Incidence and management of toxicity associated with ibrutinib and idelalisib: a practical approach. *Haematologica*, 102(10): 1629–1639.

DeAngelo, D. J., George, T. I., Linder, A., Langford, C., Perkins, C., Ma, J., Westervelt, P., Merker, J. D., Berube, C., Coutre, S., Liedtke, M., Medeiros, B., Sternberg, D., Dutreix, C., Ruffie, P. A., Corless, C., Graubert, T. J., & Gotlib, J. (2018). Efficacy and safety of midostaurin in patients with advanced systemic mastocytosis: 10-year median follow-up of a phase II trial. *Leukemia*, 32(2), 470–478.

Dees, E. C., Cohen, R. B., von Mehren, M., Stinchcombe, T. E., Liu, H., Venkatakrishnan, K., Manfredi, M., Fingert, H., Burris, H. A., & Infante, J. R. (2012). Phase I study of aurora A kinase inhibitor MLN8237 in advanced solid tumors: Safety, pharmacokinetics, pharmacodynamics, and bioavailability of two oral formulations. *Clinical Cancer Research*, 18 (17): 4775-84.

den Hollander, J., Rimpi, S., Doherty, J. R., Rudelius, M., Buck, A., Hoellein, A., Kremer, M., Graf, N., Scheerer, M., Hall, M. A., Goga, A., von Bubnoff, N., Duyster, J., Peschel, C., Cleveland, J. L., Nilsson, J.

A., & Keller, U. (2010). Aurora kinases A and B are up-regulated by Myc and are essential for maintenance of the malignant state. *Blood*, 116 (9): 1498-505.

Deng, M., Shi, Y., Chen, K., Zhao, H., Wang, Y., Xie, S., Zhao, J., Luo, Y., Fang, Z., Fan, Y., & Xu, B. (2018). CS2164 exerts an antitumor effect against human non-hodgkin's lymphomas in vitro and in vivo. *Experimental Cell Research*, 369 (2): 356-362.

Deng, M., Zhao, H., Chen, Q., Zhao, J., Shi, Y., Yu, L., Fang, Z., & Xu, B. (2019). CS2164 suppresses acute myeloid leukemia cell growth via inhibiting VEGFR2 signaling in preclinical models. *European Journal of Pharmacology*, 853: 193-200.

Dennis, M., Davies, M., Oliver, S. D'Souza, R., Pike, L., & Stockman, P. (2012). Phase I study of the aurora B kinase inhibitor barasertib (AZD1152) to assess the pharmacokinetics, metabolism and excretion in patients with acute myeloid leukemia. *Cancer Chemotherapy and Pharmacology*, 70 (3): 461-9.

Dhomen, N., & Marais, R. (2007). New insight into BRAF mutations in cancer. *Current Opinion in Genetics & Development*, 17(1), 31–39.

Dickler, M. N., Tolaney, S. M., Rugo, H. S., Cortés, J., Diéras, V., Patt, D., Wildiers, H., Hudis, C. A., O'Shaughnessy, J., Zamora, E., Yardley, D. A., Frenzel, M., Koustenis, A., & Baselga, J. (2017). MONARCH 1, A Phase II Study of Abemaciclib, a CDK4 and CDK6 Inhibitor, as a Single Agent, in Patients with Refractory HR+/HER2- Metastatic Breast Cancer. *Clinical Cancer research: an Official Journal of the American Association for Cancer Research*, 23(17), 5218–5224.

Dimopoulos, M. A., Tedeschi, A., Trotman, J., García-Sanz, R., Macdonald, D., Leblond, V., Mahe, B., Herbaux, C., Tam, C., Orsucci, L., Palomba, M. L., Matous, J. V., Shustik, C., Kastritis, E., Treon, S. P., Li, J., Salman, Z., Graef, T., Buske, C., & iNNOVATE Study Group and the European Consortium for Waldenström's Macroglobulinemia (2018). Phase 3 Trial of Ibrutinib plus Rituximab in Waldenström's Macroglobulinemia. *The New England Journal of Medicine*, 378(25), 2399–2410.

Ding, X., Huang, T., Peng, C., Ahn, K. S., Andersen, J. B., Lewinska, M., Cao, Y., Xu, G., Chen, G., Kong, B., Friess, H., Shen, S., Roberts, L. R., Wang, L., & Zou, X. (2020). Therapeutic Rationale to Target Highly Expressed Aurora kinase A Conferring Poor Prognosis in Cholangiocarcinoma. *Journal of Cancer*, 11(8), 2241–2251.

Dombi, E., Baldwin, A., Marcus, L. J., Fisher, M. J., Weiss, B., Kim, A., Whitcomb, P., Martin, S., Aschbacher-Smith, L. E., Rizvi, T. A., Wu, J., Ershler, R., Wolters, P., Therrien, J., Glod, J., Belasco, J. B., Schorry, E., Brofferio, A., Starosta, A. J., Gillespie, A., … Widemann, B. C. (2016). Activity of Selumetinib in Neurofibromatosis Type 1-Related Plexiform Neurofibromas. *The New England Journal of Medicine*, 375(26), 2550–2560.

Dong, J., Park, S. Y., Nguyen, N., Ezhilarasan, R., Martinez-Ledesma, E., Wu, S., Henry, V., Piao, Y., Tiao, N., Brunell, D., Stephan, C., Verhaak, R., Sulman, E., Balasubramaniyan, V., & de Groot, J. F. (2018). The polo-Like kinase 1 inhibitor Volasertib synergistically increases radiation efficacy in glioma stem cells. *Oncotarget*, 9 (12): 10497-10509.

Douillard, J. Y., Oliner, K. S., Siena, S., Tabernero, J., Burkes, R., Barugel, M., Humblet, Y., Bodoky, G., Cunningham, D., Jassem, J., Rivera, F., Kocákova, I., Ruff, P., Błasińska-Morawiec, M., Šmakal, M., Canon, J. L., Rother, M., Williams, R., Rong, A., Wiezorek, J., … Patterson, S. D. (2013). Panitumumab-FOLFOX4 treatment and RAS mutations in colorectal cancer. *The New England Journal of Medicine*, 369(11), 1023–1034.

Douillard, J. Y., Oliner, K. S., Siena, S., Tabernero, J., Burkes, R., Barugel, M., Humblet, Y., Bodoky, G., Cunningham, D., Jassem, J., Rivera, F., Kocákova, I., Ruff, P., Błasińska-Morawiec, M., Šmakal, M., Canon, J. L., Rother, M., Williams, R., Rong, A., Wiezorek, J., … Patterson, S. D. (2013). Panitumumab-FOLFOX4 treatment and RAS mutations in colorectal cancer. *The New England Journal of Medicine*, 369(11), 1023–1034.

Douillard, J. Y., Siena, S., Cassidy, J., Tabernero, J., Burkes, R., Barugel, M., Humblet, Y., Bodoky, G., Cunningham, D., Jassem, J., Rivera, F.,

Kocákova, I., Ruff, P., Błasińska-Morawiec, M., Šmakal, M., Canon, J. L., Rother, M., Oliner, K. S., Wolf, M., & Gansert, J. (2010). Randomized, phase III trial of panitumumab with infusional fluorouracil, leucovorin, and oxaliplatin (FOLFOX4) versus FOLFOX4 alone as first-line treatment in patients with previously untreated metastatic colorectal cancer: the PRIME study. *Journal of clinical oncology: official journal of the American Society of Clinical Oncology*, 28(31), 4697–4705.

Dreyling, M., Jurczak, W., Jerkeman, M., Silva, R. S., Rusconi, C., Trneny, M., Offner, F., Caballero, D., Joao, C., Witzens-Harig, M., Hess, G., Bence-Bruckler, I., Cho, S. G., Bothos, J., Goldberg, J. D., Enny, C., Traina, S., Balasubramanian, S., Bandyopadhyay, N., Sun, S., … Rule, S. (2016). Ibrutinib versus temsirolimus in patients with relapsed or refractory mantle-cell lymphoma: an international, randomised, open-label, phase 3 study. *Lancet (London, England)*, 387(10020), 770–778.

Dreyling, M., Santoro, A., Mollica, L., Leppä, S., Follows, G., Lenz, G., Kim, W. S., Nagler, A., Dimou, M., Demeter, J., Özcan, M., Kosinova, M., Bouabdallah, K., Morschhauser, F., Stevens, D. A., Trevarthen, D., Munoz, J., Rodrigues, L., Hiemeyer, F., Miriyala, A., … Zinzani, P. L. (2019). Long-term safety and efficacy of the PI3K inhibitor copanlisib in patients with relapsed or refractory indolent lymphoma: 2-year follow-up of the CHRONOS-1 study. *American Journal of Hematology*, 10.1002/ajh.25711. Advance online publication.

Drilon, A., Fu, S., Patel, M. R., Fakih, M., Wang, D., Olszanski, A. J., Morgensztern, D., Liu, S. V., Cho, B. C., Bazhenova, L., Rodriguez, C. P., Doebele, R. C., Wozniak, A., Reckamp, K. L., Seery, T., Nikolinakos, P., Hu, Z., Oliver, J. W., Trone, D., McArthur, K., … Ahn, M. J. (2019). A Phase I/Ib Trial of the VEGFR-Sparing Multikinase RET Inhibitor RXDX-105. *Cancer Discovery*, 9(3), 384–395.

Drilon, A., Hu, Z. I., Lai, G., & Tan, D. (2018). Targeting RET-driven cancers: lessons from evolving preclinical and clinical landscapes. *Nature reviews. Clinical Oncology*, 15(3), 150.

Drilon, A., Rekhtman, N., Arcila, M., Wang, L., Ni, A., Albano, M., Van Voorthuysen, M., Somwar, R., Smith, R. S., Montecalvo, J.,

Plodkowski, A., Ginsberg, M. S., Riely, G. J., Rudin, C. M., Ladanyi, M., & Kris, M. G. (2016). Cabozantinib in patients with advanced RET-rearranged non-small-cell lung cancer: an open-label, single-centre, phase 2, single-arm trial. *The Lancet. Oncology*, 17(12), 1653–1660.

Drilon, A., Siena, S., Ou, S. I., Patel, M., Ahn, M. J., Lee, J., Bauer, T. M., Farago, A. F., Wheler, J. J., Liu, S. V., Doebele, R., Giannetta, L., Cerea, G., Marrapese, G., Schirru, M., Amatu, A., Bencardino, K., Palmeri, L., Sartore-Bianchi, A., Vanzulli, A., … De Braud, F. G. (2017). Safety and Antitumor Activity of the Multitargeted Pan-TRK, ROS1, and ALK Inhibitor Entrectinib: Combined Results from Two Phase I Trials (ALKA-372-001 and STARTRK-1). *Cancer Discovery*, 7(4), 400–409.

Driscoll N. (2016). Idelalisib: Practical Tools for Identifying and Managing Adverse Events in Clinical Practice. *Journal of the Advanced Practitioner in Oncology*, 7(6): 604–613.

Du, Z., & Lovly, C. M. (2018). Mechanisms of receptor tyrosine kinase activation in cancer. *Molecular cancer*, 17(1), 58.

Du, Z., & Lovly, C. M. (2018). Mechanisms of receptor tyrosine kinase activation in cancer. *Molecular Cancer*, 17(1), 58.

Ducreux, M., Chamseddine, A., Laurent-Puig, P., Smolenschi, C., Hollebecque, A., Dartigues, P., Samallin, E., Boige, V., Malka, D., & Gelli, M. (2019). Molecular targeted therapy of BRAF-mutant colorectal cancer. *Therapeutic Advances in Medical Oncology*, 11, 1758835919856494.

Dummer, R., Ascierto, P. A., Gogas, H. J., Arance, A., Mandala, M., Liszkay, G., Garbe, C., Schadendorf, D., Krajsova, I., Gutzmer, R., Chiarion Sileni, V., Dutriaux, C., de Groot, J., Yamazaki, N., Loquai, C., Moutouh-de Parseval, L. A., Pickard, M. D., Sandor, V., Robert, C., & Flaherty, K. T. (2018b). Overall survival in patients with BRAF-mutant melanoma receiving encorafenib plus binimetinib versus vemurafenib or encorafenib (COLUMBUS): a multicentre, open-label, randomised, phase 3 trial. *The Lancet. Oncology*, 19(10), 1315–1327.

Dummer, R., Ascierto, P. A., Gogas, H. J., Arance, A., Mandala, M., Liszkay, G., Garbe, C., Schadendorf, D., Krajsova, I., Gutzmer, R., Chiarion-Sileni, V., Dutriaux, C., de Groot, J., Yamazaki, N., Loquai,

C., Moutouh-de Parseval, L. A., Pickard, M. D., Sandor, V., Robert, C., & Flaherty, K. T. (2018a). Encorafenib plus binimetinib versus vemurafenib or encorafenib in patients with BRAF-mutant melanoma (COLUMBUS): a multicentre, open-label, randomised phase 3 trial. *The Lancet. Oncology*, 19(5), 603–615.

Dummer, R., Schadendorf, D., Ascierto, P. A., Arance, A., Dutriaux, C., Di Giacomo, A. M., Rutkowski, P., Del Vecchio, M., Gutzmer, R., Mandala, M., Thomas, L., Demidov, L., Garbe, C., Hogg, D., Liszkay, G., Queirolo, P., Wasserman, E., Ford, J., Weill, M., Sirulnik, L. A., … Flaherty, K. (2017). Binimetinib versus dacarbazine in patients with advanced NRAS-mutant melanoma (NEMO): a multicentre, open-label, randomised, phase 3 trial. *The Lancet. Oncology*, 18(4), 435–445.

Dungo, R. T., & Keating, G. M. (2013). Afatinib: first global approval. *Drugs*, 73(13), 1503–1515.

Dutreix, C., Munarini, F., Lorenzo, S., Roesel, J., & Wang, Y. (2013). Investigation into CYP3A4-mediated drug-drug interactions on midostaurin in healthy volunteers. *Cancer Chemotherapy and Pharmacology*, 72(6), 1223–1234.

Eadie, L. N., Hughes, T. P., & White, D. L. (2014). Interaction of the Efflux Transporters ABCB1 and ABCG2 with Imatinib, Nilotinib, and Dasatinib. *Clinical Pharmacology & Therapeutics*, 95 (3): 294-306.

Eadie, L. N., Saunders, V. A., Branford, S., White, D. L., & Hughes, T. P. (2018). The new allosteric inhibitor asciminib is susceptible to resistance mediated by ABCB1 and ABCG2 overexpression *in vitro*. *Oncotarget*, 9 (17).

Eckerdt, F., Yuan, J., & Strebhardt, K. (2005). Polo-like kinases and oncogenesis. *Oncogene*, 24 (2): 267-276.

Efremov, D. G., and Laurenti, L. (2011). The Syk kinase as a therapeutic target in leukemia and lymphoma. *Expert Opinion on Investigational Drugs*, 20 (5): 623-636.

Eide, C. A., Zabriskie, M. S., Savage Stevens, S. L., Antelope, O., Vellore, N. A., Than, H., Schultz, A. R., Clair, P., Bowler, A. D., Pomicter, A. D., Yan, D., Senina, A. V., Qiang, W., Kelley, T. W., Szankasi, P., Heinrich, M. C., Tyner, J. W., Rea, D., Cayuela, J. M., Kim, D. W., …

Deininger, M. W. (2019). Combining the Allosteric Inhibitor Asciminib with Ponatinib Suppresses Emergence of and Restores Efficacy against Highly Resistant BCR-ABL1 Mutants. *Cancer Cell*, 36(4), 431–443.e5.

Elisei, R., Schlumberger, M. J., Müller, S. P., Schöffski, P., Brose, M. S., Shah, M. H., Licitra, L., Jarzab, B., Medvedev, V., Kreissl, M. C., Niederle, B., Cohen, E. E., Wirth, L. J., Ali, H., Hessel, C., Yaron, Y., Ball, D., Nelkin, B., & Sherman, S. I. (2013). Cabozantinib in progressive medullary thyroid cancer. *Journal of Clinical Oncology: Official Journal of the American Society of Clinical Oncology*, 31(29), 3639–3646.

Elli, E. M., Baratè, C., Mendicino, F., Palandri, F., & Palumbo, G. A. (2019). Mechanisms Underlying the Anti-inflammatory and Immunosuppressive Activity of Ruxolitinib. *Frontiers in Oncology*, 9: 1186.

Eltantawy, A., Vallejos, X., Sebea, E., & Evans, K. (2019). Copanlisib: An Intravenous Phosphatidylinositol 3-Kinase (PI3K) Inhibitor for the Treatment of Relapsed Follicular Lymphoma. *The Annals of Pharmacotherapy*, 53(9): 954–958.

Escamilla Gómez, V., García-Gutiérrez, V., López Corral, L., García Cadenas, I., Pérez Martínez, A., Márquez Malaver, F. J., Caballero-Velázquez, T., González Sierra, P. A., Viguria Alegría, M. C., Parra Salinas, I. M., Calderón Cabrera, C., González Vicent, M., Rodríguez Torres, N., Parody Porras, R., Ferra Coll, C., Orti, G., Valcárcel Ferreiras, D., De la Cámara L Lanzá, R., Molés, P., Velázquez-Kennedy, K., … Grupo Español de Trasplante Hematopoyético (GETH) (2020). Ruxolitinib in refractory acute and chronic graft-versus-host disease: a multicenter survey study. *Bone Marrow Transplantation*, 55(3), 641–648.

Escudier, B., Pluzanska, A., Koralewski, P., Ravaud, A., Bracarda, S., Szczylik, C., Chevreau, C., Filipek, M., Melichar, B., Bajetta, E., Gorbunova, V., Bay, J. O., Bodrogi, I., Jagiello-Gruszfeld, A., Moore, N., & AVOREN Trial investigators (2007). Bevacizumab plus interferon alfa-2a for treatment of metastatic renal cell carcinoma: a randomised, double-blind phase III trial. *Lancet (London, England)*, 370(9605), 2103–2111.

Escudier, B., Porta, C., Schmidinger, M., Rioux-Leclercq, N., Bex, A., Khoo, V., Grünwald, V., Gillessen, S., Horwich, A., & ESMO Guidelines Committee. Electronic address: clinicalguidelines@ esmo.org (2019). Renal cell carcinoma: ESMO Clinical Practice Guidelines for diagnosis, treatment and follow-up†. *Annals of oncology: official journal of the European Society for Medical Oncology*, 30(5), 706–720.

Eskazan, A. E., & Keskin, D. (2017). Radotinib and its clinical potential in chronic-phase chronic myeloid leukemia patients: an update. *Therapeutic Advances in Hematology*, 8 (9): 237-243.

Fancelli, D., Moll, J., Varasi, M., Bravo, R., Artico, R., Berta, D., Bindi, S., Cameron, A., Candiani, I., Cappella, P., Carpinelli, P., Croci, W., Forte, B., Giorgini, M. L., Klapwijk, J., Marsiglio, A., Pesenti, E., Rocchetti, M., Roletto, F., Severino, D., … Vianello, P. (2006). 1,4,5,6-tetrahydropyrrolo[3,4-c]pyrazoles: identification of a potent Aurora kinase inhibitor with a favorable antitumor kinase inhibition profile. *Journal of Medicinal Chemistry*, 49(24), 7247–7251.

Feng, G. & Wang, X. (2014). Role of spleen tyrosine kinase in the pathogenesis of chronic lymphocytic leukemia. *Leukemia & Lymphoma*, 55(12): 2699–2705.

Ferrara MG, Di Noia V, D'Argento E, Vita E, Damiano P, Cannella A, Ribelli M, Pilotto S, Milella M, Tortora G, & Bria E. Oncogene-Addicted Non-Small-Cell Lung Cancer: Treatment Opportunities and Future Perspectives. *Cancers (Basel)*. 2020;12(5):1196.

Ferrara, R., Auger, N., Auclin, E., & Besse, B. (2018). Clinical and Translational Implications of RET Rearrangements in Non-Small Cell Lung Cancer. *Journal of Thoracic Oncology: official publication of the International Association for the Study of Lung Cancer*, 13(1), 27–45.

Figg, W. D., Monga, M., Headlee, D., Shah, A., Chau, C. H., Peer, C., Messman, R., Elsayed, Y. A., Murgo, A. J., Melillo, G., Ryan, Q. C., Kalnitskiy, M., Senderowicz, A. M., Hollingshead, M., Arbuck, S. G., & Sausville, E. A. (2014). A phase I and pharmacokinetic study of oral perifosine with different loading schedules in patients with refractory neoplasms. *Cancer chemotherapy and pharmacology*, 74(5), 955–967.

Finn, R. S., Aleshin, A., & Slamon, D. J. (2016). Targeting the cyclin-dependent kinases (CDK) 4/6 in estrogen receptor-positive breast cancers. *Breast Cancer Research: BCR*, 18(1), 17.

Finn, R. S., Crown, J. P., Lang, I., Boer, K., Bondarenko, I. M., Kulyk, S. O., Ettl, J., Patel, R., Pinter, T., Schmidt, M., Shparyk, Y., Thummala, A. R., Voytko, N. L., Fowst, C., Huang, X., Kim, S. T., Randolph, S., & Slamon, D. J. (2015). The cyclin-dependent kinase 4/6 inhibitor palbociclib in combination with letrozole versus letrozole alone as first-line treatment of oestrogen receptor-positive, HER2-negative, advanced breast cancer (PALOMA-1/TRIO-18): a randomised phase 2 study. *The Lancet. Oncology*, 16(1), 25–35.

Finn, R. S., Martin, M., Rugo, H. S., Jones, S., Im, S. A., Gelmon, K., Harbeck, N., Lipatov, O. N., Walshe, J. M., Moulder, S., Gauthier, E., Lu, D. R., Randolph, S., Diéras, V., & Slamon, D. J. (2016). Palbociclib and Letrozole in Advanced Breast Cancer. *The New England Journal of Medicine*, 375(20), 1925–1936.

Flaherty, K. T., Lorusso, P. M., Demichele, A., Abramson, V. G., Courtney, R., Randolph, S. S., Shaik, M. N., Wilner, K. D., O'Dwyer, P. J., & Schwartz, G. K. (2012). Phase I, dose-escalation trial of the oral cyclin-dependent kinase 4/6 inhibitor PD 0332991, administered using a 21-day schedule in patients with advanced cancer. *Clinical Cancer Research: an Official Journal of the American Association for Cancer Research*, 18(2), 568–576.

Flaherty, K. T., Puzanov, I., Kim, K. B., Ribas, A., McArthur, G. A., Sosman, J. A., O'Dwyer, P. J., Lee, R. J., Grippo, J. F., Nolop, K., & Chapman, P. B. (2010). Inhibition of mutated, activated BRAF in metastatic melanoma. *The New England Journal of Medicine*, 363(9), 809–819.

Flaherty, K. T., Robert, C., Hersey, P., Nathan, P., Garbe, C., Milhem, M., Demidov, L. V., Hassel, J. C., Rutkowski, P., Mohr, P., Dummer, R., Trefzer, U., Larkin, J. M., Utikal, J., Dreno, B., Nyakas, M., Middleton, M. R., Becker, J. C., Casey, M., Sherman, L. J., … METRIC Study Group (2012). Improved survival with MEK inhibition in BRAF-mutated melanoma. *The New England Journal of Medicine*, 367(2), 107–114.

Flinn, I. W., Bartlett, N. L., Blum, K. A., Ardeshna, K. M., LaCasce, A. S., Flowers, C. R., Shustov, A. R., Thress, K. S., Mitchell, P., Zheng, F., Skolnik, J. M., & Friedberg, J. W. (2016). A phase II trial to evaluate the efficacy of fostamatinib in patients with relapsed or refractory diffuse large B-cell lymphoma (DLBCL). *European Journal of Cancer (Oxford, England : 1990)*, 54, 11–17.

Flinn, I. W., Hillmen, P., Montillo, M., Nagy, Z., Illés, Á., Etienne, G., Delgado, J., Kuss, B. J., Tam, C. S., Gasztonyi, Z., Offner, F., Lunin, S., Bosch, F., Davids, M. S., Lamanna, N., Jaeger, U., Ghia, P., Cymbalista, F., Portell, C. A., Skarbnik, A. P., … Stilgenbauer, S. (2018). The phase 3 DUO trial: duvelisib vs ofatumumab in relapsed and refractory CLL/SLL. *Blood*, 132(23), 2446–2455.

Flinn, I. W., Kahl, B. S., Leonard, J. P., Furman, R. R., Brown, J. R., Byrd, J. C., Wagner-Johnston, N. D., Coutre, S. E., Benson, D. M., Peterman, S., Cho, Y., Webb, H. K., Johnson, D. M., Yu, A. S., Ulrich, R. G., Godfrey, W. R., Miller, L. L., & Spurgeon, S. E. (2014). Idelalisib, a selective inhibitor of phosphatidylinositol 3-kinase-δ, as therapy for previously treated indolent non-Hodgkin lymphoma. *Blood*, 123(22), 3406–3413.

Flinn, I. W., Miller, C. B., Ardeshna, K. M., Tetreault, S., Assouline, S. E., Mayer, J., Merli, M., Lunin, S. D., Pettitt, A. R., Nagy, Z., Tournilhac, O., Abou-Nassar, K. E., Crump, M., Jacobsen, E. D., de Vos, S., Kelly, V. M., Shi, W., Steelman, L., Le, N., Weaver, D. T., … Zinzani, P. L. (2019). DYNAMO: A Phase II Study of Duvelisib (IPI-145) in Patients With Refractory Indolent Non-Hodgkin Lymphoma. *Journal of Clinical Oncology: Official Journal of the American Society of Clinical Oncology*, 37(11), 912–922.

Flinn, I. W., O'Brien, S., Kahl, B., Patel, M., Oki, Y., Foss, F. F., Porcu, P., Jones, J., Burger, J. A., Jain, N., Kelly, V. M., Allen, K., Douglas, M., Sweeney, J., Kelly, P., & Horwitz, S. (2018). Duvelisib, a novel oral dual inhibitor of PI3K-δ,γ, is clinically active in advanced hematologic malignancies. *Blood*, 131(8), 877–887.

Forero-Torres, A., Ramchandren, R., Yacoub, A., Wertheim, M. S., Edenfield, W. J., Caimi, P., Gutierrez, M., Akard, L., Escobar, C., Call, J., Persky, D., Iyer, S., DeMarini, D. J., Zhou, L., Chen, X., Dawkins, F., & Phillips, T. J. (2019). Parsaclisib, a potent and highly selective PI3Kδ inhibitor, in patients with relapsed or refractory B-cell malignancies. *Blood*, 133(16), 1742–1752.

Fouad, Y. A., & Aanei, C. (2017). Revisiting the hallmarks of cancer. *American journal of cancer research*, 7(5), 1016–1036.

Fowler, N., Jurczak, W., Cordoba Mascunano, R., Abrisqueta Costa, P., Strati, P., Yang, C., Kania, M., Kauh, J., and Ferreri, A. J. M. (2019). 1106TiP - A phase I study of HMPL-523, a selective oral anti-spleen tyrosine kinase inhibitor, in patients with relapsed or refractory lymphoma. *Annals of Oncology*, 30: v447.

Fragoulis, G. E., McInnes, I. B., & Siebert, S. (2019). JAK-inhibitors. New players in the field of immune-mediated diseases, beyond rheumatoid arthritis. *Rheumatology (Oxford, England)*, 58(Suppl 1): i43–i54.

Friedberg, J. W., Mahadevan, D., Cebula, E., Persky, D., Lossos, I., Agarwal, A. B., Jung, J., Burack, R., Zhou, X., Leonard, E. J., Fingert, H., Danaee, H., & Bernstein, S. H. (2014). Phase II Study of Alisertib, a Selective Aurora A Kinase Inhibitor, in Relapsed and Refractory Aggressive B- And T-cell non-Hodgkin Lymphomas. *Journal of Clinical Oncology*, 32 (1): 44-50.

Friedberg, J. W., Sharman, J., Sweetenham, J., Johnston, P. B., Vose, J. M., Lacasce, A., Schaefer-Cutillo, J., De Vos, S., Sinha, R., Leonard, J. P., Cripe, L. D., Gregory, S. A., Sterba, M. P., Lowe, A. M., Levy, R., & Shipp, M. A. (2010). Inhibition of Syk with fostamatinib disodium has significant clinical activity in non-Hodgkin lymphoma and chronic lymphocytic leukemia. *Blood*, 115(13), 2578–2585.

Friedberg, J. W., Sharman, J., Sweetenham, J., Johnston, P. B., Vose, J. M., LaCasce, A., Schaefer-Cutillo, J., De Vos, S., Sinha, R., Leonard, J. P., Cripe, L. D., Gregory, S. A., Sterba, M. P., Lowe, A. M., Levy, R., and Shipp, M. A. (2010). Inhibition of Syk with fostamatinib disodium has significant clinical activity in non-Hodgkin lymphoma and chronic lymphocytic leukemia. *Blood*, 115 (13): 2578-2585.

Frustaci, A. M., Tedeschi, A., Deodato, M., Zamprogna, G., Cairoli, R., & Montillo, M. (2019). Duvelisib: a new phosphoinositide-3-kinase inhibitor in chronic lymphocytic leukemia. *Future Oncology (London, England)*, 15(19), 2227–2239.

Fry, D. W., Harvey, P. J., Keller, P. R., Elliott, W. L., Meade, M., Trachet, E., Albassam, M., Zheng, X., Leopold, W. R., Pryer, N. K., & Toogood, P. L. (2004). Specific inhibition of cyclin-dependent kinase 4/6 by PD 0332991 and associated antitumor activity in human tumor xenografts. *Molecular Cancer Therapeutics*, 3(11), 1427–1438.

Fu, Z., & Wen, D. (2017). The emerging role of polo-like kinase 1 in epithelial-mesenchymal transition and tumor metastasis. *Cancers (Basel)*, 9 (10): 131.

Fukuoka, M., Wu, Y. L., Thongprasert, S., Sunpaweravong, P., Leong, S. S., Sriuranpong, V., Chao, T. Y., Nakagawa, K., Chu, D. T., Saijo, N., Duffield, E. L., Rukazenkov, Y., Speake, G., Jiang, H., Armour, A. A., To, K. F., Yang, J. C., & Mok, T. S. (2011). Biomarker analyses and final overall survival results from a phase III, randomized, open-label, first-line study of gefitinib versus carboplatin/paclitaxel in clinically selected patients with advanced non-small-cell lung cancer in Asia (IPASS). *Journal of clinical oncology: official journal of the American Society of Clinical Oncology*, 29(21), 2866–2874.

Furman, R. R., Sharman, J. P., Coutre, S. E., Cheson, B. D., Pagel, J. M., Hillmen, P., Barrientos, J. C., Zelenetz, A. D., Kipps, T. J., Flinn, I., Ghia, P., Eradat, H., Ervin, T., Lamanna, N., Coiffier, B., Pettitt, A. R., Ma, S., Stilgenbauer, S., Cramer, P., Aiello, M., … O'Brien, S. M. (2014). Idelalisib and rituximab in relapsed chronic lymphocytic leukemia. *The New England Journal of Medicine*, 370(11), 997–1007.

Gainor, J. F., & Shaw, A. T. (2013). Novel targets in non-small cell lung cancer: ROS1 and RET fusions. *The Oncologist*, 18(7), 865–875.

Garcia-Manero, G., Fenaux, P., Al-Kali, A., Baer, M. R., Sekeres, M. A., Roboz, G. J., Gaidano, G., Scott, B. L., Greenberg, P., Platzbecker, U., Steensma, D. P., Kambhampati, S., Kreuzer, K. A., Godley, L. A., Atallah, E., Collins, R., Jr, Kantarjian, H., Jabbour, E., Wilhelm, F. E., Azarnia, N., … ONTIME study investigators (2016). Rigosertib versus best supportive care for patients with high-risk myelodysplastic syndromes after failure of hypomethylating drugs (ONTIME): a randomised, controlled, phase 3 trial. *The Lancet. Oncology*, 17(4), 496–508.

Gatz, S. A., Aladowicz, E., Casanova, M., Chisholm, J. C., Kearns, P. R., Fulda, S., Geoerger, B., Schäfer, B. W., & Shipley, J. M. (2019). A Perspective on Polo-Like Kinase-1 Inhibition for the Treatment of Rhabdomyosarcomas. *Frontiers in Oncology*, 9, 1271.

Geahlen RL (2014). Getting Syk: spleen tyrosine kinase as a therapeutic target. *Trends in Pharmacological Sciences,* 35(8):414-422.

Geahlen, R. L. (2014). Getting Syk: spleen tyrosine kinase as a therapeutic target. *Trends in Pharmacological Sciences*, 35 (8): 414-422.

Gerisch, M., Schwarz, T., Lang, D., Rohde, G., Reif, S., Genvresse, I., Reschke, S., van der Mey, D., & Granvil, C. (2017). Pharmacokinetics of intravenous pan-class I phosphatidylinositol 3-kinase (PI3K) inhibitor [14C] copanlisib (BAY 80-6946) in a mass balance study in healthy male volunteers. *Cancer Chemotherapy and Pharmacology*, 80(3): 535–544.

Germann, U. A., Furey, B. F., Markland, W., Hoover, R. R., Aronov, A. M., Roix, J. J., Hale, M., Boucher, D. M., Sorrell, D. A., Martinez-Botella, G., Fitzgibbon, M., Shapiro, P., Wick, M. J., Samadani, R., Meshaw, K., Groover, A., DeCrescenzo, G., Namchuk, M., Emery, C. M., Saha, S., … Welsch, D. J. (2017). Targeting the MAPK Signaling Pathway in Cancer: Promising Preclinical Activity with the Novel Selective ERK1/2 Inhibitor BVD-523 (Ulixertinib). *Molecular Cancer Therapeutics*, 16(11), 2351–2363.

Geyer, C. E., Forster, J., Lindquist, D., Chan, S., Romieu, C. G., Pienkowski, T., Jagiello-Gruszfeld, A., Crown, J., Chan, A., Kaufman, B., Skarlos, D., Campone, M., Davidson, N., Berger, M., Oliva, C., Rubin, S. D., Stein, S., & Cameron, D. (2006). Lapatinib plus capecitabine for HER2-positive advanced breast cancer. *The New England Journal of Medicine*, 355(26), 2733–2743.

Ghia, P., Pluta, A., Wach, M., Lysak, D., Kozak, T., Simkovic, M., Kaplan, P., Kraychok, I., Illes, A., de la Serna, J., Dolan, S., Campbell, P.,

Musuraca, G., Jacob, A., Avery, E., Lee, J. H., Liang, W., Patel, P., Quah, C., & Jurczak, W. (2020). ASCEND: Phase III, Randomized Trial of Acalabrutinib Versus Idelalisib Plus Rituximab or Bendamustine Plus Rituximab in Relapsed or Refractory Chronic Lymphocytic Leukemia. *Journal of Clinical Oncology: Official Journal of the American Society of Clinical Oncology*, JCO1903355. Advance online publication.

Giannoudis, A., Davies, A., Lucas, C. M., Harris, R. J., Pirmohamed, M., & Clark, R. E. (2008). Effective dasatinib uptake may occur without human organic cation transporter 1 (hOCT1): implications for the treatment of imatinib-resistant chronic myeloid leukemia. *Blood*, 112 (8): 3348-3354.

Gianoukakis, A. G., Dutcus, C. E., Batty, N., Guo, M., & Baig, M. (2018). Prolonged duration of response in lenvatinib responders with thyroid cancer. *Endocrine-related Cancer*, 25(6), 699–704.

Gilmartin, A. G., Bleam, M, R., Groy, A., Moss, K. G., Minthorn, E. A., Kulkarni, S. G., Rominger, C. M., Erskine, S., Fisher, K. E., Yang, J., Zappacosta, F., Annan, R., Sutton, D., & Laquerre, S. G. (2011). GSK1120212 (JTP-74057) is an inhibitor of MEK activity and activation with favorable pharmacokinetic properties for sustained in vivo pathway inhibition. *Clinical Cancer Research*, 17 (5): 989-1000.

Giona, F., Mariani, S., Gnessi, L., Moleti, M. L., Rea, M., De Vellis, A., Marzella, D., Testi, A. M., & Foà, R. (2013). Bone metabolism, growth rate and pubertal development in children with chronic myeloid leukemia treated with Imatinib during puberty. *Haematologica*, 98 (3): e25-e27.

Giordano, A., Liu, Y., Armeson, K., Park, Y., Ridinger, M., Erlander, M., Reuben, J., Britten, C., Kappler, C., Yeh, E., & Ethier, S. (2019). Polo-like kinase 1 (Plk1) inhibition synergizes with taxanes in triple negative breast cancer. *PLoS One*, 14 (11): e0224420.

Girard, J., Reneau, J., Devata, S., Wilcox, R. A., Kaminski, M. S., Mercer, J., Carty, S., & Phillips, T. J. (2019). Evaluating Acalabrutinib In The Treatment Of Mantle Cell Lymphoma: Design, Development, And Place In Therapy. *OncoTargets and Therapy*, 12, 8003–8014.

Giustini, N. P., Jeong, A. R., Buturla, J., & Bazhenova, L. (2020). Advances in Treatment of Locally Advanced or Metastatic Non-Small Cell Lung Cancer: Targeted Therapy. *Clinics in Chest Medicine*, 41(2), 223–235.

Goldstein, N. I., Prewett, M., Zuklys, K., Rockwell, P., & Mendelsohn, J. (1995). Biological efficacy of a chimeric antibody to the epidermal growth factor receptor in a human tumor xenograft model. *Clinical cancer research: an official journal of the American Association for Cancer Research*, 1(11), 1311–1318.

Gopal, A. K., Kahl, B. S., de Vos, S., Wagner-Johnston, N. D., Schuster, S. J., Jurczak, W. J., Flinn, I. W., Flowers, C. R., Martin, P., Viardot, A., Blum, K. A., Goy, A. H., Davies, A. J., Zinzani, P. L., Dreyling, M., Johnson, D., Miller, L. L., Holes, L., Li, D., Dansey, R. D., … Salles, G. A. (2014). PI3Kδ inhibition by idelalisib in patients with relapsed indolent lymphoma. *The New England Journal of Medicine*, 370(11), 1008–1018.

Gordon, L. I., Kaplan, J. B., Popat, R., Burris, H. A., Ferrari, S., Madan, S., Patel, M. R., Gritti, G., El-Sharkawi, D., Chau, I., Radford, J. A., Pérez de Oteyza, J., Zinzani, P. L., Iyer, S., Townsend, W., Karmali, R., Miao, H., Proscurshim, I., Wang, S., Wu, Y., Stumpo, K., Shou, Y., Carpio, C., and Bosch, F. (2020). Phase I Study of TAK-659, an Investigational, Dual SYK/FLT3 Inhibitor, in Patients with B-Cell Lymphoma. *Clinical cancer research: an official journal of the American Association for Cancer Research*, 10.1158/1078-0432.CCR-19-3239. Advance online publication.

Gore, L., Kearns, P. R., de Martino, M. L., Lee, De Souza, C. A., Bertrand, Y., Hijiya, N., Stork, L. C., Chung, N. G., Cardos, R. C., Saikia, T., Fagioli, F., Seo, J. J., Landman-Parker, J., Lancaster, D., Place, A. E., Rabin, K. R., Sacchi, M., Swanink, R., & Zwaan, C. M. (2018). Dasatinib in Pediatric Patients with Chronic Myeloid Leukemia in Chronic Phase: Results from a Phase II Trial. *Journal of Clinical Oncology: Official Journal of the American Society of Clinical Oncology*, 36(13), 1330–1338.

Gorlick, R., Kolb, E. A., Keir, S. T., Maris, J. M., Reynolds, C. P., Kang, M. H., Carol, H., Lock, R., Billups, C. A., Kurmasheva, R. T., Houghton,

P. J., & Smith, M. A. (2014). Initial testing (Stage 1) of the polo-like kinase inhibitor Volasertib (BI 6727), by the pediatric preclinical testing program. *Pediatric Blood Cancer*, 61 (1): 158–164.

Goroshchuk, O., Kolosenko, I., Vidarsdottir, L., Azimi, A., & Palm-Apergi, C. (2019). Polo-like kinases and acute leukemia. *Oncogene*, 38 (1): 1–16.

Gotlib, J., Kluin-Nelemans, H. C., George, T. I., Akin, C., Sotlar, K., Hermine, O., Awan, F. T., Hexner, E., Mauro, M. J., Sternberg, D. W., Villeneuve, M., Huntsman Labed, A., Stanek, E. J., Hartmann, K., Horny, H. P., Valent, P., & Reiter, A. (2016). Efficacy and Safety of Midostaurin in Advanced Systemic Mastocytosis. *The New England Journal of Medicine*, 374(26), 2530–2541.

Green, S. D., & Konig, H. (2020). Treatment of acute myeloid leukemia in the era of genomics - Achievements and persisting challenges. *Frontiers in Genetics*, 11: 480.

Greenfield, G., McPherson, S., Mills, K., & McMullin, M. F. (2018). The ruxolitinib effect: understanding how molecular pathogenesis and epigenetic dysregulation impact therapeutic efficacy in myeloproliferative neoplasms. *Journal of Translational Medicine*, 16(1): 360.

Greenwell, I. B., Ip, A., & Cohen, J. B. (2017). PI3K Inhibitors: Understanding Toxicity Mechanisms and Management. *Oncology (Williston Park, N.Y.)*, 31(11): 821–828.

Grégoire, V., Lefebvre, J. L., Licitra, L., Felip, E., & EHNS-ESMO-ESTRO Guidelines Working Group (2010). Squamous cell carcinoma of the head and neck: EHNS-ESMO-ESTRO Clinical Practice Guidelines for diagnosis, treatment and follow-up. *Annals of oncology: official journal of the European Society for Medical Oncology*, 21 Suppl 5, v184–v186.

Gribben, J. G., Bosch, F., Cymbalista, F., Geisler, C. H., Ghia, P., Hillmen, P., Moreno, C., & Stilgenbauer, S. (2018). Optimising outcomes for patients with chronic lymphocytic leukaemia on ibrutinib therapy: European recommendations for clinical practice. *British Journal of Haematology*, 180(5), 666–679.

Gritsko, T. M., Coppola, D., Paciga, J. E., Yang, L., Sun, M., Shelley, S. A., Fiorica, J. V., Nicosia, S. V., & Cheng, J. Q. (2003). Activation and overexpression of centrosome kinase BTAK/Aurora-A in human ovarian cancer. *Clinical Cancer Research: an Official Journal of the American Association for Cancer Research*, 9(4), 1420–1426.

Gross, A. M., Wolters, P. L., Dombi, E., Baldwin, A., Whitcomb, P., Fisher, M. J., Weiss, B., Kim, A., Bornhorst, M., Shah, A. C., Martin, S., Roderick, M. C., Pichard, D. C., Carbonell, A., Paul, S. M., Therrien, J., Kapustina, O., Heisey, K., Clapp, D. W., Zhang, C., … Widemann, B. C. (2020). Selumetinib in Children with Inoperable Plexiform Neurofibromas. *The New England Journal of Medicine*, 382(15), 1430–1442.

Gross, S., Rahal, R., Stransky, N., Lengauer, C., & Hoeflich, K. P. (2015). Targeting cancer with kinase inhibitors. *The Journal of Clinical Investigation*, 125(5), 1780–1789.

Grundy, M., Seedhouse, C., Shang, S.; Richardson, J: Russell, N., & Pallis, M. (2010). The FLT3 internal tandem duplication mutation is a secondary target of the aurora B kinase inhibitor AZD1152-HQPA in acute myelogenous leukemia cells. *Molecular Cancer Therapeutics*, 9 (3): 661-72.

Guidetti, A., Carlo-Stella, C., Locatelli, S. L., Malorni, W., Mortarini, R.,Viviani, S., Russo, D., Marchianò, A., Sorasio, R., Dodero, A., Farina, L., Giordano, L., Di Nicola, M., Anichini, A., Corradini, P., & Gianni, A. M. (2014). Phase II study of perifosine and sorafenib dual-targeted therapy in patients with relapsed or refractory lymphoproliferative diseases. *Clinical cancer research: an official journal of the American Association for Cancer Research*, 20(22), 5641–5651.

Gumireddy, K., Reddy, M. V. R., Cosenza, Boominathan, R., Baker, S. J., Papathi, N., Jiang, J., Holland, J. & Reddy E. P. (2005). ON01910, a non-ATP-competitive small molecule inhibitor of Plk1, is a potent anticancer agent. *Cancer Cell*, 7 (3): 275-86.

Guo, A., Lu, P., Coffey, G., Conley, P., Pandey, A., and Wang, Y. L. (2017). Dual SYK/JAK inhibition overcomes ibrutinib resistance in chronic lymphocytic leukemia: Cerdulatinib, but not ibrutinib, induces apoptosis of tumor cells protected by the microenvironment. *Oncotarget*, 8 (8): 12953-12967.

Guo, R., Schreyer, M., Chang, J. C., Rothenberg, S. M., Henry, D., Cotzia, P., Kris, M. G., Rekhtman, N., Young, R. J., Hyman, D. M., & Drilon, A. (2019). Response to Selective RET Inhibition With LOXO-292 in a Patient With RET Fusion-Positive Lung Cancer With Leptomeningeal Metastases. *JCO Precision Oncology*, 3, 10.1200/PO.19.00021.

Hamlin, P. A., Flinn, I. W., Wagner-Johnston, N., Burger, J. A., Coffey, G. P., Conley, P. B., Michelson, G., Leeds, J. M., Der, K., Kim, Y., Sabalvaro-Torres, A., Birrell, M., Pandey, A., Curnutte, J. T., and Patel, M. R. (2019). Efficacy and safety of the dual SYK/JAK inhibitor cerdulatinib in patients with relapsed or refractory B-cell malignancies: Results of a phase I study. *American Journal of Hematology*, 94 (4): E90-E93.

Hanahan, D., & Weinberg, R. A. (2000). The hallmarks of cancer. *Cell*, 100(1), 57–70.

Hanahan, D., & Weinberg, R. A. (2011). Hallmarks of cancer: the next generation. *Cell*, 144(5), 646–674.

Hancox, U., Cosulich, S., Hanson, L., Trigwell, C., Lenaghan, C., Ellston, R., Dry, H., Crafter, C., Barlaam, B., Fitzek, M., Smith, P. D., Ogilvie, D., D'Cruz, C., Castriotta, L., Wedge, S. R., Ward, L., Powell, S., Lawson, M., Davies, B. R., Harrington, E. A., … Barry, S. T. (2015). Inhibition of PI3Kβ signaling with AZD8186 inhibits growth of PTEN-deficient breast and prostate tumors alone and in combination with docetaxel. *Molecular Cancer Therapeutics*, 14(1): 48–58.

Hao, Z., & Kota, V. (2015). Volasertib for AML: Clinical use and patient consideration. *OncoTargets and Therapy,* 8: 1761-1771.

Harari, P. M., Harris, J., Kies, M. S., Myers, J. N., Jordan, R. C., Gillison, M. L., Foote, R. L., Machtay, M., Rotman, M., Khuntia, D., Straube, W., Zhang, Q., & Ang, K. (2014). Postoperative chemoradiotherapy and cetuximab for high-risk squamous cell carcinoma of the head and neck: Radiation Therapy Oncology Group RTOG-0234. *Journal of clinical oncology: official journal of the American Society of Clinical Oncology*, 32(23), 2486–2495.

Harrison, C. N., Kiladjian, J., Al-Ali, H. K., Gisslinger, H., Waltzman, R. J., Stalbovskaya, V., Barbui, T., & Barosi, G. (2011). Results of a randomized study of the JAK inhibitor ruxolitinib (INC424) versus best available therapy (BAT) in primary myelofibrosis (PMF), post-polycythemia vera-myelofibrosis (PPV-MF) or post-essential thrombocythemia-myelofibrosis (PET-MF). *J Clin Oncol,* 29 (18 supplement):LBA6501.

Harrison, C. N., Mead, A. J., Panchal, A., Fox, S., Yap, C., Gbandi, E., Houlton, A., Alimam, S., Ewing, J., Wood, M., Chen, F., Coppell, J., Panoskaltsis, N., Knapper, S., Ali, S., Hamblin, A., Scherber, R., Dueck, A. C., Cross, N., Mesa, R., … McMullin, M. F. (2017b). Ruxolitinib vs best available therapy for ET intolerant or resistant to hydroxycarbamide. *Blood*, 130(17), 1889–1897.

Harrison, C. N., Schaap, N., Vannucchi, A. M., Kiladjian, J. J., Tiu, R. V., Zachee, P., Jourdan, E., Winton, E., Silver, R. T., Schouten, H. C., Passamonti, F., Zweegman, S., Talpaz, M., Lager, J., Shun, Z., & Mesa, R. A. (2017a). Janus kinase-2 inhibitor fedratinib in patients with myelofibrosis previously treated with ruxolitinib (JAKARTA-2): a single-arm, open-label, non-randomised, phase 2, multicentre study. *The Lancet. Haematology*, 4(7), e317–e324.

Harrison, C., & Vannucchi, A. M. (2012). Ruxolitinib: a potent and selective Janus kinase 1 and 2 inhibitor in patients with myelofibrosis. An update for clinicians. *Therapeutic Advances in Hematology*, 3(6): 341–354.

Harrison. C., Schaap, N., Vannucchi, A., Kiladjian, J. J., Passamonti, F., Zweegman, S., Talpaz, M., Verstovsek, S., Gerike, T., Rose, S., Zhang, J., Berry, T., Brownstein, C., & Mesa, R (2019). Fedratinib induces spleen responses in patients with Myeloproliferative Neoplasm (MPN)-associated intermediate- or high-risk myelofibrosis (MF) resistant or intolerant to ruxolitinib: an updated analysis of the phase II JAKARTA2 study. *Clinical Lymphoma, Myeloma and Leukemia*, 19 (supplement 1): S356.

Hauschild, A., Grob, J. J., Demidov, L. V., Jouary, T., Gutzmer, R., Millward, M., Rutkowski, P., Blank, C. U., Miller, W. H., Jr, Kaempgen, E., Martín-Algarra, S., Karaszewska, B., Mauch, C., Chiarion-Sileni, V., Martin, A. M., Swann, S., Haney, P., Mirakhur, B., Guckert, M. E., Goodman, V., … Chapman, P. B. (2012). Dabrafenib in BRAF-mutated metastatic melanoma: a multicentre, open-label, phase 3 randomised controlled trial. *Lancet (London, England)*, 380(9839), 358–365.

Hess, G., Herbrecht, R., Romaguera, J., Verhoef, G., Crump, M., Gisselbrecht, C., Laurell, A., Offner, F., Strahs, A., Berkenblit, A., Hanushevsky, O., Clancy, J., Hewes, B., Moore, L., & Coiffier, B. (2009). Phase III study to evaluate temsirolimus compared with investigator's choice therapy for the treatment of relapsed or refractory mantle cell lymphoma. *Journal of Clinical Oncology: Official Journal of the American Society of Clinical Oncology*, 27(23), 3822–3829.

Hillmen, P., Rawstron, A. C., Brock, K., Muñoz-Vicente, S., Yates, F. J., Bishop, R., Boucher, R., MacDonald, D., Fegan, C., McCaig, A., Schuh, A., Pettitt, A., Gribben, J. G., Patten, P., Devereux, S., Bloor, A., Fox, C. P., Forconi, F., & Munir, T. (2019). Ibrutinib Plus Venetoclax in Relapsed/Refractory Chronic Lymphocytic Leukemia: The CLARITY Study. *Journal of clinical oncology: Official Journal of the American Society of Clinical Oncology*, 37(30), 2722–2729.

Hiwase, D. K., Saunders, V., Hewett, D., Frede, A., Zrim, S., Dang, P., Eadie, L., To, L. B., Melo, J., Kumar, S., Hughes, T. P., & White, D. L. (2008). Dasatinib Cellular Uptake and Efflux in Chronic Myeloid Leukemia Cells: Therapeutic Implications. *Clinical Cancer Research*, 14 (12): 3881-3888.

Hochhaus, A., Larson, R. A., Guilhot, F., Radich, J. P., Branford, S., Hughes, T. P., Baccarani, M., Deininger, M. W., Cervantes, F., Fujihara, S., Ortmann, C.-E., Menssen, H. D., Kantarjian, H., O'Brien, S. G., & Druker, B. J. (2017). Long-Term Outcomes of Imatinib Treatment for Chronic Myeloid Leukemia. *New England Journal of Medicine*, 376 (10): 917-927.

Holohan, C., Van Schaeybroeck, S., Longley, D. B., & Johnston, P. G. (2013). Cancer drug resistance: an evolving paradigm. *Nature reviews. Cancer*, 13(10), 714–726.

Hölzel, M., Bovier, A., & Tüting, T. (2013). Plasticity of tumour and immune cells: a source of heterogeneity and a cause for therapy resistance?. *Nature reviews. Cancer*, 13(5), 365–376.

Hortobagyi, G. N., Stemmer, S. M., Burris, H. A., Yap, Y. S., Sonke, G. S., Paluch-Shimon, S., Campone, M., Blackwell, K. L., André, F., Winer, E. P., Janni, W., Verma, S., Conte, P., Arteaga, C. L., Cameron, D. A., Petrakova, K., Hart, L. L., Villanueva, C., Chan, A., Jakobsen, E., ... O'Shaughnessy, J. (2016). Ribociclib as First-Line Therapy for HR-Positive, Advanced Breast Cancer. *The New England Journal of Medicine*, 375(18), 1738–1748.

Hosseini, A., Gharibi, T., Marofi, F., Javadian, M., Babaloo, Z., & Baradaran, B. (2020). Janus kinase inhibitors: A therapeutic strategy for cancer and autoimmune diseases. *Journal of Cellular Physiology*, 235(9): 5903–5924.

Huang S., Nastoupil L. J., Guo H., Bell, T., Ahmed, M., Li, C. J., Wang, J., Liu, Y., Zhang, V., Kim, C. R., Boyle, J. N., Lorence, E. A., Lam, L. T., Chen, Z., Zhang, H., Shuttleworth, S. J., Nomie, K., Wang, M., Zhang, L. (2016). Pre-Clinical Evaluation of the PI3K-p110β/δ Inhibitor KA2237 in Mantle Cell Lymphoma. *Blood*, 128 (22): 1837.

Hughes, T. P., Mauro, M. J., Cortes, J. E., Minami, H., Rea, D., DeAngelo, D. J., Breccia, M., Goh, Y.-T., Talpaz, M., Hochhaus, A., le Coutre, P., Ottmann, O., Heinrich, M. C., Steegmann, J. L., Deininger, M. W. N., Janssen, J. J. W. M., Mahon, F.-X., Minami, Y., Yeung, D., ... Kim, D.-W. (2019). Asciminib in Chronic Myeloid Leukemia after ABL Kinase Inhibitor Failure. *New England Journal of Medicine*, 381 (24): 2315-2326.

Hurwitz, H., Fehrenbacher, L., Novotny, W., Cartwright, T., Hainsworth, J., Heim, W., Berlin, J., Baron, A., Griffing, S., Holmgren, E., Ferrara, N., Fyfe, G., Rogers, B., Ross, R., & Kabbinavar, F. (2004). Bevacizumab plus irinotecan, fluorouracil, and leucovorin for metastatic colorectal cancer. *The New England Journal of Medicine*, 350(23), 2335–2342.

Hyman, D. M., Puzanov, I., Subbiah, V., Faris, J. E., Chau, I., Blay, J. Y., Wolf, J., Raje, N. S., Diamond, E. L., Hollebecque, A., Gervais, R., Elez-Fernandez, M. E., Italiano, A., Hofheinz, R. D., Hidalgo, M., Chan, E., Schuler, M., Lasserre, S. F., Makrutzki, M., Sirzen, F., … Baselga, J. (2015). Vemurafenib in Multiple Nonmelanoma Cancers with BRAF V600 Mutations. *The New England Journal of Medicine*, 373(8), 726–736.

Ikeda, K., Kudo, M., Kawazoe, S., Osaki, Y., Ikeda, M., Okusaka, T., Tamai, T., Suzuki, T., Hisai, T., Hayato, S., Okita, K., & Kumada, H. (2017). Phase 2 study of lenvatinib in patients with advanced hepatocellular carcinoma. *Journal of Gastroenterology*, 52(4), 512–519.

Infante, J. R., Cassier, P. A., Gerecitano, J. F., Witteveen, P. O., Chugh, R., Ribrag, V., Chakraborty, A., Matano, A., Dobson, J. R., Crystal, A. S., Parasuraman, S., & Shapiro, G. I. (2016). A Phase I Study of the Cyclin-Dependent Kinase 4/6 Inhibitor Ribociclib (LEE011) in Patients with Advanced Solid Tumors and Lymphomas. *Clinical Cancer Research: an Official Journal of the American Association for Cancer Research*, 22(23), 5696–5705.

Infante, J. R., Fecher, L. A., Falchook, G. S., Nallapareddy, S., Gordon, M. S., Becerra, C., DeMarini, D. J., Cox, D. S., Xu, Y., Morris, S. R., Peddareddigari, V. G., Le, N. T., Hart, L., Bendell, J. C., Eckhardt, G., Kurzrock, R., Flaherty, K., Burris, H. A., 3rd, & Messersmith, W. A. (2012). Safety, pharmacokinetic, pharmacodynamic, and efficacy data for the oral MEK inhibitor trametinib: a phase 1 dose-escalation trial. *The Lancet. Oncology*, 13(8), 773–781.

Ivanova, E. S., Tatarskiy, V. V., Yastrebova, M. A., Khamidullina, A. I., Shunaev, A. V., Kalinina, A. A., Zeifman, A. A., Novikov, F. N., Dutikova, Y. V., Chilov, G. G., & Shtil, A. A. (2019). PF-114, a novel selective inhibitor of BCR-ABL tyrosine kinase, is a potent inducer of apoptosis in chronic myelogenous leukemia cells. *International Journal of Oncology*, 55: 289-297.

Jabbarzadeh Kaboli, P., Salimian, F., Aghapour, S., Xiang, S., Zhao, Q., Li, M., Wu, X., Du, F., Zhao, Y., Shen, J., Cho, C. H., & Xiao, Z. (2020). Akt-targeted therapy as a promising strategy to overcome drug resistance in breast cancer - A comprehensive review from chemotherapy to immunotherapy. *Pharmacological research*, 156, 104806.

Jabbour, E. (2016). Chronic myeloid leukemia: First-line drug of choice. *American Journal of Hematology*, 91 (1): 59-66.

Jabbour, E., & Kantarjian, H. (2018). Chronic myeloid leukemia: 2018 update on diagnosis, therapy and monitoring. *American Journal of Hematology*, 93 (3): 442-459.

Jacobsen, A., Bosch, L. J. W., Martens-de Kemp, S. R., Carvalho, B., Sillars-Hardebol, A. H., Dobson, R. J., de Rinaldis E., Meijer, G. A., Abeln, S., Heringa, J., Fijneman, R. J. A., and Feenstra, K. A. (2018). Aurora kinase A (AURKA) interaction with Wnt and Ras-MAPK signalling pathways in colorectal cancer. Sci Rep, 8 (1): 7522. Kanagal-Shamanna, R., Lehman, N. L., O'Donnell, J. P., Lim, M. S., Schultz, D. S., Chitale, D. A., Bueso-Ramos, C. E., Medeiros, L. J., and Inamdar, K. V. (2013). Differential expression of aurora-A kinase in T-cell lymphomas. *Modern Pathology*, 26 (5): 640-7.

Jain, N., Keating, M., Thompson, P., Ferrajoli, A., Burger, J., Borthakur, G., Takahashi, K., Estrov, Z., Fowler, N., Kadia, T., Konopleva, M., Alvarado, Y., Yilmaz, M., DiNardo, C., Bose, P., Ohanian, M., Pemmaraju, N., Jabbour, E., Sasaki, K., Kanagal-Shamanna, R., … Wierda, W. (2019). Ibrutinib and Venetoclax for First-Line Treatment of CLL. *The New England Journal of Medicine,* 380(22), 2095–2103.

Jänne, P. A., Wang, X., Socinski, M. A., Crawford, J., Stinchcombe, T. E., Gu, L., Capelletti, M., Edelman, M. J., Villalona-Calero, M. A., Kratzke, R., Vokes, E. E., & Miller, V. A. (2012). Randomized phase II trial of erlotinib alone or with carboplatin and paclitaxel in patients who were never or light former smokers with advanced lung adenocarcinoma: CALGB 30406 trial. *Journal of clinical oncology: official journal of the American Society of Clinical Oncology*, 30(17), 2063–2069.

Jerkeman, M., Eskelund, C. W., Hutchings, M., Räty, R., Wader, K. F., Laurell, A., Toldbod, H., Pedersen, L. B., Niemann, C. U., Dahl, C., Kuitunen, H., Geisler, C. H., Grønbæk, K., & Kolstad, A. (2018). Ibrutinib, lenalidomide, and rituximab in relapsed or refractory mantle cell lymphoma (PHILEMON): a multicentre, open-label, single-arm, phase 2 trial. *The Lancet. Haematology*, 5(3), e109–e116.

Jhiang S. M. (2000). The RET proto-oncogene in human cancers. *Oncogene*, 19(49), 5590–5597.

Jiang, N., Dai, Q., Su, X., Fu, J., Feng, X., & Peng, J. (2020). Role of PI3K/AKT pathway in cancer: the framework of malignant behavior. *Molecular biology reports*, 47(6), 4587–4629.

Jiao, Q., Bi, L., Ren, Y., Song, S., Wang, Q., & Wang, Y. S. (2018). Advances in studies of tyrosine kinase inhibitors and their acquired resistance. *Molecular Cancer*, 17(1), 36.

Jin, F., Robeson, M., Zhou, H., Moyer, C., Wilbert, S., Murray, B., & Ramanathan, S. (2015). Clinical drug interaction profile of idelalisib in healthy subjects. *Journal of Clinical Pharmacology*, 55(8), 909–919.

John Mascarenhas, J., Kremyanskaya, M., Hoffman, R., Bose, P., Talpaz, M., Harrison, C. N., Gupta, V., Leber, B., Sirhan, S., Kabir, S., Senderowicz, A., Shao, J., Mertz, J., Trojer, P., & Verstovsek, S. (2019). MANIFEST, a Phase 2 Study of CPI-0610, a Bromodomain and Extraterminal Domain Inhibitor (BETi), As Monotherapy or "Add-on" to Ruxolitinib, in Patients with Refractory or Intolerant Advanced Myelofibrosis. *Blood*, 134 (Supplement_1): 670.

Johnston, S., Martin, M., Di Leo, A., Im, S. A., Awada, A., Forrester, T., Frenzel, M., Hardebeck, M. C., Cox, J., Barriga, S., Toi, M., Iwata, H., & Goetz, M. P. (2019). MONARCH 3 final PFS: a randomized study of abemaciclib as initial therapy for advanced breast cancer. *NPJ Breast Cancer*, 5, 5.

Jonasova, A., Luger, S. M., Al-Kali, A., Valcarcel, D., Woodman, R. C., Adesanya, A. R., Azarnia, N., Parris, M., Warlick, E. D., Jedrzejczak, W. W., Díez-Campelo, M., & Garcia-Manero, G. (2019). The Inspire Study in higher-risk Myelodysplastic Syndrome (HR-MDS): A novel Phase 3 Study adaptive design for hematological malignancies in adults. *Blood*, 134 (Supplement_1): 4249.

Jones J., Wach M., Robak T., Brown, J. R., Menter, A. R., Ysebaert, E. V., Wagner-Johnston, N. D., Polikoff, J., Salman, H. S., Taylor, K. M., Coutre, S., Spurgeon, S., E., F., Kendall, S. D., Flinn, I., Dreiling, L.,

Dubowy, R., Cho, Y., Peterman, S., & Owen, C. (2015) Results of a phase III randomized, controlled study evaluating the efficacy and safety of idelalisib (IDELA) in combination with ofatumumab (OFA) for previously treated chronic lymphocytic leukemia (CLL). *Journal of Clinical Oncology*, 33(15): 7023-7023.

Kabbinavar, F. F., Hambleton, J., Mass, R. D., Hurwitz, H. I., Bergsland, E., & Sarkar, S. (2005). Combined analysis of efficacy: the addition of bevacizumab to fluorouracil/leucovorin improves survival for patients with metastatic colorectal cancer. *Journal of clinical oncology: official journal of the American Society of Clinical Oncology*, 23(16), 3706–3712.

Kaley, T. J., Panageas, K. S., Mellinghoff, I. K., Nolan, C., Gavrilovic, I. T., DeAngelis, L. M., Abrey, L. E., Holland, E. C., & Lassman, A. B. (2019). Phase II trial of an AKT inhibitor (perifosine) for recurrent glioblastoma. *Journal of neuro-oncology*, 144(2), 403–407.

Kanhaiya, K., Czeizler, E., Gratie, C., & Petre, I. (2017). Controlling Directed Protein Interaction Networks in Cancer. *Scientific Reports*, 7(1), 10327.

Kantarjian, H. M., Shah, N. P., Cortes, J. E., Baccarani, M., Agarwal, M. B., Undurraga, M. S., Wang, J., Kassack Ipiña, J. J., Kim, D.-W., Ogura, M., Pavlovsky, C., Junghanss, C., Milone, J. H., Nicolini, F. E., Robak, T., Van Droogenbroeck, J., Vellenga, E., Bradley-Garelik, M. B., Zhu, C., & Hochhaus, A. (2012). Dasatinib or Imatinib in newly diagnosed chronic-phase chronic myeloid leukemia: 2-year follow-up from a randomized phase 3 trial (DASISION). *Blood*, 119 (5): 1123-1129.

Kaplan, J. B., Bixby, D. L., Morris, J. C., Frankfurt, O., Altman, J., Wise-Draper, T., Burke, P. W., Collins, S., Kannan, K., Wang, L., Faucette, S., Lee, B., Shou, Y., Levis, M. J., and Pratz, K. W. (2016). a Phase 1b/2 Study of TAK-659, an Investigational Dual SYK and FLT-3 Inhibitor, in Patients (Pts) with Relapsed or Refractory Acute Myelogenous Leukemia (R/R AML). *Blood*, 128 (22): 2834-2834.

Kaplan, J. B., Gordon, L. I., Infante, J. R., Popat, R., Rambaldi, A., Madan, S., Patel, M. R., Gritti, G., Ng, C.-H., Chau, I., Radford, J. A., Oteyza, J. P., Zinzani, P. L., PharmD, S. F., Sheldon-Waniga, E., Williams, M.,

Stumpo, K., Shou, Y., Carpio, C., Bosch, F. (2016). Updated Results from a Phase 1 Study of TAK-659, an Investigational and Reversible SYK Inhibitor, in Patients (Pts) with Advanced Solid Tumor or Lymphoma Malignancies. *Blood*, 128 (22): 624.

Kato, S., Subbiah, V., Marchlik, E., Elkin, S. K., Carter, J. L., & Kurzrock, R. (2017). RET Aberrations in Diverse Cancers: Next-Generation Sequencing of 4,871 Patients. *Clinical Cancer Research: an Official Journal of the American Association for Cancer Research*, 23(8), 1988–1997.

Kawakami, M., Mustachio, L. M., Zheng, L., Chen, Y., Rodriguez-Canales, J., Mino, B., Kurie, J. M., Roszik, J., Villalobos, P. A., Thu, K. L., Silvester, J., Cescon, D. W., Wistuba, I. I., Mak, T. W., Liu, X., & Dmitrovsky, E. (2018). Polo-like kinase 4 inhibition produces polyploidy and apoptotic death of lung cancers. *Proceedings of the National Academy of Sciences of the United States of America*, 115(8), 1913–1918.

Ke, X., & Shen, L. Molecular targeted therapy of cancer: The progress and future. (2017). *Frontiers in Laboratory Medicine*, 1(2), 69–75.

Keane, N. A., Glavey, S. V., Krawczyk, J., & O'Dwyer, M. (2014). AKT as a therapeutic target in multiple myeloma. *Expert opinion on therapeutic targets*, 18(8), 897–915.

Khan, J., Ezan, F., Crémet, J. Y., Fautrel, A., Gilot, D., Lambert, M., Benaud, C., Troadec, M.-B., & Prigent, C. (2011). Overexpression of active Aurora-C kinase results in cell transformation and tumour formation. *PLoS One*, 6 (10): e26512.

Khan, M., Lin, J., Liao, G., Tian, Y., Liang, Y., Li, R., Liu, M., & Yuan, Y. (2019) ALK Inhibitors in the Treatment of ALK Positive NSCLC. *Frontiers in Oncology*, 8:557.

Khoury, H. J., Cortes, J. E., Kantarjian, H. M., Gambacorti-Passerini, C. B., Baccarani, M., Kim, D.-W., Zaritskey, A., Countouriotis, A., Besson, N., Leip, E., Kelly, V., & Brummendorf, T. H. (2012). Bosutinib is active in chronic phase chronic myeloid leukemia after imatinib and dasatinib and/or nilotinib therapy failure. *Blood*, 119 (15): 3403-3412.

Kiladjian, J. J., Zachee, P., Hino, M., Pane, F., Masszi, T., Harrison, C. N., Mesa, R., Miller, C. B., Passamonti, F., Durrant, S., Griesshammer, M., Kirito, K., Besses, C., Moiraghi, B., Rumi, E., Rosti, V., Blau, I. W., Francillard, N., Dong, T., Wroclawska, M., … Verstovsek, S. (2020). Long-term efficacy and safety of ruxolitinib versus best available therapy in polycythaemia vera (RESPONSE): 5-year follow up of a phase 3 study. *The Lancet. Haematology*, 7(3), e226–e237.

Kim, D. W., Tiseo, M., Ahn, M. J., Reckamp, K. L., Hansen, K. H., Kim, S. W., Huber, R. M., West, H. L., Groen, H., Hochmair, M. J., Leighl, N. B., Gettinger, S. N., Langer, C. J., Paz-Ares Rodríguez, L. G., Smit, E. F., Kim, E. S., Reichmann, W., Haluska, F. G., Kerstein, D., & Camidge, D. R. (2017). Brigatinib in Patients with Crizotinib-Refractory Anaplastic Lymphoma Kinase-Positive Non-Small-Cell Lung Cancer: A Randomized, Multicenter Phase II Trial. *Journal of Clinical Oncology: Official Journal of the American Society of Clinical Oncology*, 35(22), 2490–2498.

Kim, D. W., Ahn, M. J., Shi, Y., Martino De Pas, T., Yang, P. C., RielyLucio Crinò, G. J., Evans, T. L., Liu, X., Han, J. Y., Salgia, R., Moro-Sibilot, D., Ou, S. H. I., Gettinger, S. N., Wu, Y. L., Lanzalone, S., Polli, A., Iyer, S., & Shaw, A. T. (2012) Results of a global phase II study with crizotinib in advanced ALK-positive nonsmall cell lung cancer (NSCLC). *Journal of Clinical Oncology,* 30(Suppl. 15):7533.

Kim, H. (2019). Development of BTK inhibitors for the treatment of B-cell malignancies. *Archives of Pharmacal Research,* 42:171–181.

Kim, S. H., Menon, H., Jootar, S., Saikia, T., Kwak, J. Y., Sohn, S. K., Park, J. S., Jeong, S. H., Kim, H. J., Kim, Y. K., Oh, S. J., Kim, H., Zang, D. Y., Chung, J. S., Shin, H. J., Do, Y. R., Kim, J. A., Kim, D. Y., Choi, C. W., Park, S., … Kim, D. W. (2014). Efficacy and safety of radotinib in chronic phase chronic myeloid leukemia patients with resistance or intolerance to BCR-ABL1 tyrosine kinase inhibitors. *Haematologica*, 99(7), 1191–1196.

Knowles, P. P., Murray-Rust, J., Kjaer, S., Scott, R. P., Hanrahan, S., Santoro, M., Ibáñez, C. F., & McDonald, N. Q. (2006). Structure and chemical inhibition of the RET tyrosine kinase domain. *The Journal of Biological Chemistry*, 281(44), 33577–33587.

Koh, H. M., Jang, B. G., Hyun, C. L., Kim, Y. S., Hyun, J. W., Chang, W, Y., & Maeng, Y. E. (2017). Aurora kinase a is a prognostic marker in colorectal adenocarcinoma. *Journal of Pathology and Translational Medicine*, 51 (1): 32-39.

Kudo, M., Finn, R. S., Qin, S., Han, K. H., Ikeda, K., Piscaglia, F., Baron, A., Park, J. W., Han, G., Jassem, J., Blanc, J. F., Vogel, A., Komov, D., Evans, T., Lopez, C., Dutcus, C., Guo, M., Saito, K., Kraljevic, S., Tamai, T., … Cheng, A. L. (2018). Lenvatinib versus sorafenib in first-line treatment of patients with unresectable hepatocellular carcinoma: a randomised phase 3 non-inferiority trial. *Lancet (London, England)*, 391(10126), 1163–1173.

Kuiatse, I., Baladandayuthapani, V., Lin, H. Y., Thomas, S. K., Bjorklund, C. C., Weber, D. M., Wang, M., Shah, J. J., Zhang, X.-D., Jones, R. J., Ansell, S. M., Yang, G., Treon, S. P., and Orlowski, R. Z. (2015). Targeting the Spleen Tyrosine Kinase with Fostamatinib as a Strategy against Waldenström Macroglobulinemia. *Clinical cancer research: an official journal of the American Association for Cancer Research*, 21(11), 2538–2545.

Kurzrock, R., Sherman, S. I., Ball, D. W., Forastiere, A. A., Cohen, R. B., Mehra, R., Pfister, D. G., Cohen, E. E., Janisch, L., Nauling, F., Hong, D. S., Ng, C. S., Ye, L., Gagel, R. F., Frye, J., Müller, T., Ratain, M. J., & Salgia, R. (2011). Activity of XL184 (Cabozantinib), an oral tyrosine kinase inhibitor, in patients with medullary thyroid cancer. *Journal of Clinical Oncology: Official Journal of the American Society of Clinical Oncology*, 29(19), 2660–2666.

Kushner, B. H., Cheung, N. V., Modak, S., Becher, O. J., Basu, E. M., Roberts, S. S., Kramer, K., & Dunkel, I. J. (2017). A phase I/Ib trial targeting the Pi3k/Akt pathway using perifosine: Long-term progression-free survival of patients with resistant neuroblastoma. *International journal of cancer*, 140(2), 480–484.

Kwak, E. L., Bang, Y. J., Camidge, D. R., Shaw, A. T., Solomon, B., Maki, R. G., Ou, S. H., Dezube, B. J., Jänne, P. A., Costa, D. B., Varella-

Garcia, M., Kim, W. H., Lynch, T. J., Fidias, P., Stubbs, H., Engelman, J. A., Sequist, L. V., Tan, W., Gandhi, L., Mino-Kenudson, M., … Iafrate, A. J. (2010). Anaplastic lymphoma kinase inhibition in non-small-cell lung cancer. *The New England Journal of Medicine,* 363(18), 1693–1703.

Kwak, J. Y., Kim, S. H., Oh, S. J., Zang, D. Y., Kim, H., Kim, J. A., Do, Y. R., Kim, H. J., Park, J. S., Choi, C. W., Lee, W. S., Mun, Y. C., Kong, J. H., Chung, J. S., Shin, H. J., Kim, D. Y., Park, J., Jung, C. W., Bunworasate, U., Comia, N. S., Jootar, S., Reksodiputro, H., Caguioa, P. B., Lee, S. E., & Kim, D. W. (2017). Phase III clinical trial (RERISE study) results of Efficacy and safety of radotinib compared with Imatinib in newly diagnosed chronic phase chronic myeloid leukemia. *Clinical Cancer Research*: clincanres.0957.2017.

Lam, B., Arikawa, Y., Cramlett, J., Dong, Q., de Jong, R., Feher, V., Grimshaw, C. E., Farrell, P. J., Hoffman, I. D., Jennings, A., Jones, B., Matuszkiewicz, J., Miura, J., Miyake, H., Natala, S. R., Shi, L., Takahashi, M., Taylor, E., Wyrick, C., Yano, J., Zalevsky, J., and Nie, Z. (2016). Discovery of TAK-659 an orally available investigational inhibitor of Spleen Tyrosine Kinase (SYK). *Bioorganic & Medicinal Chemistry Letters*, 26 (24): 5947-5950.

Lampson, B. L., & Brown, J. R. (2017). PI3Kδ-selective and PI3Kα/δ-combinatorial inhibitors in clinical development for B-cell non-Hodgkin lymphoma. *Expert Opinion on Investigational Drugs*, 26(11): 1267–1279.

Landel, I., Quambusch, L., Depta, L., & Rauh, D. (2020). Spotlight on AKT: Current Therapeutic Challenges. *ACS medicinal chemistry letters*, 11(3), 225–227.

Laplante, M., & Sabatini, D. M. (2012). mTOR Signaling. *Cold Spring Harbor Perspectives in Biology*, 4(2), a011593.

Larsen, J. T., Shanafelt, T. D., Leis, J. F., LaPlant, B., Call, T., Pettinger, A., Hanson, C., Erlichman, C., Habermann, T. M., Reeder, C., Nikcevich, D., Bowen, D., Conte, M., Boysen, J., Secreto, C., Lesnick, C., Tschumper, R., Jelinek, D., Kay, N. E., & Ding, W. (2017). Akt inhibitor MK-2206 in combination with bendamustine and rituximab in relapsed or refractory chronic lymphocytic leukemia: Results from the N1087 alliance study. *American journal of hematology*, 92(8), 759–763.

Larson, R. A., Mandrekar, S. J., Sanford, B. L., Laumann, K., Geyer, S. M., Bloomfield, C. D., Thiede, C., Prior, T. W., Dohner, K., Marcucci, G., Lo Coco, F., Klisovic, R. B., Wei, A., Sierra, J., Sanz, M. A., Brandwein, J. M., de Witte, T. M. M., Niederwieser, D., Appelbaum, F. R., Medeiros, B. C., Tallman, M. S., Krauter, J., Schlenk, R. F., Ganser, A., Serve, H., Ehninger, G., Amadori, S., Döhner, H., & Stone, R. M. (2017). An Analysis of Maintenance Therapy and Post-Midostaurin Outcomes in the International Prospective Randomized, Placebo-Controlled, Double-Blind Trial (CALGB 10603/RATIFY [Alliance]) for Newly Diagnosed Acute Myeloid Leukemia (AML) Patients with FLT3 Mutations. *Blood*, 130 (Supplement 1): 145.

Layton, T., Stalens, C., Gunderson, F., Goodison, S., and Silletti, S. (2009). Syk Tyrosine Kinase Acts as a Pancreatic Adenocarcinoma Tumor Suppressor by Regulating Cellular Growth and Invasion. *The American Journal of Pathology*, 175 (6): 2625-2636.

Lee, M. G., & Nurse, P. (1987). Complementation used to clone a human homologue of the fission yeast cell cycle control gene cdc2. *Nature*, 327(6117), 31–35.

Lee, S. H., Lee, J. K., Ahn, M. J., Kim, D. W., Sun, J. M., Keam, B., Kim, T. M., Heo, D. S., Ahn, J. S., Choi, Y. L., Min, H. S., Jeon, Y. K., & Park, K. (2017). Vandetanib in pretreated patients with advanced non-small cell lung cancer-harboring RET rearrangement: a phase II clinical trial. *Annals of Oncology: Official Journal of the European Society for Medical Oncology*, 28(2), 292–297.

Lefebvre, J. L., Pointreau, Y., Rolland, F., Alfonsi, M., Baudoux, A., Sire, C., de Raucourt, D., Malard, O., Degardin, M., Tuchais, C., Blot, E., Rives, M., Reyt, E., Tourani, J. M., Geoffrois, L., Peyrade, F., Guichard, F., Chevalier, D., Babin, E., Lang, P., … Bardet, E. (2013). Induction chemotherapy followed by either chemoradiotherapy or bioradiotherapy for larynx preservation: the TREMPLIN randomized phase II study. *Journal of clinical oncology : official journal of the American Society of Clinical Oncology*, 31(7), 853–859.

Lemmon, M. A., & Schlessinger, J. (2010). Cell signaling by receptor tyrosine kinases. *Cell*, 141(7), 1117–1134.

Lens, S. M. A., Voest, E. E., & Medema, R. H. (2010). Shared and Separate Functions of Polo-Like Kinases and Aurora Kinases in Cancer. *Nature Reviews Cancer*, 10 (12): 825-41.

Lenz, H. J., Ahn, D. H., Rindinger, M., Erlander, M. G., & Barzi, A. (2020). A phase Ib/II study of onvansertib (PCM-075) in combination with FOLFIRI and bevacizumab for second-line treatment of metastatic colorectal cancer (mCRC) in patients with a KRAS mutation. *Journal of Clinical Oncology*, 38(Suppl 4): TPS265.

Levis, M., Smith, C., Litzow, M., Perl, A., Altman, J., James, A., Kadokura, T., Sargent, B., Yuen, G., Lu, Z., Liu, C., Nagase, I., & Bahceci, E. (2017). Drug-drug interaction potential of gilteritinib in healthy subjects and patients with relapsed/refractory acute myeloid leukemia. *EHA Learn Center*, Abstract E940.

Li, D., Zhu, J., Firozi, P. F., Abbruzzese, J. L., Evans, D. B., Cleary, K., Friess, H., & Sen, S. (2003). Overexpression of oncogenic STK15/BTAK/Aurora A kinase in human pancreatic cancer. *Clinical Cancer Research*, 9 (3): 991-997.

Li, G. G., Somwar, R., Joseph, J., Smith, R. S., Hayashi, T., Martin, L., Franovic, A., Schairer, A., Martin, E., Riely, G. J., Harris, J., Yan, S., Wei, G., Oliver, J. W., Patel, R., Multani, P., Ladanyi, M., & Drilon, A. (2017). Antitumor Activity of RXDX-105 in Multiple Cancer Types with RET Rearrangements or Mutations. *Clinical Cancer Research: an Official Journal of the American Association for Cancer Research*, 23(12), 2981–2990.

Lin J. J., Riely G. J., & Shaw A. T. (2017). Targeting ALK: Precision Medicine Takes on Drug Resistance. *Cancer Discovery*, 7(2):137-155.

Lin, C., Wang, S., Xie, W., Chang, J., & Gan, Y. (2015). The RET fusion gene and its correlation with demographic and clinicopathological features of non-small cell lung cancer: a meta-analysis. *Cancer Biology & Therapy*, 16(7), 1019–1028.

Liu, D. & Mamorska-Dyga, A. (2017). Syk inhibitors in clinical development for hematological malignancies. *Journal of Hematology & Oncology*, 10:145-152.

Liu, D., and Mamorska-Dyga, A. (2017). Syk inhibitors in clinical development for hematological malignancies. *Journal of Hematology & Oncology*, 10 (1): 145.

Liu, X. (2015). Targeting Polo-like kinases: A promising therapeutic Approach for cancer treatment. *Translational Oncology*, 8 (3): 185-195.

Liu, X., Wang, G., Yan, X., Qiu, H., Min, P., Wu, M., Tang, C., Zhang, F., Tang, Q., Zhu, S., Qiu, M., Zhuang, W., Fang, D. D., Zhou, Z., Yang, D., & Zhai, Y. (2019). Preclinical development of HQP1351, a multikinase inhibitor targeting a broad spectrum of mutant KIT kinases, for the treatment of imatinib-resistant gastrointestinal stromal tumors. *Cell & Bioscience*, 9 (1): 88.

Liu, Y., Fang, B., Jiang, J., & Wang, P. (2016). Clinical efficacy and safety of high-dose Imatinib for chronic myeloid leukemia patients: An updated meta-analysis. *Journal of Cancer Research and Therapeutics*, 12 (5): 23-26.

Liu, Z. G., Yi, W., Tao, Y. L., Chan, H. C., Zeng, M. S., & Xia, Y. F. (2012). Aurora-A is an efficient marker for predicting poor prognosis in human nasopharyngeal carcinoma with aggressive local invasion: 208 cases with a 10-year follow-up from a single institution. *Oncology Letters*, 3 (6): 1237-1244.

Long, G. V., Hauschild, A., Santinami, M., Atkinson, V., Mandalà, M., Chiarion-Sileni, V., Larkin, J., Nyakas, M., Dutriaux, C., Haydon, A., Robert, C., Mortier, L., Schachter, J., Schadendorf, D., Lesimple, T., Plummer, R., Ji, R., Zhang, P., Mookerjee, B., Legos, J., … Kirkwood, J. M. (2017). Adjuvant Dabrafenib plus Trametinib in Stage III BRAF-Mutated Melanoma. *The New England Journal of Medicine*, 377(19), 1813–1823.

Long, G. V., Stroyakovskiy, D., Gogas, H., Levchenko, E., de Braud, F., Larkin, J., Garbe, C., Jouary, T., Hauschild, A., Grob, J. J., Chiarion-Sileni, V., Lebbe, C., Mandalà, M., Millward, M., Arance, A., Bondarenko, I., Haanen, J. B., Hansson, J., Utikal, J., Ferraresi, V., …

Flaherty, K. (2015). Dabrafenib and trametinib versus dabrafenib and placebo for Val600 BRAF-mutant melanoma: a multicentre, double-blind, phase 3 randomised controlled trial. *Lancet (London, England)*, 386(9992), 444–451.

Long, L., Luo, Y., Hou, Z. J., Ma, H. J., Long, Z. J., Tu, G. C., Huang, L. J., Liu, Q., & Lu G. (2018). Synthesis and biological evaluation of aurora kinases inhibitors based on n-trisubstituted pyrimidine scaffold. *European Journal of Medicinal Chemistry*, 145: 805-812.

Lorusso, P. M., Adjei, A. A., Varterasian, M., Gadgeel, S., Reid, J., Mitchell, D. Y., Hanson, L., DeLuca, P., Bruzek, L., Piens, J., Asbury, P., Becelaere, K. V., Herrera, R., Sebolt-Leopold, J. & Meyer, M. B. (2005). Phase I and pharmacodynamic study of the oral MEK inhibitor CI-1040 in patients with advanced malignancies. *Journal of Clinical Oncology*, 23 (23): 5281-93.

Lovly, C. M., Heuckmann, J. M., de Stanchina, E., Chen, H., Thomas, R. K., Liang, C., & Pao, W. (2011). Insights into ALK-driven cancers revealed through development of novel ALK tyrosine kinase inhibitors. *Cancer Research*, 71(14), 4920–4931.

Löwenberg, B., Muus, P., Ossenkoppele, G., Rousselot, P., Cahn, J. Y., Ifrah, N., Martinelli, G., Amadori, S., Berman, E., Sonneveld, P., Jongen-Lavrencic, M., Rigaudeau, S., Stockman, P., Goudie, A., Faderl, S., Jabbour, E., & Kantarjian, H. (2011). Phase 1/2 study to assess the safety, efficacy, and pharmacokinetics of barasertib (AZD1152) in patients with advanced acute myeloid leukemia. *Blood*, 118 (23): 6030-6036.

Lowery, D. M., Lim, D., & Yaffe, M. B. (2005). Structure and function of Polo-like kinases. *Oncogene*, 24 (2): 248-59.

Lucena-Araujo, A. R., de Oliveira, F. M., Leite-Cueva, S. D., dos Santos, G. A., Falcao, R. P., & Rego, E. M. (2011). High expression of AURKA and AURKB is associated with unfavorable cytogenetic abnormalities and high white blood cell count in patients with acute myeloid leukemia. *Leukemia Research*, 35 (2): 260-264.

Lussana, F., Cattaneo, M., Rambaldi, A., & Squizzato, A. (2018). Ruxolitinib-associated infections: A systematic review and meta-analysis. *American Journal of Hematology*, 93(3): 339–347.

Ma, J., Xing, W., Coffey, G., Dresser, K., Lu, K., Guo, A., Raca, G., Pandey, A., Conley, P., Yu, H., and Wang, Y. L. (2015). Cerdulatinib, a novel dual SYK/JAK kinase inhibitor, has broad anti-tumor activity in both ABC and GCB types of diffuse large B cell lymphoma. *Oncotarget*, 6 (41): 43881-96.

Macedo, L. T., da Costa Lima, A. B., & Sasse, A. D. (2012). Addition of bevacizumab to first-line chemotherapy in advanced colorectal cancer: a systematic review and meta-analysis, with emphasis on chemotherapy subgroups. *BMC cancer*, 12, 89.

Madanat, Y. F., Smith, M. R., Almasan, A., & Hill, B. T. (2016). Idelalisib therapy of indolent B-cell malignancies: chronic lymphocytic leukemia and small lymphocytic or follicular lymphomas. *Blood and Lymphatic Cancer: Targets and Therapy*, 6: 1–6.

Maddocks, K., Christian, B., Jaglowski, S., Flynn, J., Jones, J. A., Porcu, P., Wei, L., Jenkins, C., Lozanski, G., Byrd, J. C., & Blum, K. A. (2015). A phase 1/1b study of rituximab, bendamustine, and ibrutinib in patients with untreated and relapsed/refractory non-Hodgkin lymphoma. *Blood*, 125(2), 242–248.

Makker, V., Rasco, D., Vogelzang, N. J., Brose, M. S., Cohn, A. L., Mier, J., Di Simone, C., Hyman, D. M., Stepan, D. E., Dutcus, C. E., Schmidt, E. V., Guo, M., Sachdev, P., Shumaker, R., Aghajanian, C., & Taylor, M. (2019). Lenvatinib plus pembrolizumab in patients with advanced endometrial cancer: an interim analysis of a multicentre, open-label, single-arm, phase 2 trial. *The Lancet. Oncology*, 20(5), 711–718.

Manfredi, M. G., Ecsedy, J. A., Meetze, K. A., Balani, S. K., Burenkova, O., Chen, W., Galvin, K. M., Hoar, K. M., Huck, J. J., LeRoy, P. J., Ray, E. T., Sells, T. B., Stringer, B., Stroud, S. G., Vos, T. J., Weatherhead, G. S., Wysong, D. R., Zhang, M., Bolen, J. B., & Claiborne, C. F. (2007). Antitumor activity of MLN8054, an orally active small-molecule inhibitor of Aurora A kinase. *Proceedings of the National Academy of Sciences of the United States of America*, 104(10), 4106–4111.

Manley, P. W., Cowan-Jacob, S. W., Buchdunger, E., Fabbro, D., Fendrich, G., Furet, P., Meyer, T., & Zimmermann, J. (2002). Imatinib: a selective tyrosine kinase inhibitor. *European Journal of Cancer*, 38: S19-S27.

Manning, G., Whyte, D. B., Martinez, R., Hunter, T., & Sudarsanam, S. (2002). The protein kinase complement of the human genome. *Science (New York, N.Y.)*, 298(5600), 1912–1934.

Marchetti, A., Felicioni, L., Malatesta, S., Grazia Sciarrotta, M., Guetti, L., Chella, A., Viola, P., Pullara, C., Mucilli, F., & Buttitta, F. (2011). Clinical features and outcome of patients with non-small-cell lung cancer harboring BRAF mutations. *Journal of Clinical Oncology: Official Journal of the American Society of Clinical Oncology*, 29(26), 3574–3579.

Markham A. (2020). Selpercatinib: First Approval. *Drugs*, 10.1007/s40265-020-01343-7. Advance online publication.

Markham, M. J., Wachter, K., Agarwal, N., Bertagnolli, M. M., Chang, S. M., Dale, W., Diefenbach, C., Rodriguez-Galindo, C., George, D. J., Gilligan, T. D., Harvey, R. D., Johnson, M. L., Kimple, R. J., Knoll, M. A., LoConte, N., Maki, R. G., Meisel, J. L., Meyerhardt, J. A., Pennell, N. A., Rocque, G. B., … Westin, S. N. (2020). Clinical Cancer Advances 2020: Annual Report on Progress against Cancer From the American Society of Clinical Oncology. *Journal of Clinical Oncology: Official Journal of the American Society of Clinical Oncology,* 38(10), 1081.

Marsola, A. P. Z. C., Simões, B. P., Palma, L. C., Berzoti-Coelho, M. G., Burin, S. M., & de Castro, F. A. (2018). Expression of Hippo signaling pathway and aurora kinase genes in chronic myeloid leukemia. *Medical Oncology*, 35 (3): 26.

Martin, P., Bartlett, N. L., Blum, K. A., Park, S., Maddocks, K., Ruan, J., Ridling, L., Dittus, C., Chen, Z., Huang, X., Inghirami, G., DiLiberto, M., Chen-Kiang, S., & Leonard, J. P. (2019). A phase 1 trial of ibrutinib plus palbociclib in previously treated mantle cell lymphoma. *Blood*, 133(11), 1201–1204.

Mascarenhas, J., & Hoffman, R. (2012). Ruxolitinib: the first FDA approved therapy for the treatment of myelofibrosis. *Clinical Cancer Research*, 18(11): 3008–3014.

Masoud, V., & Pagès, G. (2017). Targeted therapies in breast cancer: New challenges to fight against resistance. *World Journal of Clinical Oncology*, 8(2), 120–134.

Mato, A. R., Hill, B. T., Lamanna, N., Barr, P. M., Ujjani, C. S., Brander, D. M., Howlett, C., Skarbnik, A. P., Cheson, B. D., Zent, C. S., Pu, J. J., Kiselev, P., Foon, K., Lenhart, J., Henick Bachow, S., Winter, A. M., Cruz, A. L., Claxton, D. F., Goy, A., Daniel, C., ... Nabhan, C. (2017). Optimal sequencing of ibrutinib, idelalisib, and venetoclax in chronic lymphocytic leukemia: results from a multicenter study of 683 patients. *Annals of Oncology: Official Journal of the European Society for Medical Oncology*, 28(5), 1050–1056.

Mato, A. R., Nabhan, C., Barr, P. M., Ujjani, C. S., Hill, B. T., Lamanna, N., Skarbnik, A. P., Howlett, C., Pu, J. J., Sehgal, A. R., Strelec, L. E., Vandegrift, A., Fitzpatrick, D. M., Zent, C. S., Feldman, T., Goy, A., Claxton, D. F., Bachow, S. H., Kaur, G., Svoboda, J., ... Evens, A. M. (2016). Outcomes of CLL patients treated with sequential kinase inhibitor therapy: a real world experience. *Blood*, 128(18), 2199–2205.

Matsubara, N., Naito, Y., Nakano, K., Fujiwara, Y., Ikezawa, H., Yusa, W., Namiki, M., Okude, T., & Takahashi, S. (2018). Lenvatinib in combination with everolimus in patients with advanced or metastatic renal cell carcinoma: A phase 1 study. *International Journal of Urology: official journal of the Japanese Urological Association*, 25(11), 922–928.

Maughan, T. S., Adams, R. A., Smith, C. G., Meade, A. M., Seymour, M. T., Wilson, R. H., Idziaszczyk, S., Harris, R., Fisher, D., Kenny, S. L., Kay, E., Mitchell, J. K., Madi, A., Jasani, B., James, M. D., Bridgewater, J., Kennedy, M. J., Claes, B., Lambrechts, D., Kaplan, R., ... MRC COIN Trial Investigators (2011). Addition of cetuximab to oxaliplatin-based first-line combination chemotherapy for treatment of advanced colorectal cancer: results of the randomised phase 3 MRC COIN trial. *Lancet (London, England)*, 377(9783), 2103–2114.

Maximov, P. Y., Lee, T. M., & Jordan, V. C. (2013). The discovery and development of selective estrogen receptor modulators (SERMs) for clinical practice. *Current Clinical Pharmacology*, 8(2), 135–155.

McAdoo, S. P., and Tam, F. W. K. (2011). Fostamatinib Disodium. *Drugs of the future*, 36 (4): 273-273.

McKeage, K. (2015). Ruxolitinib: A Review in Polycythaemia Vera. *Drugs*, 75(15): 1773–1781.

McLornan, D. P., Khan, A. A., & Harrison, C. N. (2015). Immunological Consequences of JAK Inhibition: Friend or Foe?. *Current Hematologic Malignancy Reports*, 10(4): 370–379.

Meenakshi Sundaram, D. N., Jiang, X., Brandwein, J. M., Valencia-Serna, J., Remant, K. C., & Uludağ, H. (2019). Current outlook on drug resistance in chronic myeloid leukemia (CML) and potential therapeutic options. *Drug Discovery Today*, 24 (7): 1355-1369.

Melichar, B., Adenis, A., Lockhart, A. C., Bennouna, J., Dees, E. C., Kayaleh, O., Obermannova, R., DeMichele, A., Zatloukal, P., Zhang, B., Ullmann, C. D., & Schusterbauer, C. (2015). Safety and activity of alisertib, an investigational aurora kinase A inhibitor, in patients with breast cancer, small-cell lung cancer, non-small-cell lung cancer, head and neck squamous-cell carcinoma, and gastro-oesophageal adenocarcinoma: a five-arm phase 2 study. *The Lancet. Oncology*, 16(4), 395–405.

Mensah, F. A., Blaize, J. P., & Bryan, L. J. (2018). Spotlight on copanlisib and its potential in the treatment of relapsed/refractory follicular lymphoma: evidence to date. *OncoTargets and Therapy*, 11: 4817–4827.

Mian, A. A., Rafiei, A., Haberbosch, I., Zeifman, A., Titov, I., Stroylov, V., Metodieva, A., Stroganov, O., Novikov, F., Brill, B., Chilov, G., Hoelzer, D., Ottmann, O. G., & Ruthardt, M. (2015). PF-114, a potent and selective inhibitor of native and mutated BCR/ABL is active against Philadelphia chromosome-positive (Ph+) leukemias harboring the T315I mutation. *Leukemia*, 29(5), 1104–1114.

Miller, K., Wang, M., Gralow, J., Dickler, M., Cobleigh, M., Perez, E. A., Shenkier, T., Cella, D., & Davidson, N. E. (2007). Paclitaxel plus bevacizumab versus paclitaxel alone for metastatic breast cancer. *The New England journal of medicine,* 357(26), 2666–2676.

Minden, M. D., Stock, W, Crosswell, H., Siegel, R. D., Chun, P., Abella, S., He, J., Eng, C., & Douer, D. (2015). A Phase 1b, Open-Label, Dose Escalation and Expansion Study Evaluating the Safety and Efficacy of Entospletinib (GS-9973) with Vincristine and Dexamethasone in Adult Subjects with Relapsed or Refractory Acute Lymphoid Leukemia (ALL). *Blood*, 126 (23): 4866.

Minden, M. D., Stock, W., Crosswell, H., Siegel, R. D., Chun, P., Abella, S., He, J., Eng, C., and Douer, D. (2015). A Phase 1b, Open-Label, Dose Escalation and Expansion Study Evaluating the Safety and Efficacy of Entospletinib (GS-9973) with Vincristine and Dexamethasone in Adult Subjects with Relapsed or Refractory Acute Lymphoid Leukemia (ALL). *Blood*, 126 (23): 4866-4866.

Mócsai, A., Ruland, J., & Tybulewicz, V. L. J. (2010). The SYK tyrosine kinase: a crucial player in diverse biological functions. *Nature Reviews Immunology*, 10 (6): 387-402.

Mok, T. S., Wu, Y. L., Thongprasert, S., Yang, C. H., Chu, D. T., Saijo, N., Sunpaweravong, P., Han, B., Margono, B., Ichinose, Y., Nishiwaki, Y., Ohe, Y., Yang, J. J., Chewaskulyong, B., Jiang, H., Duffield, E. L., Watkins, C. L., Armour, A. A., & Fukuoka, M. (2009). Gefitinib or carboplatin-paclitaxel in pulmonary adenocarcinoma. *The New England Journal of Medicine*, 361(10), 947–957.

Moore, M. J., Goldstein, D., Hamm, J., Figer, A., Hecht, J. R., Gallinger, S., Au, H. J., Murawa, P., Walde, D., Wolff, R. A., Campos, D., Lim, R., Ding, K., Clark, G., Voskoglou-Nomikos, T., Ptasynski, M., Parulekar, W., & National Cancer Institute of Canada Clinical Trials Group (2007). Erlotinib plus gemcitabine compared with gemcitabine alone in patients with advanced pancreatic cancer: a phase III trial of the National Cancer Institute of Canada Clinical Trials Group. *Journal of clinical oncology: official journal of the American Society of Clinical Oncology*, 25(15), 1960–1966.

Moreno, C., Greil, R., Demirkan, F., Tedeschi, A., Anz, B., Larratt, L., Simkovic, M., Samoilova, O., Novak, J., Ben-Yehuda, D., Strugov, V.,

Gill, D., Gribben, J. G., Hsu, E., Lih, C. J., Zhou, C., Clow, F., James, D. F., Styles, L., & Flinn, I. W. (2019). Ibrutinib plus obinutuzumab versus chlorambucil plus obinutuzumab in first-line treatment of chronic lymphocytic leukaemia (iLLUMINATE): a multicentre, randomised, open-label, phase 3 trial. *The Lancet. Oncology*, 20(1), 43–56.

Morris, S. W., Kirstein, M. N., Valentine, M. B., Dittmer, K. G., Shapiro, D. N., Saltman, D. L., & Look, A. T. (1994). Fusion of a kinase gene, ALK, to a nucleolar protein gene, NPM, in non-Hodgkin's lymphoma. *Science (New York, N.Y.)*, 263(5151), 1281–1284.

Mortlock, A. A., Foote, K. M., Heron, N. M., Jung, F. H., Pasquet, G., Lohmann, J. J., Warin, N., Renaud, F., De Savi, C., Roberts, N. J., Johnson, T., Dousson, C. B., Hill, G. B., Perkins, D., Hatter, G., Wilkinson, R. W., Wedge, S. R., Heaton, S. P., Odedra, R., Keen, N. J., … Green, S. (2007). Discovery, synthesis, and in vivo activity of a new class of pyrazoloquinazolines as selective inhibitors of aurora B kinase. *Journal of Medicinal Chemistry*, 50(9), 2213–2224.

Motzer, R. J., Hutson, T. E., Glen, H., Michaelson, M. D., Molina, A., Eisen, T., Jassem, J., Zolnierek, J., Maroto, J. P., Mellado, B., Melichar, B., Tomasek, J., Kremer, A., Kim, H. J., Wood, K., Dutcus, C., & Larkin, J. (2015). Lenvatinib, everolimus, and the combination in patients with metastatic renal cell carcinoma: a randomised, phase 2, open-label, multicentre trial. *The Lancet. Oncology*, 16(15), 1473–1482.

Mullally, A., Hood, J., Harrison, C., & Mesa, R. (2020). Fedratinib in myelofibrosis. *Blood Advances*, 4(8): 1792–1800.

Muller R. (2019). JAK inhibitors in 2019, synthetic review in 10 points. *European Journal of Internal Medicine*, 66: 9–17.

Mulligan L. M. (2014). RET revisited: expanding the oncogenic portfolio. *Nature reviews. Cancer*, 14(3), 173–186.

Munir, T., Brown, J. R., O'Brien, S., Barrientos, J. C., Barr, P. M., Reddy, N. M., Coutre, S., Tam, C. S., Mulligan, S. P., Jaeger, U., Kipps, T. J., Moreno, C., Montillo, M., Burger, J. A., Byrd, J. C., Hillmen, P., Dai, S., Szoke, A., Dean, J. P., & Woyach, J. A. (2019). Final analysis from RESONATE: Up to six years of follow-up on ibrutinib in patients with previously treated chronic lymphocytic leukemia or small lymphocytic lymphoma. *American Journal of Hematology*, 94(12), 1353–1363.

Muranen, T., Selfors, L. M., Worster, D. T., Iwanicki, M. P., Song, L., Morales, F. C., Gao, S., Mills, G. B., & Brugge, J. S. (2012). Inhibition of PI3K/mTOR leads to adaptive resistance in matrix-attached cancer cells. *Cancer Cell*, 21(2), 227–239.

Murugan, A. K., Dong, J., Xie, J. & Xing, M. (2009). MEK1 mutations, but not ERK2 mutations, occur in melanomas and colon carcinomas, but none in thyroid carcinomas. *Cell Cycle*, 8 (13): 2122-4.

Nagar, B., Hantschel, O., Young, M. A., Scheffzek, K., Veach, D., Bornmann, W., Clarkson, B., Superti-Furga, G., & Kuriyan, J. (2003). Structural basis for the autoinhibition of c-Abl tyrosine kinase. *Cell*, 112 (6): 859-71.

Nair, K. S., & Cheson, B. (2016). The role of idelalisib in the treatment of relapsed and refractory chronic lymphocytic leukemia. *Therapeutic Advances in Hematology*, 7(2): 69–84.

Nakagawa, K., Garon, E. B., Seto, T., Nishio, M., Ponce Aix, S., Paz-Ares, L., Chiu, C. H., Park, K., Novello, S., Nadal, E., Imamura, F., Yoh, K., Shih, J. Y., Au, K. H., Moro-Sibilot, D., Enatsu, S., Zimmermann, A., Frimodt-Moller, B., Visseren-Grul, C., Reck, M., … RELAY Study Investigators (2019). Ramucirumab plus erlotinib in patients with untreated, EGFR-mutated, advanced non-small-cell lung cancer (RELAY): a randomised, double-blind, placebo-controlled, phase 3 trial. *The Lancet. Oncology*, 20(12), 1655–1669.

Nastoupil, L. J., Lunning, M. A., Vose, J. M., Schreeder, M. T., Siddiqi, T., Flowers, C. R., Cohen, J. B., Burger, J. A., Wierda, W. G., O'Brien, S., Sportelli, P., Miskin, H. P., Purdom, M. A., Weiss, M. S., & Fowler, N. H. (2019). Tolerability and activity of ublituximab, umbralisib, and ibrutinib in patients with chronic lymphocytic leukaemia and non-Hodgkin lymphoma: a phase 1 dose escalation and expansion trial. *The Lancet. Haematology*, 6(2), e100–e109.

Navada, S. C., & Silverman, L. R. (2016). The safety and efficacy of Rigosertib in the treatment of myelodysplastic syndromes. *Expert Review of Anticancer Therapy*, 16 (8): 805-10.

Nazha, A., Sekeres, M. A., Komrokji, R., Steensma, D. P., Kantarjian, H., Roboz, G., Fenaux, P., Prebet, T., Azarnia, N., Zbyszewski, P. S., Fruchtman, S. M., Santini, V., Silverman, L. R., Platzbecker, U., & Garcia-Manero, G. (2017). Validation of a post-Hypomethylating agent failure prognostic model in Myelodysplastic Syndromes patients treated in a randomized controlled Phase III Trial of Rigosertib vs. Best Supportive Care. *Blood Cancer Journal*, 7 (12): 644.

Nelson, V., Ziehr, J., Agulnik, M., & Johnson, M. (2013). Afatinib: emerging next-generation tyrosine kinase inhibitor for NSCLC. *OncoTargets and therapy*, 6, 135–143.

Neul, C., Schaeffeler, E., Sparreboom, A., Laufer, S., Schwab, M., & Nies, A. T. (2016). Impact of Membrane Drug Transporters on Resistance to Small-Molecule Tyrosine Kinase Inhibitors. *Trends in Pharmacological Sciences*, 37 (11): 904-932.

Neuman L. L., Ward, R., Arnold, D., Combs, D. L., Gruver, D., Hill, W., Kunjom, J. M., Miller, L. L. & Fox, J. A. (2016). First-in-Human Phase 1a Study of the Safety, Pharmacokinetics, and Pharmacodynamics of the Noncovalent Bruton Tyrosine Kinase (BTK) Inhibitor SNS-062 in Healthy Subjects. *Blood*, 128(22): 2032.

Nguyen, T., Parker, R., Hawkins, E., Holkova, B., Yazbeck, V., Kolluri, A., Kmieciak, M., Rahmani, M., & Grant, S. (2017). Synergistic interactions between PLK1 and HDAC inhibitors in non-Hodgkin's lymphoma cells occur in vitro and in vivo and proceed through multiple mechanisms. *Oncotarget*, 8 (19): 31478-31493.

Nikolaev, S. I., Rimoldi, D., Iseli, C., Valsesia, A., Robyr, D., Gehrig, C., Harshman, K., Guipponi, M., Bukach, O., Zoete, V., Michielin, O., Muehlethaler, K., Speiser, D., Beckmann, J. S., Xenarios, I., Halazonetis, T. D., Jongeneel, C. V., Stevenson, B. J., & Antonarakis, S. E. (2011). Exome sequencing identifies recurrent somatic MAP2K1 and MAP2K2 mutations in melanoma. *Nature Genetics*, 44 (2): 133-9.

Norman, P. (2014). Spleen tyrosine kinase inhibitors: a review of the patent literature 2010 – 2013. *Expert Opinion on Therapeutic Patents*, 24 (5): 573-595.

Nwizu, T., Kanteti, R., Kawada, I., Rolle, C., Vokes, E. E., & Salgia, R. (2011). Crizotinib (PF02341066) as a ALK /MET inhibitor- Special Emphasis as a Therapeutic Drug against Lung Cancer. *Drugs of the future,* 36(2), 91–99.

O'Brien, S. G., Guilhot, F., Larson, R. A., Gathmann, I., Baccarani, M., Cervantes, F., Cornelissen, J. J., Fischer, T., Hochhaus, A., Hughes, T., Lechner, K., Nielsen, J. L., Rousselot, P., Reiffers, J., Saglio, G., Shepherd, J., Simonsson, B., Gratwohl, A., Goldman, J. M., Kantarjian, H., … IRIS Investigators (2003). Imatinib compared with interferon and low-dose cytarabine for newly diagnosed chronic-phase chronic myeloid leukemia. *The New England Journal of Medicine*, 348(11), 994–1004.

O'Brien, S. M., Lamanna, N., Kipps, T. J., Flinn, I., Zelenetz, A. D., Burger, J. A., Keating, M., Mitra, S., Holes, L., Yu, A. S., Johnson, D. M., Miller, L. L., Kim, Y., Dansey, R. D., Dubowy, R. L., & Coutre, S. E. (2015). A phase 2 study of idelalisib plus rituximab in treatment-naïve older patients with chronic lymphocytic leukemia. *Blood*, 126(25), 2686–2694.

O'Brien, S., Furman, R. R., Coutre, S. E., Sharman, J. P., Burger, J. A., Blum, K. A., Grant, B., Richards, D. A., Coleman, M., Wierda, W. G., Jones, J. A., Zhao, W., Heerema, N. A., Johnson, A. J., Izumi, R., Hamdy, A., Chang, B. Y., Graef, T., Clow, F., Buggy, J. J., … Byrd, J. C. (2014). Ibrutinib as initial therapy for elderly patients with chronic lymphocytic leukaemia or small lymphocytic lymphoma: an open-label, multicentre, phase 1b/2 trial. *The Lancet. Oncology*, 15(1), 48–58.

O'Brien, S., Furman, R. R., Coutre, S., Flinn, I. W., Burger, J. A., Blum, K., Sharman, J., Wierda, W., Jones, J., Zhao, W., Heerema, N. A., Johnson, A. J., Luan, Y., James, D. F., Chu, A. D., & Byrd, J. C. (2018). Single-agent ibrutinib in treatment-naïve and relapsed/refractory chronic lymphocytic leukemia: a 5-year experience. *Blood*, 131(17), 1910–1919.

O'Brien, S., Hillmen, P., Coutre, S., Barr, P. M., Fraser, G., Tedeschi, A., Burger, J. A., Dilhuydy, M. S., Hess, G., Moreno, C., Cramer, P., Liu, E., Chang, S., Vermeulen, J., Styles, L., Howes, A., James, D. F., Patel,

K., Graef, T., & Valentino, R. (2018). Safety Analysis of Four Randomized Controlled Studies of Ibrutinib in Patients With Chronic Lymphocytic Leukemia/Small Lymphocytic Lymphoma or Mantle Cell Lymphoma. *Clinical Lymphoma, Myeloma & Leukemia*, 18(10), 648–657.e15.

O'Brien, S., Jones, J. A., Coutre, S. E., Mato, A. R., Hillmen, P., Tam, C., Österborg, A., Siddiqi, T., Thirman, M. J., Furman, R. R., Ilhan, O., Keating, M. J., Call, T. G., Brown, J. R., Stevens-Brogan, M., Li, Y., Clow, F., James, D. F., Chu, A. D., Hallek, M., … Stilgenbauer, S. (2016). Ibrutinib for patients with relapsed or refractory chronic lymphocytic leukaemia with 17p deletion (RESONATE-17): a phase 2, open-label, multicentre study. *The Lancet. Oncology*, 17(10), 1409–1418.

O'Connor, O. A., Özcan, M., Jacobsen, E. D., Roncero, J. M., Trotman, J., Demeter, J., Masszi, T., Pereira, J., Ramchandren, R., Beaven, A., Caballero, D., Horwitz, S. M., Lennard, A., Turgut, M., Hamerschlak, N., d'Amore, F. A., Foss, F., Kim, W. S., Leonard, J. P., Zinzani, P. L., … Lumiere Study Investigators (2019). Randomized Phase III Study of Alisertib or Investigator's Choice (Selected Single Agent) in Patients With Relapsed or Refractory Peripheral T-Cell Lymphoma. *Journal of Clinical Oncology: Official Journal of the American Society of Clinical Oncology*, 37(8), 613–623.

O'Hare, T., Shakespeare, W. C., Zhu, X., Eide, C. A., Rivera, V. M., Wang, F., Adrian, L. T., Zhou, T., Huang, W. S., Xu, Q., Metcalf, C. A., 3rd, Tyner, J. W., Loriaux, M. M., Corbin, A. S., Wardwell, S., Ning, Y., Keats, J. A., Wang, Y., Sundaramoorthi, R., Thomas, M., … Clackson, T. (2009). AP24534, a pan-BCR-ABL inhibitor for chronic myeloid leukemia, potently inhibits the T315I mutant and overcomes mutation-based resistance. *Cancer Cell*, 16(5), 401–412.

Ohren, J. F., Chen, H., Pavlovsky, A., Whitehead, C., Zhang, E., Kuffa, P., Yan, C., McConnell, P., Spessard, C., Banotai, C., Mueller, W. T., Delaney, A., Omer, C., Sebolt-Leopold, J., Dudley, D. T., Leung, I. K., Flamme, C., Warmus, J., Kaufman, M., Barrett, S., … Hasemann, C. A. (2004). Structures of human MAP kinase kinase 1 (MEK1) and MEK2 describe novel noncompetitive kinase inhibition. *Nature Structural & Molecular Biology*, 11(12), 1192–1197.

Oki Y., Haverkos B., Zain J. M., Lechowicz, M. J., Devata, S., Korman, N. J., Ramchandren, R., Pinter-Brown, L. C., Barde, P. J., Nair, A., Huen, A. (2018). Tenalisib, a dual PI3K δ/γ inhibitor: Safety and efficacy results from an on-going phase I/Ib study in relapsed/refractory T-cell lymphoma. *Journal of Clinical Oncology* 36(15): 7510-7510.

Otto, T., & Sicinski, P. (2017). Cell cycle proteins as promising targets in cancer therapy. *Nature reviews. Cancer*, 17(2), 93–115.

Ou, S. I., Zhu, V. W., & Nagasaka, N., Catalog of 5' Fusion Partners in ALK-positive NSCLC Circa 2020. *JTO Clinical and Research Reports*, 1:100015.

Özgür Yurttaş, N., & Eşkazan, A. E. (2020). Novel therapeutic approaches in chronic myeloid leukemia. *Leukemia Research*, 91: 106337.

Papadopoulos, N., & Lennartsson, J. (2018). The PDGF/PDGFR pathway as a drug target. *Molecular aspects of medicine*, 62, 75–88.

Pardanani, A., Harrison, C., Cortes, J. E., Cervantes, F., Mesa, R. A., Milligan, D., Masszi, T., Mishchenko, E., Jourdan, E., Vannucchi, A. M., Drummond, M. W., Jurgutis, M., Kuliczkowski, K., Gheorghita, E., Passamonti, F., Neumann, F., Patki, A., Gao, G., & Tefferi, A. (2015). Safety and Efficacy of Fedratinib in Patients with Primary or Secondary Myelofibrosis: A Randomized Clinical Trial. *JAMA oncology*, 1(5), 643–651.

Park, S. R., Speranza, G., Piekarz, R., Wright, J. J., Kinders, R. J., Wang, L., Pfister, T., Trepel, J. B., Lee, M. J., Alarcon, S., Steinberg, S. M., Collins, J., Doroshow, J. H., and Kummar, S. (2013). A multi-histology trial of fostamatinib in patients with advanced colorectal, non-small cell lung, head and neck, thyroid, and renal cell carcinomas, and pheochromocytomas. *Cancer Chemotherapy and Pharmacology*, 71 (4): 981-90.

Patel, A. B., O'Hare, T., & Deininger, M. W. (2017). Mechanisms of Resistance to ABL Kinase Inhibition in Chronic Myeloid Leukemia and the Development of Next Generation ABL Kinase Inhibitors. *Hematology Oncology clinics of North America*, 31 (4): 589-612.

Pellegrino, R., Calvisi, D. F., Ladu, S., Ehemann, V., Staniscia, T., Evert, M., Dombrowski, F., Schirmacher, P., & Longerich, T. (2010). Oncogenic and Tumor Suppressive Roles of Polo-like kinases in human hepatocellular carcinoma. *Hepatology*, 51 (3): 857-868.

Perez, E. A., Romond, E. H., Suman, V. J., Jeong, J. H., Davidson, N. E., Geyer, C. E., Jr, Martino, S., Mamounas, E. P., Kaufman, P. A., & Wolmark, N. (2011). Four-year follow-up of trastuzumab plus adjuvant chemotherapy for operable human epidermal growth factor receptor 2-positive breast cancer: joint analysis of data from NCCTG N9831 and NSABP B-31. *Journal of clinical oncology: official journal of the American Society of Clinical Oncology*, 29(25), 3366–3373.

Perez, E. A., Romond, E. H., Suman, V. J., Jeong, J. H., Sledge, G., Geyer, C. E., Jr, Martino, S., Rastogi, P., Gralow, J., Swain, S. M., Winer, E. P., Colon-Otero, G., Davidson, N. E., Mamounas, E., Zujewski, J. A., & Wolmark, N. (2014). Trastuzumab plus adjuvant chemotherapy for human epidermal growth factor receptor 2-positive breast cancer: planned joint analysis of overall survival from NSABP B-31 and NCCTG N9831. *Journal of clinical oncology: official journal of the American Society of Clinical Oncology*, 32(33), 3744–3752.

Perl, A. E., Martinelli, G., Cortes, J. E., Neubauer, A., Berman, E., Paolini, S., Montesinos, P., Baer, M. R., Larson, R. A., Ustun, C., Fabbiano, F., Erba, H. P., Di Stasi, A., Stuart, R., Olin, R., Kasner, M., Ciceri, F., Chou, W. C., Podoltsev, N., Recher, C., … Levis, M. J. (2019). Gilteritinib or Chemotherapy for Relapsed or Refractory FLT3-Mutated AML. *The New England Journal of Medicine*, 381(18), 1728–1740.

Petrich, A. M., Gordon, L. I., Infante, J. R., Madan, S., Giles, F. J., Nimeiri, H. S., Kaplan, J. B., Stumpo, K., Zhang, B., Faucette, S., Shou, Y., and Shih, K. C. (2015). Phase 1 Dose-Escalation Study of TAK-659, an Investigational SYK Inhibitor, in Patients (Pts) with Advanced Solid Tumor or Lymphoma Malignancies. *Blood*, 126 (23): 2693-2693.

Piccart-Gebhart, M. J., Procter, M., Leyland-Jones, B., Goldhirsch, A., Untch, M., Smith, I., Gianni, L., Baselga, J., Bell, R., Jackisch, C., Cameron, D., Dowsett, M., Barrios, C. H., Steger, G., Huang, C. S., Andersson, M., Inbar, M., Lichinitser, M., Láng, I., Nitz, U., …

Herceptin Adjuvant (HERA) Trial Study Team (2005). Trastuzumab after adjuvant chemotherapy in HER2-positive breast cancer. *The New England Journal of Medicine*, 353(16), 1659–1672.

Pietrantonio, F., Cremolini, C., Petrelli, F., Di Bartolomeo, M., Loupakis, F., Maggi, C., Antoniotti, C., de Braud, F., Falcone, A., & Iacovelli, R. (2015). First-line anti-EGFR monoclonal antibodies in panRAS wild-type metastatic colorectal cancer: A systematic review and meta-analysis. *Critical reviews in oncology/hematology*, 96(1), 156–166.

Pirker, R., Pereira, J. R., Szczesna, A., von Pawel, J., Krzakowski, M., Ramlau, R., Vynnychenko, I., Park, K., Yu, C. T., Ganul, V., Roh, J. K., Bajetta, E., O'Byrne, K., de Marinis, F., Eberhardt, W., Goddemeier, T., Emig, M., Gatzemeier, U., & FLEX Study Team (2009). Cetuximab plus chemotherapy in patients with advanced non-small-cell lung cancer (FLEX): an open-label randomised phase III trial. *Lancet (London, England)*, 373(9674), 1525–1531.

Planchard D., Mazieres J., Riely G. J., Rudin C. M., Barlesi F., Quoix E. A., Souquet, P. J., Socinski, M. A., Switzky, J., Ma, B., Goodman, V. L., Carson, S. W., Curtis, C. M., Streit, M. R. W., Johnson, B. E. (2013). Interim results of phase II study BRF113928 of dabrafenib in BRAF V600E mutation–positive non-small cell lung cancer (NSCLC) patients. *Journal of Clinical Oncolology,* 31(15_suppl):8009.

Planchard, D., Besse, B., Groen, H., Souquet, P. J., Quoix, E., Baik, C. S., Barlesi, F., Kim, T. M., Mazieres, J., Novello, S., Rigas, J. R., Upalawanna, A., D'Amelio, A. M., Jr, Zhang, P., Mookerjee, B., & Johnson, B. E. (2016a). Dabrafenib plus trametinib in patients with previously treated BRAF(V600E)-mutant metastatic non-small cell lung cancer: an open-label, multicentre phase 2 trial. *The Lancet. Oncology*, 17(7), 984–993.

Planchard, D., Kim, T. M., Mazieres, J., Quoix, E., Riely, G., Barlesi, F., Souquet, P. J., Smit, E. F., Groen, H. J., Kelly, R. J., Cho, B. C., Socinski, M. A., Pandite, L., Nase, C., Ma, B., D'Amelio, A., Jr, Mookerjee, B., Curtis, C. M., Jr, & Johnson, B. E. (2016b). Dabrafenib in patients with BRAF(V600E)-positive advanced non-small-cell lung cancer: a single-arm, multicentre, open-label, phase 2 trial. *The Lancet. Oncology*, 17(5), 642–650.

Planchard, D., Popat, S., Kerr, K., Novello, S., Smit, E. F., Faivre-Finn, C., Mok, T. S., Reck, M., Van Schil, P. E., Hellmann, M. D., Peters, S., & ESMO Guidelines Committee. Electronic address: clinicalguidelines @esmo.org (2018). Metastatic non-small cell lung cancer: ESMO Clinical Practice Guidelines for diagnosis, treatment and follow-up. *Annals of Oncology: Official Journal of the European Society for Medical Oncology*, 29 Suppl 4, iv192–iv237.

Planchard, D., Popat, S., Kerr, K., Novello, S., Smit, E. F., Faivre-Finn, C., Mok, T. S., Reck, M., Van Schil, P. E., Hellmann, M. D., & Peters, S. (2019). Correction to: "Metastatic non-small cell lung cancer: ESMO Clinical Practice Guidelines for diagnosis, treatment and follow-up." *Annals of Oncology: Official Journal of the European Society for Medical Oncology*, 30(5), 863–870.

Planchard, D., Smit, E. F., Groen, H. J. M., Mazieres, J., Besse, B., Helland, A., Giannone, V., D'Amelio Jr, A. M., Zhang, P., Mookerjee, B., & Johnson, B. E. (2017). Dabrafenib plus Trametinib in patients with previously untreated BRAF V600E-mutant metastatic non-small-cell lung cancer: An open-label, phase 2 trial. *The Lancet. Oncology*, 18 (10): 1307-1316.

Pratz, K., Levis, M. J., Morris, J. C., Trisha Wise-Draper, T., Levy, M., Bixby, D. L., Burke, P., Hernandez, D., Stumpo, K., Kannan, K., Sheldon-Waniga, E., Wang, S., Zhang, S., Shou, Y., Altman, MD, J. K., Kaplan, J., Frankfurt, O. (2017). A Phase (ph) 1b/2 Study of TAK-659, an Investigational Dual FLT-3 and SYK Inhibitor, in Patients (Pts) with Relapsed or Refractory Acute Myelogenous Leukemia (R/R AML). *Blood*, 130 (Supplement 1): 2622.

Pujade-Lauraine, E., Selle, F., Weber, B., Ray-Coquard, I. L., Vergote, I., Sufliarsky, J., Del Campo, J. M., Lortholary, A., Lesoin, A., Follana, P., Freyer, G., Pardo, B., Vidal, L., Tholander, B., Gladieff, L., Sassi, M., Garin-Chesa, P., Nazabadioko, S., Marzin, K., Pilz, K., … Joly, F. (2016). Volasertib Versus Chemotherapy in Platinum-Resistant or -Refractory Ovarian Cancer: A Randomized Phase II Groupe des

Investigateurs Nationaux pour l'Etude des Cancers de l'Ovaire Study. *Journal of Clinical Oncology: Official Journal of the American Society of Clinical Oncology*, 34(7), 706–713.

Puła, B., Gołos, A., Górniak, P., & Jamroziak, K (2019). Overcoming Ibrutinib Resistance in Chronic Lymphocytic Leukemia. *Cancers*, 11:1834-1858.

Purroy, N., Carabia, J., Abrisqueta, P., Egia, L., Aguiló, M., Carpio, C., Palacio, C., Crespo, M., and Bosch, F. (2017). Inhibition of BCR signaling using the Syk inhibitor TAK-659 prevents stroma-mediated signaling in chronic lymphocytic leukemia cells. *Oncotarget*, 8 (1): 742-756.

Pushpam, D., & Bakhshi, S. (2020). Pharmacology of tyrosine kinase inhibitors in chronic myeloid leukemia; a clinician's perspective. *DARU Journal of Pharmaceutical Sciences*, 28 (1): 371-385.

Puttini, M., Coluccia, A. M. L., Boschelli, F., Cleris, L., Marchesi, E., Donella-Deana, A., Ahmed, S., Redaelli, S., Piazza, R., Magistroni, V., Andreoni, F., Scapozza, L., Formelli, F., & Gambacorti-Passerini, C. (2006). In vitro and In vivo Activity of SKI-606, a Novel Src-Abl Inhibitor, against Imatinib-Resistant Bcr-Abl+ Neoplastic Cells. *Cancer Research*, 66 (23): 11314-11322.

Qi, J., Gao, X., Zhong, X., Zhang, N., Wang, R., Zhang, H., Pan, T., Liu, X., Yao, Y., Wu, Q., Niu, M., & Xu, K. (2019). Selective inhibition of Aurora A and B kinases effectively induces cell cycle arrest in t(8;21) acute myeloid leukemia. *Biomedicine & pharmacotherapy*, 117, 109113.

Qi, W. X., Shen, Z., Lin, F., Sun, Y. J., Min, D. L., Tang, L. N., He, A. N., & Yao, Y. (2013). Incidence and risk of hypertension with vandetanib in cancer patients: a systematic review and meta-analysis of clinical trials. *British Journal of Clinical Pharmacology*, 75(4), 919–930.

Qin, S., Li, J., Wang, L., Xu, J., Cheng, Y., Bai, Y., Li, W., Xu, N., Lin, L. Z., Wu, Q., Li, Y., Yang, J., Pan, H., Ouyang, X., Qiu, W., Wu, K., Xiong, J., Dai, G., Liang, H., Hu, C., … Liu, T. (2018). Efficacy and Tolerability of First-Line Cetuximab Plus Leucovorin, Fluorouracil, and Oxaliplatin (FOLFOX-4) Versus FOLFOX-4 in Patients with RAS

Wild-Type Metastatic Colorectal Cancer: The Open-Label, Randomized, Phase III TAILOR Trial. *Journal of clinical oncology: official journal of the American Society of Clinical Oncology*, 36(30), 3031–3039.

Raedler L. A. (2015). Jakafi (Ruxolitinib): First FDA-Approved Medication for the Treatment of Patients with Polycythemia Vera. *American Health & Drug Benefits*, 8(Spec Feature): 75–79.

Ramanathan, S., Di Paolo, J. A., Jin, F., Shao, L., Sharma, S., Robeson, M., and Kearney, B. P. (2017). Pharmacokinetics, Pharmacodynamics, and Safety of Entospletinib, a Novel pSYK Inhibitor, Following Single and Multiple Oral Dosing in Healthy Volunteers. *Clinical Drug Investigation*, 37 (2): 195-205.

Ramanathan, S., Jin, F., Sharma, S., & Kearney, B. P. (2016). Clinical Pharmacokinetic and Pharmacodynamic Profile of Idelalisib. *Clinical Pharmacokinetics*, 55(1): 33–45.

Rawlings, J. S., Rosler, K. M., & Harrison, D. A. (2004). The JAK/STAT signaling pathway. *Journal of cell science,* 117(Pt 8): 1281–1283.

Rea, D. (2015). Management of adverse events associated with tyrosine kinase inhibitors in chronic myeloid leukemia. *Annals of Hematology*, 94 (2): 149-158.

Recio, Carlota. 2018. "JAK, an Oncokinase in Hematological Cancer." In *Tyrosine Kinases as Druggable Targets in Cancer,* edited by Huan Ren, 1-25. *IntechOpen*.

Reckamp, K. L., Infante, J. R., Blumenschein, G. R., Wakelee, H., Carter, C. A., Gockerman, J. P., Lovly, C., Dukart, G., Harrow, K., Liang, C., Gibbons, J. J., & Horn, L. (2016) Phase I/II trial of X-396, a novel anaplastic lymphoma kinase (ALK) inhibitor, in patients with ALKþ non-small cell lung cancer (NSCLC). *Journal of Thoracic Oncology*, 11(suppl):S36–37.

Redaelli, S., Mologni, L., Rostagno, R., Piazza, R., Magistroni, V., Ceccon, M., Viltadi, M., Flynn, D., & Gambacorti-Passerini, C. (2012). Three novel patient-derived BCR/ABL mutants show different sensitivity to second and third generation tyrosine kinase inhibitors. *American Journal of Hematology*, 87 (11): E125-E128.

Reindl, W., Yuan, J., Krämer, A., Strebhardt, K., & Berg, T. (2008). Inhibition of polo-like kinase 1 by blocking polo-box domain-dependent protein-protein interactions. *Chemistry & Biology*, 15(5), 459–466..

Ren, X., Pan, X., Zhang, Z., Wang, D., Lu, X., Li, Y., Wen, D., Long, H., Luo, J., Feng, Y., Zhuang, X., Zhang, F., Liu, J., Leng, F., Lang, X., Bai, Y., She, M., Tu, Z., Pan, J., & Ding, K. (2013). Identification of GZD824 as an Orally Bioavailable Inhibitor That Targets Phosphorylated and Nonphosphorylated Breakpoint Cluster Region–Abelson (Bcr-Abl) Kinase and Overcomes Clinically Acquired Mutation-Induced Resistance against Imatinib. *Journal of Medicinal Chemistry,* 56 (3): 879-894.

Ribas, A., Gonzalez, R., Pavlick, A., Hamid, O., Gajewski, T. F., Daud, A., Flaherty, L., Logan, T., Chmielowski, B., Lewis, K., Kee, D., Boasberg, P., Yin, M., Chan, I., Musib, L., Choong, N., Puzanov, I., & McArthur, G. A. (2014). Combination of vemurafenib and cobimetinib in patients with advanced BRAF(V600)-mutated melanoma: A phase 1b study. *The Lancet Oncology*, 15 (9): 954-65.

Ribas, A., Kim, K. B., Schuchter, L. M., Gonzalez, R., Pavlick, A. C., Weber, J. S., McArthur, G. A., Hutson, T. E., Flaherty, K. T., Moschos, J. S., Lawrence, D. P., Hersey, P., Kefford, R. F., Chmielowski, B., Puzanov, I., Li, J., Nolop, K. B., Lee, R. J., Joe, A. K., Sosman, J. A. (2011). BRIM-2: An open-label, multicenter phase II study of vemurafenib in previously treated patients with BRAF V600E mutation-positive metastatic melanoma. *Journal of Clinical Oncology*, 29: 15_suppl (May 20, 2011) 8509-8509.

Rice, K. D., Aay, N., Anand, N. K., Blazey, C. M., Bowles, O. J., Bussenius, J., Costanzo, S., Curtis, J. K., Defina, S. C., Dubenko, L., Engst, S., Joshi, A. A., Kennedy, A. R., Kim, A. I., Koltun, E. S., Lougheed, J. C., Manalo, J. C., Martini, J. F., Nuss, J. M., Peto, C. J., … Johnston, S. (2012). Novel Carboxamide-Based Allosteric MEK Inhibitors: Discovery and Optimization Efforts toward XL518 (GDC-0973). *ACS Medicinal Chemistry Letters*, 3(5), 416–421.

Rikova, K., Guo, A., Zeng, Q., Possemato, A., Yu, J., Haack, H., Nardone, J., Lee, K., Reeves, C., Li, Y., Hu, Y., Tan, Z., Stokes, M., Sullivan, L.,

Mitchell, J., Wetzel, R., Macneill, J., Ren, J. M., Yuan, J., Bakalarski, C. E., … Comb, M. J. (2007). Global survey of phosphotyrosine signaling identifies oncogenic kinases in lung cancer. *Cell*, 131(6), 1190–1203.

Robert, C., Flaherty, K., Nathan, P., Hersey, P., Garbe, C., Milhem, M., Demidov, L., Mohr, P., Hassel, J. C., Rutkowski, P., Dummer, R., Utikal, J., Kiecker, F., Larkin, J., D'Amelio, A., Jr, Mookerjee, B., & Schadendorf, D. (2019). Five-year outcomes from a phase 3 METRIC study in patients with BRAF V600 E/K-mutant advanced or metastatic melanoma. *European Journal of Cancer (Oxford, England: 1990)*, 109, 61–69.

Robert, C., Grob, J. J., Stroyakovskiy, D., Karaszewska, B., Hauschild, A., Levchenko, E., Chiarion Sileni, V., Schachter, J., Garbe, C., Bondarenko, I., Gogas, H., Mandalá, M., Haanen, J., Lebbé, C., Mackiewicz, A., Rutkowski, P., Nathan, P. D., Ribas, A., Davies, M. A., Flaherty, K. T., … Long, G. V. (2019b). Five-Year Outcomes with Dabrafenib plus Trametinib in Metastatic Melanoma. *The New England Journal of Medicine*, 381(7), 626–636.

Robert, C., Karaszewska, B., Schachter, J., Rutkowski, P., Mackiewicz, A., Stroiakovski, D., Lichinitser, M., Dummer, R., Grange, F., Mortier, L., Chiarion-Sileni, V., Drucis, K., Krajsova, I., Hauschild, A., Lorigan, P., Wolter, P., Long, G. V., Flaherty, K., Nathan, P., Ribas, A., … Schadendorf, D. (2015). Improved overall survival in melanoma with combined dabrafenib and trametinib. *The New England Journal of Medicine*, 372(1), 30–39.

Robert, N. J., Diéras, V., Glaspy, J., Brufsky, A. M., Bondarenko, I., Lipatov, O. N., Perez, E. A., Yardley, D. A., Chan, S. Y., Zhou, X., Phan, S. C., & O'Shaughnessy, J. (2011). RIBBON-1: randomized, double-blind, placebo-controlled, phase III trial of chemotherapy with or without bevacizumab for first-line treatment of human epidermal growth factor receptor 2-negative, locally recurrent or metastatic breast cancer. *Journal of clinical oncology: official journal of the American Society of Clinical Oncology*, 29(10), 1252–1260.

Rodgers, S. J., Ferguson, D. T., Mitchell, C. A., & Ooms, L. M. (2017). Regulation of PI3K effector signalling in cancer by the phosphoinositide phosphatases. *Bioscience Reports*, 37(1): BSR20160432.

Rodrigues, D. A., Sagrillo, F. S., & Fraga, C. (2019). Duvelisib: A 2018 Novel FDA-Approved Small Molecule Inhibiting Phosphoinositide 3-Kinases. *Pharmaceuticals (Basel, Switzerland)*, 12(2): 69.

Rogers, K. A., Huang, Y., Ruppert, A. S., Awan, F. T., Hoffman, C., Maddocks, K. J., Reid, M., Woyach, J. A. Whitlow, T., Jones, J. A., Byrd, J. C.(2018). Phase 2 study of combination obinutuzumab, ibrutinib, and venetoclax in treatment-naïve and relapsed/refractory chronic lymphocytic leukemia. *Blood*, 132(Suppl 1): 693.

Rogers, K. A., Huang, Y., Ruppert, A. S., Awan, F. T., Heerema, N. A., Hoffman, C., Lozanski, G., Maddocks, K. J., Moran, M. E., Reid, M. A., Lucas, M., Woyach, J. A., Whitlow, W. T., Jones, J. A., & Byrd, J. C. (2018a). Phase 1b study of obinutuzumab, ibrutinib, and venetoclax in relapsed and refractory chronic lymphocytic leukemia. *Blood*, 132(15), 1568–1572.

Rolf, M. G., Curwen, J. O., Veldman-Jones, M., Eberlein, C., Wang, J., Harmer, A., Hellawell, C. J., & Braddock, M. (2015). In vitro pharmacological profiling of R406 identifies molecular targets underlying the clinical effects of fostamatinib. *Pharmacology Research & Perspectives*, 3(5), e00175.

Romond, E. H., Perez, E. A., Bryant, J., Suman, V. J., Geyer, C. E., Jr, Davidson, N. E., Tan-Chiu, E., Martino, S., Paik, S., Kaufman, P. A., Swain, S. M., Pisansky, T. M., Fehrenbacher, L., Kutteh, L. A., Vogel, V. G., Visscher, D. W., Yothers, G., Jenkins, R. B., Brown, A. M., Dakhil, S. R., … Wolmark, N. (2005). Trastuzumab plus adjuvant chemotherapy for operable HER2-positive breast cancer. *The New England Journal of Medicine*, 353(16), 1673–1684.

Rosell, R., Carcereny, E., Gervais, R., Vergnenegre, A., Massuti, B., Felip, E., Palmero, R., Garcia-Gomez, R., Pallares, C., Sanchez, J. M., Porta, R., Cobo, M., Garrido, P., Longo, F., Moran, T., Insa, A., De Marinis, F., Corre, R., Bover, I., Illiano, A., … Spanish Lung Cancer Group in collaboration with Groupe Français de Pneumo-Cancérologie and

Associazione Italiana Oncologia Toracica (2012). Erlotinib versus standard chemotherapy as first-line treatment for European patients with advanced EGFR mutation-positive non-small-cell lung cancer (EURTAC): a multicentre, open-label, randomised phase 3 trial. *The Lancet. Oncology*, 13(3), 239–246.

Rosen, A. C., Wu, S., Damse, A., Sherman, E., & Lacouture, M. E. (2012). Risk of rash in cancer patients treated with vandetanib: systematic review and meta-analysis. *The Journal of Clinical Endocrinology and Metabolism*, 97(4), 1125–1133.

Roskoski R., Jr (2019). Properties of FDA-approved small molecule protein kinase inhibitors. *Pharmacological Research*, 144, 19–50.

Roskoski R., Jr (2020). Properties of FDA-approved small molecule protein kinase inhibitors: A 2020 update. *Pharmacological Research*, 152, 104609.

Ross, J. S., Ali, S. M., Fasan, O., Block, J., Pal, S., Elvin, J. A., Schrock, A. B., Suh, J., Nozad, S., Kim, S., Jeong Lee, H., Sheehan, C. E., Jones, D. M., Vergilio, J. A., Ramkissoon, S., Severson, E., Daniel, S., Fabrizio, D., Frampton, G., Miller, V. A., … Gay, L. M. (2017). ALK Fusions in a Wide Variety of Tumor Types Respond to Anti-ALK Targeted Therapy. *The Oncologist*, 22(12), 1444–1450.

Rothenstein, J. M., & Chooback, N. (2018). ALK inhibitors, resistance development, clinical trials. *Current oncology (Toronto, Ont.),* 25(Suppl 1), S59–S67.

Ruan, J. (2019). Molecular profiling and management of mantle cell lymphoma. *Hematology. American Society of Hematology. Education Program,* 2019(1):30-40.

Rubner, S., Schubert, S., & Berg, T. (2019). Poloxin-2HT+: Changing the hydrophobic tag of Poloxin-2HT increases Plk1 degradation and apoptosis induction in tumor cells. *Organic & Biomolecular Chemistry*, 17 (12): 3113-3117.

Rudolph, D., Steegmaier, M., Hoffmann, M., Grauert, M., Baum, A., Quant, J., Haslinger, C., Garin-Chesa, P., and Adolf, G. R. (2009). BI 6727, a polo-like kinase inhibitor with improved pharmacokinetic profile and broad antitumor activity. *Clinical Cancer Research*, 15 (9): 3094-3102.

Rule, S., Diels, J., Healy, N., Iraqi, W., Aschan, J., & Wildgust, M. (2016). Real-world experience of ibrutinib in >700 patients with mantle-cell lymphoma: data from a global named patient program. *Haematologica*, 101(s1): 279.

Rusnak, D. W., Affleck, K., Cockerill, S. G., Stubberfield, C., Harris, R., Page, M., Smith, K. J., Guntrip, S. B., Carter, M. C., Shaw, R. J., Jowett, A., Stables, J., Topley, P., Wood, E. R., Brignola, P. S., Kadwell, S. H., Reep, B. R., Mullin, R. J., Alligood, K. J., Keith, B. R., … Lackey, K. (2001). The characterization of novel, dual ErbB-2/EGFR, tyrosine kinase inhibitors: potential therapy for cancer. *Cancer research*, 61(19), 7196–7203.

Sacha, T., & Saglio, G. (2018). Nilotinib in the treatment of chronic myeloid leukemia. *Future Oncology*, 15 (9): 953-965.

Saglio, G., Kim, D. W., Issaragrisil, S., le Coutre, P., Etienne, G., Lobo, C., Pasquini, R., Clark, R. E., Hochhaus, A., Hughes, T. P., Gallagher, N., Hoenekopp, A., Dong, M., Haque, A., Larson, R. A., & Kantarjian, H. M. (2010). Nilotinib versus Imatinib for Newly Diagnosed Chronic Myeloid Leukemia. *New England Journal of Medicine*, 362 (24): 2251-2259.

Saito, H., Fukuhara, T., Furuya, N., Watanabe, K., Sugawara, S., Iwasawa, S., Tsunezuka, Y., Yamaguchi, O., Okada, M., Yoshimori, K., Nakachi, I., Gemma, A., Azuma, K., Kurimoto, F., Tsubata, Y., Fujita, Y., Nagashima, H., Asai, G., Watanabe, S., Miyazaki, M., … Maemondo, M. (2019). Erlotinib plus bevacizumab versus erlotinib alone in patients with EGFR-positive advanced non-squamous non-small-cell lung cancer (NEJ026): interim analysis of an open-label, randomised, multicentre, phase 3 trial. *The Lancet. Oncology*, 20(5), 625–635.

Salles, G., Schuster, S. J., de Vos, S., Wagner-Johnston, N. D., Viardot, A., Blum, K. A., Flowers, C. R., Jurczak, W. J., Flinn, I. W., Kahl, B. S., Martin, P., Kim, Y., Shreay, S., Will, M., Sorensen, B., Breuleux, M., Zinzani, P. L., & Gopal, A. K. (2017). Efficacy and safety of idelalisib in patients with relapsed, rituximab- and alkylating agent-refractory follicular lymphoma: a subgroup analysis of a phase 2 study. *Haematologica*, 102(4), e156–e159.

Saltz, L. B., Clarke, S., Díaz-Rubio, E., Scheithauer, W., Figer, A., Wong, R., Koski, S., Lichinitser, M., Yang, T. S., Rivera, F., Couture, F., Sirzén, F., & Cassidy, J. (2008). Bevacizumab in combination with oxaliplatin-based chemotherapy as first-line therapy in metastatic colorectal cancer: a randomized phase III study. *Journal of clinical oncology: official journal of the American Society of Clinical Oncology*, 26(12), 2013–2019.

Sandler, A., Gray, R., Perry, M. C., Brahmer, J., Schiller, J. H., Dowlati, A., Lilenbaum, R., & Johnson, D. H. (2006). Paclitaxel-carboplatin alone or with bevacizumab for non-small-cell lung cancer. *The New England journal of medicine*, 355(24), 2542–2550.

Sanhaji, M., Kreis, N.-N., Zimmer, B., Berg, T., Louwen, F., & Yuan, J. (2012). p53 is not directly relevant to the response of Polo-like kinase 1 inhibitors. *Cell Cycle*, 11 (3): 543-53.

Sant'Antonio, E., Bonifacio, M., Breccia, M., & Rumi, E. (2019). A journey through infectious risk associated with ruxolitinib. *British Journal of Haematology*, 187(3): 286–295.

Santini, V. (2019). How I Treat MDS After Hypomethylating Agent Failure. *Blood*, 133 (6): 521-529.

Sanz-Garcia, E., Argiles, G., Elez, E., & Tabernero, J. (2017). BRAF mutant colorectal cancer: prognosis, treatment, and new perspectives. *Annals of Oncology: Official Journal of the European Society for Medical Oncology*, 28(11), 2648–2657.

Sappal, J., Theisen, M., Xiang, Z., Tirrell, S., Christmas, R., Yu, J., Zhang, M., & Kannan, K. (2018). TAK-659, a SYK kinase inhibitor, demonstrates preclinical antitumor activity in solid tumor model. *Cancer Research*, 78 (13 Supplement): 3844.

Sarmento-Ribeiro, A. B., Scorilas, A., Gonçalves, A. C., Efferth, T., & Trougakos, I. P. (2019). The emergence of drug resistance to targeted cancer therapies: Clinical evidence. *Drug resistance updates*, 47, 100646.

Sarmento-Ribeiro, A. B., Ribeiro, A. I. L., Gonçalves, A. C., Carda, J. P. (2013). Molecular and Cellular Characterization of Chronic

Lymphocytic Leukemia: Prognostic Implications. *Horizons in Cancer Research*, 52, 141–164.

Saura, C., Roda, D., Roselló, S., Oliveira, M., Macarulla, T., Pérez-Fidalgo, J. A., Morales-Barrera, R., Sanchis-García, J. M., Musib, L., Budha, N., Zhu, J., Nannini, M., Chan, W. Y., Sanabria Bohórquez, S. M., Meng, R. D., Lin, K., Yan, Y., Patel, P., Baselga, J., Tabernero, J., … Cervantes, A. (2017). A First-in-Human Phase I Study of the ATP-Competitive AKT Inhibitor Ipatasertib Demonstrates Robust and Safe Targeting of AKT in Patients with Solid Tumors. *Cancer discovery*, 7(1), 102–113.

Saussele, S., Richter, J., Guilhot, J., Gruber, F. X., Hjorth-Hansen, H., Almeida, A., Janssen, J., Mayer, J., Koskenvesa, P., Panayiotidis, P., Olsson-Strömberg, U., Martinez-Lopez, J., Rousselot, P., Vestergaard, H., Ehrencrona, H., Kairisto, V., Machová Poláková, K., Müller, M. C., Mustjoki, S., Berger, M. G., … EURO-SKI investigators (2018). Discontinuation of tyrosine kinase inhibitor therapy in chronic myeloid leukaemia (EURO-SKI): a prespecified interim analysis of a prospective, multicentre, non-randomised, trial. The Lancet. Oncology, 19(6), 747–757.Savage, D. G., and Antman, K. H. (2002). Imatinib Mesylate — A New Oral Targeted Therapy. *The New England Journal of Medicine*, 346 (9): 683-693.

Schlumberger, M., Jarzab, B., Cabanillas, M. E., Robinson, B., Pacini, F., Ball, D. W., McCaffrey, J., Newbold, K., Allison, R., Martins, R. G., Licitra, L. F., Shah, M. H., Bodenner, D., Elisei, R., Burmeister, L., Funahashi, Y., Ren, M., O'Brien, J. P., & Sherman, S. I. (2016). A Phase II Trial of the Multitargeted Tyrosine Kinase Inhibitor Lenvatinib (E7080) in Advanced Medullary Thyroid Cancer. *Clinical Cancer Research: an Official Journal of the American Association for Cancer Research*, 22(1), 44–53.

Schlumberger, M., Tahara, M., Wirth, L. J., Robinson, B., Brose, M. S., Elisei, R., Habra, M. A., Newbold, K., Shah, M. H., Hoff, A. O., Gianoukakis, A. G., Kiyota, N., Taylor, M. H., Kim, S. B., Krzyzanowska, M. K., Dutcus, C. E., de las Heras, B., Zhu, J., & Sherman, S. I. (2015). Lenvatinib versus placebo in radioiodine-refractory thyroid cancer. *The New England Journal of Medicine*, 372(7), 621–630.

Schoepfer, J., Jahnke, W., Berellini, G., Buonamici, S., Cotesta, S., Cowan-Jacob, S. W., Dodd, S., Drueckes, P., Fabbro, D., Gabriel, T., Groell, J. M., Grotzfeld, R. M., Hassan, A. Q., Henry, C., Iyer, V., Jones, D., Lombardo, F., Loo, A., Manley, P. W., Pellé, X., … Furet, P. (2018). Discovery of Asciminib (ABL001), an Allosteric Inhibitor of the Tyrosine Kinase Activity of BCR-ABL1. *Journal of Medicinal Chemistry*, 61(18), 8120–8135.

Schöffski, P., Cresta, S., Mayer, I. A., Wildiers, H., Damian, S., Gendreau, S., Rooney, I., Morrissey, K. M., Spoerke, J. M., Ng, V. W., Singel, S. M., & Winer, E. (2018). A phase Ib study of pictilisib (GDC-0941) in combination with paclitaxel, with and without bevacizumab or trastuzumab, and with letrozole in advanced breast cancer. *Breast Cancer Research: B*CR, 20(1), 109.

Scholl, C., Gilliland, D. G., & Fröhling, S. (2008). Deregulation of signaling pathways in acute myeloid leukemia. *Seminars in Oncology*, 35(4), 336–345.

Schrank, Z., Chhabra, G., Lin, L., Iderzorig, T., Osude, C., Khan, N., Kuckovic, A., Singh, S., Miller, R. J., & Puri, N. (2018). Current Molecular-Targeted Therapies in NSCLC and Their Mechanism of Resistance. *Cancers*, 10(7), 224.

Schwartz, G. K., Carvajal, R. D., Midgley, R., Rodig, S. J., Stockman, P. K., Ataman, O., Wilson, D., Das, S., & Shapiro G. I. (2013). Phase I study of barasertib (AZD1152), a selective inhibitor of aurora B kinase, in patients with advanced solid tumors. *Investigational New Drugs*, 31 (2): 370-80.

Schwartz, G. K., LoRusso, P. M., Dickson, M. A., Randolph, S. S., Shaik, M. N., Wilner, K. D., Courtney, R., & O'Dwyer, P. J. (2011). Phase I study of PD 0332991, a cyclin-dependent kinase inhibitor, administered in 3-week cycles (Schedule 2/1). *British Journal of Cancer*, 104(12), 1862–1868.

Seoane, J., & Capdevila, J. (2018). The right compound for the right target: tackling RET. *Annals of Oncology: Official Journal of the European Society for Medical Oncology*, 29(8), 1623–1625.

Sequist, L. V., Yang, J. C., Yamamoto, N., O'Byrne, K., Hirsh, V., Mok, T., Geater, S. L., Orlov, S., Tsai, C. M., Boyer, M., Su, W. C., Bennouna, J., Kato, T., Gorbunova, V., Lee, K. H., Shah, R., Massey, D., Zazulina, V., Shahidi, M., & Schuler, M. (2013). Phase III study of afatinib or cisplatin plus pemetrexed in patients with metastatic lung adenocarcinoma with EGFR mutations. *Journal of clinical oncology: official journal of the American Society of Clinical Oncology*, 31(27), 3327–3334.

Seshacharyulu, P., Ponnusamy, M. P., Haridas, D., Jain, M., Ganti, A. K., & Batra, S. K. (2012). Targeting the EGFR signaling pathway in cancer therapy. *Expert Opinion on Therapeutic Targets*, 16(1), 15–31.

Sever, R., & Brugge, J. S. (2015). Signal transduction in cancer. *Cold Spring Harbor Perspectives in Medicine*, 5(4), a006098.

Shah, A., Bloomquist, E., Tang, S., Fu, W., Bi, Y., Liu, Q., Yu, J., Zhao, P., Palmby, T. R., Goldberg, K. B., Chang, C., Patel, P., Alebachew, E., Tilley, A., Pierce, W. F., Ibrahim, A., Blumenthal, G. M., Sridhara, R., Beaver, J. A., & Pazdur, R. (2018). FDA Approval: Ribociclib for the Treatment of Postmenopausal Women with Hormone Receptor-Positive, HER2-Negative Advanced or Metastatic Breast Cancer. *Clinical Cancer Research: an Official Journal of the American Association for Cancer Research*, 24(13), 2999–3004.

Shah, H. A., Fischer, J. H., Venepalli, N. K., Danciu, O. C., Christian, S., Russell, M. J., Liu, l. C., Zacny, J. P., & Dudek, A. Z. (2019). Phase I study of aurora A kinase inhibitor alisertib (MLN8237) in combination with selective VEGFR inhibitor pazopanib for therapy of advanced solid tumors. *American Journal of Clinical Oncology*, 42 (5): 413-420.

Shanafelt, T. D., Wang, X. V., Kay, N. E., Hanson, C. A., O'Brien, S., Barrientos, J., Jelinek, D. F., Braggio, E., Leis, J. F., Zhang, C. C., Coutre, S. E., Barr, P. M., Cashen, A. F., Mato, A. R., Singh, A. K., Mullane, M. P., Little, R. F., Erba, H., Stone, R. M., Litzow, M., … Tallman, M. (2019). Ibrutinib-Rituximab or Chemoimmunotherapy for

Chronic Lymphocytic Leukemia. *The New England Journal of Medicine*, 381(5), 432–443.

Shanafelt, T. D., Wang, X. V., Kay, N. E., Hanson, C. A., O'Brien, S., Barrientos, J., Jelinek, D. F., Braggio, E., Leis, J. F., Zhang, C. C., Coutre, S. E., Barr, P. M., Cashen, A. F., Mato, A. R., Singh, A. K., Mullane, M. P., Little, R. F., Erba, H., Stone, R. M., … Tallman, M. (2019). Ibrutinib-Rituximab or Chemoimmunotherapy for Chronic Lymphocytic Leukemia. *The New England Journal of Medicine*, 381(5), 432–443.

Shariati, M., & Meric-Bernstam, F. (2019). Targeting AKT for cancer therapy. *Expert opinion on investigational drugs*, 28(11), 977–988.

Sharma, G. G., Mota, I., Mologni, L., Patrucco, E., Gambacorti-Passerini, C., & Chiarle, R. (2018). Tumor Resistance against ALK Targeted Therapy-Where It Comes From and Where It Goes. *Cancers*, 10(3), 62.

Sharman, J. P., Banerji, V., Fogliatto, L. M., Herishanu, Y., Munir, T., Walewska, R., Follows, G., Karlsson, K., Ghia, P., Corbett, G., Walker, P., Egyed, M., Jurczak, W., Salles, G., Janssens, A., Cymbalista, F., Wierda, W. G. Coutre, S., Pagel, J. M., …Byrd, J. C. (2019). ELEVATE TN: Phase 3 Study of Acalabrutinib Combined with Obinutuzumab (O) or Alone Vs O Plus Chlorambucil (Clb) in Patients (Pts) with Treatment-Naïve Chronic Lymphocytic Leukemia (CLL). *Blood*, 134 (Supplement_1): 31.

Sharman, J. P., Klein, L. M., Boxer, M., Kolibaba, K. S., Abella, S., Eng, C., He, J., Hu, J., Yasenchak, A. A. (2015). Phase 2 Trial of Entospletinib (GS-9973), a Selective Syk Inhibitor, in Indolent Non-Hodgkin's Lymphoma (iNHL). *Blood*, 126 (23): 1545.

Sharman, J. P., Kolibaba, K. S., Shustov, A. R., Giever, T. A., Klein, L. M. Nay, D., Rado, T. A., Saleh, A., Zhang, D., Shi, W., Forero, A., Assouline S. (2016). Results of a Phase 2 Trial Evaluating Efficacy and Safety of Entospletinib (GS-9973) in Patients with Mantle Cell Lymphoma. *Blood*, 128(22): 2963.

Sharman, J., and Di Paolo, J. (2016). Targeting B-cell receptor signaling kinases in chronic lymphocytic leukemia: the promise of entospletinib. *Therapeutic Advances in Hematology*, 7 (3): 157-170.

Sharman, J., Hawkins, M., Kolibaba, K., Boxer, M., Klein, L., Wu, M., Hu, J., Abella, S., & Yasenchak, C. (2015). An open-label phase 2 trial of entospletinib (GS-9973), a selective spleen tyrosine kinase inhibitor, in chronic lymphocytic leukemia. *Blood*, 125(15), 2336–2343.

Sharman, J., Hawkins, M., Kolibaba, K., Boxer, M., Klein, L., Wu, M., Hu, J., Abella, S., and Yasenchak, C. (2015). An open-label phase 2 trial of entospletinib (GS-9973), a selective spleen tyrosine kinase inhibitor, in chronic lymphocytic leukemia. *Blood*, 125 (15): 2336-43.

Sharman, J., Kabadi, S., Clark, J., Amirian, E. S., Andorsky, D. J. (2018). Treatment Patterns and Outcomes of 159 Ibrutinib-Treated MCL Patients in the United States: A Retrospective Electronic Medical Record Database and Chart Review Study. *Blood*, 132 (Supplement 1): 4163.

Shaw A. T., Kim T. M., Crinò L., Gridelli C., Kiura K., Liu G., Novello S., Bearz A., Gautschi O., Mok T., Nishio M., Scagliotti G., Spigel D. R., Deudon S., Zheng C., Pantano S., Urban P., Massacesi C., Viraswami-Appanna K., Felip E. (2017) Ceritinib versus chemotherapy in patients with ALK-rearranged non-small-cell lung cancer previously given chemotherapy and crizotinib (ASCEND-5): a randomised, controlled, open-label, phase 3 trial. *The Lancet. Oncology*, 18(7):874-886.

Shaw, A. T., Hsu, P. P., Awad, M. M., & Engelman, J. A. (2013). Tyrosine kinase gene rearrangements in epithelial malignancies. *Nature reviews. Cancer*, 13(11), 772–787.

Shaw, A. T., Kim, D. W., Nakagawa, K., Seto, T., Crinó, L., Ahn, M. J., De Pas, T., Besse, B., Solomon, B. J., Blackhall, F., Wu, Y. L., Thomas, M., O'Byrne, K. J., Moro-Sibilot, D., Camidge, D. R., Mok, T., Hirsh, V., Riely, G. J., Iyer, S., Tassell, V., … Jänne, P. A. (2013). Crizotinib versus chemotherapy in advanced ALK-positive lung cancer. *The New England journal of medicine*, 368(25), 2385–2394.

Shaw, A. T., Yeap, B. Y., Mino-Kenudson, M., Digumarthy, S. R., Costa, D. B., Heist, R. S., Solomon, B., Stubbs, H., Admane, S., McDermott, U., Settleman, J., Kobayashi, S., Mark, E. J., Rodig, S. J., Chirieac, L. R., Kwak, E. L., Lynch, T. J., & Iafrate, A. J. (2009). Clinical features and outcome of patients with non-small-cell lung cancer who harbor

EML4-ALK. *Journal of Clinical Oncology: Official Journal of the American Society of Clinical Oncology*, 27(26), 4247–4253.

Shi Y. (2009). Serine/threonine phosphatases: mechanism through structure. *Cell*, 139(3), 468–484.

Shirley M. (2017). Olaratumab: First Global Approval. *Drugs*, 77(1), 107–112.

Siddiqi, T., Frankel, P., Beumer J. H., Kiesel, B. F., Christner, S., Ruel, C., Song, J. Y., Chen, R., Kelly, K. R., Ailawadhi, S., Kaesberg, P., Popplewell, L., Puverel, S., Piekarz, R., Forman, S. J., and Newman, E. M. (2019). Phase 1 study of the Aurora kinase A inhibitor alisertib (MLN8237) combined with the histone deacetylase inhibitor vorinostat in lymphoid malignancies. *Leukemia & Lymphoma*, 61(2):309-317.

Simkens, L. H., van Tinteren, H., May, A., ten Tije, A. J., Creemers, G. J., Loosveld, O. J., de Jongh, F. E., Erdkamp, F. L., Erjavec, Z., van der Torren, A. M., Tol, J., Braun, H. J., Nieboer, P., van der Hoeven, J. J., Haasjes, J. G., Jansen, R. L., Wals, J., Cats, A., Derleyn, V. A., Honkoop, A. H., … Koopman, M. (2015). Maintenance treatment with capecitabine and bevacizumab in metastatic colorectal cancer (CAIRO3): a phase 3 randomised controlled trial of the Dutch Colorectal Cancer Group. *Lancet (London, England)*, 385(9980), 1843–1852.

Siveen, K. S., Prabhu, K. S., Achkar, I. W., Kuttikrishnan, S., Shyam, S., Khan, A. Q., Merhi, M., Dermime, S., & Uddin, S. (2018). Role of Non Receptor Tyrosine Kinases in Hematological Malignances and its Targeting by Natural Products. *Molecular cancer*, 17(1), 31.

Skinner, M., Philp, K., Lengel, D., Coverley, L., Lamm Bergström, E., Glaves, P., Musgrove, H., Prior, H., Braddock, M., Huby, R., Curwen, J. O., Duffy, P., & Harmer, A. R. (2014). The contribution of VEGF signalling to fostamatinib-induced blood pressure elevation. *British Journal of Pharmacology*, 171(9), 2308–2320.

Slamon, D. J., Neven, P., Chia, S., Fasching, P. A., De Laurentiis, M., Im, S. A., Petrakova, K., Bianchi, G. V., Esteva, F. J., Martín, M., Nusch, A., Sonke, G. S., De la Cruz-Merino, L., Beck, J. T., Pivot, X., Vidam, G., Wang, Y., Rodriguez Lorenc, K., Miller, M., Taran, T., …

Jerusalem, G. (2018). Phase III Randomized Study of Ribociclib and Fulvestrant in Hormone Receptor-Positive, Human Epidermal Growth Factor Receptor 2-Negative Advanced Breast Cancer: MONALEESA-3. *Journal of Clinical Oncology: Official Journal of the American Society of Clinical Oncology*, 36(24), 2465–2472.

Sledge, G. W., Jr, Toi, M., Neven, P., Sohn, J., Inoue, K., Pivot, X., Burdaeva, O., Okera, M., Masuda, N., Kaufman, P. A., Koh, H., Grischke, E. M., Frenzel, M., Lin, Y., Barriga, S., Smith, I. C., Bourayou, N., & Llombart-Cussac, A. (2017). MONARCH 2: Abemaciclib in Combination with Fulvestrant in Women With HR+/HER2- Advanced Breast Cancer Who Had Progressed While Receiving Endocrine Therapy. *Journal of Clinical Oncology: Official Journal of the American Society of Clinical Oncology*, 35(25), 2875–2884.

Smith, I., Procter, M., Gelber, R. D., Guillaume, S., Feyereislova, A., Dowsett, M., Goldhirsch, A., Untch, M., Mariani, G., Baselga, J., Kaufmann, M., Cameron, D., Bell, R., Bergh, J., Coleman, R., Wardley, A., Harbeck, N., Lopez, R. I., Mallmann, P., Gelmon, K., … HERA study team (2007). 2-year follow-up of trastuzumab after adjuvant chemotherapy in HER2-positive breast cancer: a randomised controlled trial. *Lancet (London, England)*, 369(9555), 29–36.

Smyth, E. C., Verheij, M., Allum, W., Cunningham, D., Cervantes, A., Arnold, D., & ESMO Guidelines Committee (2016). Gastric cancer: ESMO Clinical Practice Guidelines for diagnosis, treatment and follow-up. *Annals of oncology: official journal of the European Society for Medical Oncology*, 27(suppl 5), v38–v49.

Soda, M., Choi, Y. L., Enomoto, M., Takada, S., Yamashita, Y., Ishikawa, S., Fujiwara, S., Watanabe, H., Kurashina, K., Hatanaka, H., Bando, M., Ohno, S., Ishikawa, Y., Aburatani, H., Niki, T., Sohara, Y., Sugiyama, Y., & Mano, H. (2007). Identification of the transforming EML4-ALK fusion gene in non-small-cell lung cancer. *Nature*, 448(7153), 561–566.

Soleymani Fard, S., Sotoudeh, M., Yazdanbod, M., Ghavamzadeh, A., Malekzadeh, R., Yaghmaie, M., Mousavi, S. A., Ghaffari, S. H., & Alimoghaddam, K. (2019). Evaluation of the Association between

Androgen Receptor and AURKA and Its Prognostic Value in Gastric Cancer. *International journal of hematology-oncology and stem cell research,* 13(4), 174–182.

Solomon, B. J., Besse, B., Bauer, T. M., Felip, E., Soo, R. A., Camidge, D. R., Chiari, R., Bearz, A., Lin, C. C., Gadgeel, S. M., Riely, G. J., Tan, E. H., Seto, T., James, L. P., Clancy, J. S., Abbattista, A., Martini, J. F., Chen, J., Peltz, G., Thurm, H., ... Shaw, A. T. (2018). Lorlatinib in patients with ALK-positive non-small-cell lung cancer: results from a global phase 2 study. *The Lancet. Oncology*, 19(12), 1654–1667.

Solomon, B. J., Mok, T., Kim, D. W., Wu, Y. L., Nakagawa, K., Mekhail, T., Felip, E., Cappuzzo, F., Paolini, J., Usari, T., Iyer, S., Reisman, A., Wilner, K. D., Tursi, J., Blackhall, F., & PROFILE 1014 Investigators (2014). First-line crizotinib versus chemotherapy in ALK-positive lung cancer. *The New England Journal of Medicine*, 371(23), 2167–2177.

Song, M., Bode, A. M., Dong, Z., & Lee, M. H. (2019). AKT as a Therapeutic Target for Cancer. *Cancer research*, 79(6), 1019–1031.

Song, Y., Zhou, K., Zou, D., Zhou, J., Hu, J., Yang, H., Zhang, H., Ji, J., Xu, W., Jin, J., Lv, F., Feng, R., Gao, S., Zhou, D., Guo, H., Wang, A., Elstrom, R., Huang, J., Novotny, W., ... Zhu, J. (2019). Zanubrutinib in patients with relapsed/refractory mantle cell lymphoma. *Hematological Oncology*, 37: 45-46.

Soria, J. C., Tan, D., Chiari, R., Wu, Y. L., Paz-Ares, L., Wolf, J., Geater, S. L., Orlov, S., Cortinovis, D., Yu, C. J., Hochmair, M., Cortot, A. B., Tsai, C. M., Moro-Sibilot, D., Campelo, R. G., McCulloch, T., Sen, P., Dugan, M., Pantano, S., Branle, F., ... de Castro, G., Jr (2017). First-line ceritinib versus platinum-based chemotherapy in advanced ALK-rearranged non-small-cell lung cancer (ASCEND-4): a randomised, open-label, phase 3 study. *Lancet (London, England)*, 389(10072), 917–929.

Sorich, M. J., Wiese, M. D., Rowland, A., Kichenadasse, G., McKinnon, R. A., & Karapetis, C. S. (2015). Extended RAS mutations and anti-EGFR monoclonal antibody survival benefit in metastatic colorectal cancer: a meta-analysis of randomized, controlled trials. *Annals of oncology:*

official journal of the European Society for Medical Oncology, 26(1), 13–21.

Soverini, S., Hochhaus, A., Nicolini, F. E., Gruber, F., Lange, T., Saglio, G., Pane, F., Müller, M. C., Ernst, T., Rosti, G., Porkka, K., Baccarani, M., Cross, N. C. P., & Martinelli, G. (2011). BCR-ABL kinase domain mutation analysis in chronic myeloid leukemia patients treated with tyrosine kinase inhibitors: recommendations from an expert panel on behalf of European LeukemiaNet. *Blood*, 118 (5): 1208-1215.

Spagnuolo, A., Maione, P., & Gridelli, C. (2018). Evolution in the treatment landscape of non-small cell lung cancer with ALK gene alterations: from the first- to third-generation of ALK inhibitors. *Expert Opinion on Emerging Drugs*, 23(3), 231–241.

Spencer, A., Yoon, S. S., Harrison, S. J., Morris, S. R., Smith, D. A., Brigandi, R. A., Gauvin, J., Kumar, R., Opalinska, J. B., & Chen, C. (2014). The novel AKT inhibitor afuresertib shows favorable safety, pharmacokinetics, and clinical activity in multiple myeloma. *Blood*, 124(14), 2190–2195.

Spriano, F., Tarantelli, C., Gaudio, E., Gerlach, M. M., Priebe, V., Cascione, L., Bernasconi, E., Targa, A., Mascia, M., Dirnhofer, S., Stathis, A., Zucca, E., & Bertoni, F. (2019). Single and combined BTK and PI3Kδ inhibition with acalabrutinib and ACP-319 in pre-clinical models of aggressive lymphomas. *British Journal of Haematology*, 187(5), 595–601.

Stephens, D. M., & Byrd, J. C. (2019). How I manage ibrutinib intolerance and complications in patients with chronic lymphocytic leukemia. *Blood*, 133(12), 1298–1307.

Stone, R. M., Mandrekar, S. J., Sanford, B. L., Laumann, K., Geyer, S., Bloomfield, C. D., Thiede, C., Prior, T. W., Döhner, K., Marcucci, G., Lo-Coco, F., Klisovic, R. B., Wei, A., Sierra, J., Sanz, M. A., Brandwein, J. M., de Witte, T., Niederwieser, D., Appelbaum, F. R., Medeiros, B. C., … Döhner, H. (2017). Midostaurin plus Chemotherapy for Acute Myeloid Leukemia with a FLT3 Mutation. *The New England Journal of Medicine*, 377(5), 454–464.

Stone, R. M., Wang, E. S., Goldberg, A. D., Sweet, K. L., Fathi, A. T., Liu, H., & Messahel B. (2019) Crenolanib versus midostaurin combined with induction and consolidation chemotherapy in newly diagnosed FLT3 mutated AML. *Journal of Clinical Oncology* 37, no. 15_suppl.

Subbiah, V., Gainor, J. F., Rahal, R., Brubaker, J. D., Kim, J. L., Maynard, M., Hu, W., Cao, Q., Sheets, M. P., Wilson, D., Wilson, K. J., DiPietro, L., Fleming, P., Palmer, M., Hu, M. I., Wirth, L., Brose, M. S., Ou, S. I., Taylor, M., Garralda, E., … Evans, E. K. (2018). Precision Targeted Therapy with BLU-667 for RET-Driven Cancers. *Cancer discovery*, 8(7), 836–849.

Sullivan, R. J., Infante, J. R., Janku, F., Wong, D., Sosman, J. A., Keedy, V., Patel, M. R., Shapiro, G. I., Mier, J. W., Tolcher, A. W., Wang-Gillam, A., Sznol, M., Flaherty, K., Buchbinder, E., Carvajal, R. D., Varghese, A. M., Lacouture, M. E., Ribas, A., Patel, S. P., DeCrescenzo, G. A., … Li, B. T. (2018). First-in-Class ERK1/2 Inhibitor Ulixertinib (BVD-523) in Patients with MAPK Mutant Advanced Solid Tumors: Results of a Phase I Dose-Escalation and Expansion Study. *Cancer Discovery*, 8(2), 184–195.

Sun, Y., Yang, L., Hao, X., Liu, Y., Zhang, J., Ning, Z., & Shi, Y. (2019). Phase I dose-escalation study of chiauranib, a novel angiogenic, mitotic, and chronic inflammation inhibitor, in patients with advanced solid tumors. *Journal of Hematology & Oncology*, 12(1), 9.

Swain, S. M., Kim, S. B., Cortés, J., Ro, J., Semiglazov, V., Campone, M., Ciruelos, E., Ferrero, J. M., Schneeweiss, A., Knott, A., Clark, E., Ross, G., Benyunes, M. C., & Baselga, J. (2013). Pertuzumab, trastuzumab, and docetaxel for HER2-positive metastatic breast cancer (CLEOPATRA study): overall survival results from a randomised, double-blind, placebo-controlled, phase 3 study. *The Lancet. Oncology*, 14(6), 461–471.

Swain, S. M., Miles, D., Kim, S. B., Im, Y. H., Im, S. A., Semiglazov, V., Ciruelos, E., Schneeweiss, A., Loi, S., Monturus, E., Clark, E., Knott, A., Restuccia, E., Benyunes, M. C., Cortés, J., & CLEOPATRA study group (2020). Pertuzumab, trastuzumab, and docetaxel for HER2-positive metastatic breast cancer (CLEOPATRA): end-of-study results from a double-blind, randomised, placebo-controlled, phase 3 study. *The Lancet. Oncology*, 21(4), 519–530.

Sweet, K., Hazlehurst, L., Sahakian, E., Powers, J., Nodzon, L., Kayali, F., Hyland, K., Nelson, A., & Pinilla-Ibarz, J. (2018). A phase I clinical trial of ruxolitinib in combination with Nilotinib in chronic myeloid leukemia patients with molecular evidence of disease. *Leukemia Research*, 74: 89-96.

Syed, Y. Y. (2020). Zanubrutinib: First Approval. *Drugs*, 80(1): 91- 97.

Takahashi, T., Sonobe, M., Kobayashi, M., Yoshizawa, A., Menju, T., Nakayama, E., Mino, N., Iwakiri, S., Sato, K., Miyahara, R., Okubo, K., Manabe, T., & Date, H. (2010). Clinicopathologic features of non-small-cell lung cancer with EML4-ALK fusion gene. *Annals of Surgical Oncology*, 17(3), 889–897.

Tam, C. S., Anderson, M. A., Pott, C., Agarwal, R., Handunnetti, S., Hicks, R. J., Burbury, K., Turner, G., Di Iulio, J., Bressel, M., Westerman, D., Lade, S., Dreyling, M., Dawson, S. J., Dawson, M. A., Seymour, J. F., & Roberts, A. W. (2018). Ibrutinib plus Venetoclax for the Treatment of Mantle-Cell Lymphoma. *The New England Journal of Medicine*, 378(13), 1211–1223.

Tam, C., Wang, M., Simpson, D., Opat, S., Cull, G., Munoz, J., Phillips, T. J., Kim, W., Atwal, S., Wei, R., Huang, J., Elstrom, R., Trotman J. (2019). Updated safety and efficacy data in the phase 1 trial of patients with Mantle Cell Lymphoma (MCL) treated with Bruton Tyrosine Kinase (BTK) inhibitor zanubrutinib (BGB-3111). *Hematol Oncol*, 37: 245-247.

Tan, J., Xu, W., Lei, L., Liu, H., Wang, H., Cao, X., and Xu, M. (2020). Inhibition of aurora kinase A by alisertib reduces cell proliferation and induces apoptosis and autophagy in HuH-6 human hepatoblastoma cells. *Onco Targets and Therapy*, 13: 3953-3963.

Tap, W. D., Jones, R. L., Van Tine, B. A., Chmielowski, B., Elias, A. D., Adkins, D., Agulnik, M., Cooney, M. M., Livingston, M. B., Pennock, G., Hameed, M. R., Shah, G. D., Qin, A., Shahir, A., Cronier, D. M., Ilaria, R., Jr, Conti, I., Cosaert, J., & Schwartz, G. K. (2016). Olaratumab and doxorubicin versus doxorubicin alone for treatment of soft-tissue sarcoma: an open-label phase 1b and randomised phase 2 trial. *Lancet (London, England)*, 388(10043), 488–497.

Tchekmedyian, V., Sherman, E. J., Dunn, L., Tran, C., Baxi, S., Katabi, N., Antonescu, C. R., Ostrovnaya, I., Haque, S. S., Pfister, D. G., & Ho, A. L. (2019). Phase II Study of Lenvatinib in Patients With Progressive, Recurrent or Metastatic Adenoid Cystic Carcinoma. *Journal of Clinical Oncology: Official Journal of the American Society of Clinical Oncology*, 37(18), 1529–1537.

Tefferi, A., & Pardanani, A. (2011). Serious adverse events during ruxolitinib treatment discontinuation in patients with myelofibrosis. *Mayo Clinic Proceedings*, 86(12): 1188–1191.

Ten Hacken, E., & Burger, J. A. (2016). Microenvironment interactions and B-cell receptor signaling in Chronic Lymphocytic Leukemia: Implications for disease pathogenesis and treatment. *Biochimica et Biophysica Acta*, 1863(3), 401–413.

Thoma, G., Smith, A. B., van Eis, M. J., Vangrevelinghe, E., Blanz, J., Aichholz, R., Littlewood-Evans, A., Lee, C. C., Liu, H., and Zerwes, H.-G. (2015). Discovery and Profiling of a Selective and Efficacious Syk Inhibitor. *Journal of Medicinal Chemistry*, 58 (4): 1950-1963.

Thomas D. Rodgers, T. D., &Reagan, P. M. (2018). Targeting the B-cell receptor pathway: a review of current and future therapies for non-Hodgkin's lymphoma. *Expert Opinion on Emerging Drugs*, 23(2): 111-122.

Timme, N., Han, Y., Liu, S., Yosief, H. O., García, H. D., Bei, Y., Klironomos, F., MacArthur, I. C., Szymansky, A., von Stebut, J., Bardinet, V., Dohna, C., Künkele, A., Rolff, J., Hundsdörfer, P., Lissat, A., Seifert, G., Eggert, A., Schulte, J. H., Zhang, W., and Henssen, A. G. (2020). Small-molecule dual PLK1 and BRD4 inhibitors are active against preclinical models of pediatric solid tumors. *Translational Oncology*, 13 (2): 221-232.

Tolaney SM, Lin NU, Thornton D, Klise S, Costigan TM, Turner PK, et al. (2017). Abemaciclib for the treatment of brain metastases (BM) secondary to hormone receptor positive (HR+), HER2 negative breast cancer. *Journal of Clinical Oncology*, 35(15_suppl):1019.

Torkamani, A., Verkhivker, G., & Schork, N. J. (2009). Cancer driver mutations in protein kinase genes. *Cancer letters*, 281(2), 117–127.

Tremblay, D., & Mascarenhas, J. (2018). Pacritinib to treat myelofibrosis patients with thrombocytopenia. *Expert Review of Hematology*, 11(9): 707–714.

Treon, S. P., Gustine, J., Meid, K., Bantilan, K. S., Dubeau, T. E., Severns, P., Yang, G., Xu, L. L., Patterson, C. J., Ghobrial, I. M., Laubach, J. P., Hunter, Z. R., Castillo, J. J., Palomba, M. L., Advani, R. H. (2018). Ibrutinib Monotherapy in Symptomatic, Treatment-Naïve Patients with Waldenström Macroglobulinemia. *J Clin Oncol.*, 36(27):2755-2761.

Treon, S. P., Meid, K., Gustine, J., et al. (2017). Long-Term Follow-up of Previously Treated Patients Who Received Ibrutinib for Symptomatic Waldenström's Macroglobulinemia: Update of Pivotal Clinical Trial. *Blood,* 130(Supplement 1): 2766.

Treon, S. P., Tripsas, C. K., Meid, K., Warren, D., Varma, G., Green, R., Argyropoulos, K. V., Yang, G., Cao, Y., Xu, L., Patterson, C. J., Rodig, S., Zehnder, J. L., Aster, J. C., Harris, N. L., Kanan, S., Ghobrial, I., Castillo, J. J., Laubach, J. P., Hunter, Z. R., … Advani, R. H. (2015). Ibrutinib in previously treated Waldenström's macroglobulinemia. *The New England Journal of Medicine*, 372(15), 1430–1440.

Tripathy, D., Im, S. A., Colleoni, M., Franke, F., Bardia, A., Harbeck, N., Hurvitz, S. A., Chow, L., Sohn, J., Lee, K. S., Campos-Gomez, S., Villanueva Vazquez, R., Jung, K. H., Babu, K. G., Wheatley-Price, P., De Laurentiis, M., Im, Y. H., Kuemmel, S., El-Saghir, N., Liu, M. C., … Lu, Y. S. (2018). Ribociclib plus endocrine therapy for premenopausal women with hormone-receptor-positive, advanced breast cancer (MONALEESA-7): a randomised phase 3 trial. *The Lancet. Oncology*, 19(7), 904–915.

Tsintarakis, A., & Zafiropoulos, A. (2017). Oncogenic Kinases in Cancer. In *eLS*, John Wiley & Sons, Ltd (Ed.). doi: 10.1002/9780470015902.a0006051.pub3.

Tsou, J. H., Chang, K. C., Chang-Liao, P. Y., Yang, S. T., Lee, C. T., Chen, Y. P., Lee, Y. C., Lin, B. W., Lee, J. C., Shen, M. R., Chuang, C. K., Chang, W. C., Wang, J. M., & Hung, L. Y. (2011). Aberrantly expressed

AURKC enhances the transformation and tumourigenicity of epithelial cells. *The Journal of Pathology*, 225(2), 243–254.

Twu, N. F., Yuan, C. C., Yen, M. S., Lai, C. R., Chao, K. C., Wang, P. H., Wu, H. H., & Chen, Y. J. (2009). Expression of Aurora kinase A and B in normal and malignant cervical tissue: high Aurora A kinase expression in squamous cervical cancer. *European Journal of Obstetrics, Gynecology, and Reproductive Biology*, 142(1), 57–63.

UK CLL Forum (2016). Ibrutinib for relapsed/refractory chronic lymphocytic leukemia: a UK and Ireland analysis of outcomes in 315 patients. *Haematologica*, 101(12): 1563–1572.

Umehara, K., Huth, F., Jin, Y., Schiller, H., Aslanis, V., Heimbach, T., & He, H. (2019). Drug-drug interaction (DDI) assessments of ruxolitinib, a dual substrate of CYP3A4 and CYP2C9, using a verified physiologically based pharmacokinetic (PBPK) model to support regulatory submissions. *Drug metabolism and personalized therapy*, 34(2): /j/dmdi.2019.34.issue-2/dmpt-2018-0042/dmpt-2018-0042.xml.

Umene, K., Yanokura, M., Banno, K., Irie, H., Adachi, M., Iida, M., Nakamura, K., Nogami, Y., Masuda, K., Kobayashi, Y., Tominaga, E., & Aoki, D. (2015). Aurora kinase A has a significant role as a therapeutic target and clinical biomarker in endometrial cancer. *International Journal of Oncology*, 46(4), 1498–1506.

Unger, C., Berdel, W., Hanauske, A. R., Sindermann, H., Engel, J., & Mross, K. (2010). First-time-in-man and pharmacokinetic study of weekly oral perifosine in patients with solid tumours. *European journal of cancer (Oxford, England: 1990)*, 46(5), 920–925.

Urata, Y., Katakami, N., Morita, S., Kaji, R., Yoshioka, H., Seto, T., Satouchi, M., Iwamoto, Y., Kanehara, M., Fujimoto, D., Ikeda, N., Murakami, H., Daga, H., Oguri, T., Goto, I., Imamura, F., Sugawara, S., Saka, H., Nogami, N., Negoro, S., … Nakanishi, Y. (2016). Randomized Phase III Study Comparing Gefitinib With Erlotinib in Patients With Previously Treated Advanced Lung Adenocarcinoma: WJOG 5108L. *Journal of clinical oncology : official journal of the American Society of Clinical Oncology*, 34(27), 3248–3257.

Vainchenker, W., Leroy, E., Gilles, L., Marty, C., Plo, I., & Constantinescu, S. N. (2018). JAK inhibitors for the treatment of myeloproliferative neoplasms and other disorders. *F1000Research,* 7: 82.

Van Cutsem, E., Cervantes, A., Nordlinger, B., Arnold, D., & ESMO Guidelines Working Group (2014). Metastatic colorectal cancer: ESMO Clinical Practice Guidelines for diagnosis, treatment and follow-up. *Annals of oncology: official journal of the European Society for Medical Oncology*, 25 Suppl 3, iii1–iii9.

Van Cutsem, E., Köhne, C. H., Láng, I., Folprecht, G., Nowacki, M. P., Cascinu, S., Shchepotin, I., Maurel, J., Cunningham, D., Tejpar, S., Schlichting, M., Zubel, A., Celik, I., Rougier, P., & Ciardiello, F. (2011). Cetuximab plus irinotecan, fluorouracil, and leucovorin as first-line treatment for metastatic colorectal cancer: updated analysis of overall survival according to tumor KRAS and BRAF mutation status. *Journal of clinical oncology: official journal of the American Society of Clinical Oncology*, 29(15), 2011–2019.

van de Weerdt, B. C. M., & Medema, R. H. (2006). Polo-like kinases: A team in control of the division. *Cell Cycle*, 5 (8): 853-64.

Van den Bossche, J., Domen, A., Peeters, M., Deben, C., De Pauw, I., Jacobs, J., De Bruycker, S., Specenier, P., Pauwels, P., Vermorken, J. B., Lardon, F., & Wouters, A. (2019). Radiosensitization of non-small cell lung cancer cells by the Plk1 inhibitor Volasertib is dependent on the p53 status. *Cancers (Basel)*, 11 (12): 1893.

Van Ummersen, L., Binger, K., Volkman, J., Marnocha, R., Tutsch, K., Kolesar, J., Arzoomanian, R., Alberti, D., & Wilding, G. (2004). A phase I trial of perifosine (NSC 639966) on a loading dose/maintenance dose schedule in patients with advanced cancer. *Clinical cancer research: an official journal of the American Association for Cancer Research*, 10(22), 7450–7456.

Vannucchi, A. M., Kiladjian, J. J., Griesshammer, M., Masszi, T., Durrant, S., Passamonti, F., Harrison, C. N., Pane, F., Zachee, P., Mesa, R., He, S., Jones, M. M., Garrett, W., Li, J., Pirron, U., Habr, D., & Verstovsek, S. (2015). Ruxolitinib versus standard therapy for the treatment of polycythemia vera. *The New England Journal of Medicine*, 372(5): 426–435.

Venook, A. P., Niedzwiecki, D., Lenz, H. J., Innocenti, F., Fruth, B., Meyerhardt, J. A., Schrag, D., Greene, C., O'Neil, B. H., Atkins, J. N., Berry, S., Polite, B. N., O'Reilly, E. M., Goldberg, R. M., Hochster, H. S., Schilsky, R. L., Bertagnolli, M. M., El-Khoueiry, A. B., Watson, P., Benson, A. B., 3rd, … Blanke, C. (2017). Effect of First-Line Chemotherapy Combined With Cetuximab or Bevacizumab on Overall Survival in Patients With KRAS Wild-Type Advanced or Metastatic Colorectal Cancer: A Randomized Clinical Trial. *JAMA*, 317(23), 2392–2401.

Verbeke, D., Gielen, O., Jacobs, K., Boeckx, N., De Keersmaecker, K., Maertens, J., Uyttebroeck, A., Segers, H., & Cools, J. (2019). Ruxolitinib Synergizes With Dexamethasone for the Treatment of T-cell Acute Lymphoblastic Leukemia. *Hema Sphere*, 3(6), e310.

Vermorken, J. B., Mesia, R., Rivera, F., Remenar, E., Kawecki, A., Rottey, S., Erfan, J., Zabolotnyy, D., Kienzer, H. R., Cupissol, D., Peyrade, F., Benasso, M., Vynnychenko, I., De Raucourt, D., Bokemeyer, C., Schueler, A., Amellal, N., & Hitt, R. (2008). Platinum-based chemotherapy plus cetuximab in head and neck cancer. *The New England Journal of Medicine*, 359(11), 1116–1127.

Verstovsek, S., Kantarjian, H. M., Estrov, Z., Cortes, J. E., Thomas, D. A., Kadia, T., Pierce, S., Jabbour, E., Borthakur, G., Rumi, E., Pungolino, E., Morra, E., Caramazza, D., Cazzola, M., & Passamonti, F. (2012). Long-term outcomes of 107 patients with myelofibrosis receiving JAK1/JAK2 inhibitor ruxolitinib: survival advantage in comparison to matched historical controls. *Blood*, 120(6), 1202–1209.

Verstovsek, S., Kantarjian, H., Mesa, R. A., Pardanani, A. D., Cortes-Franco, J., Thomas, D. A., Estrov, Z., Fridman, J. S., Bradley, E. C., Erickson-Viitanen, S., Vaddi, K., Levy, R., and Tefferi, A. (2010). Safety and efficacy of INCB018424, a JAK1 and JAK2 inhibitor, in myelofibrosis. *The New England Journal of Medicine,* 363(12): 1117–1127.

Verstovsek, S., Mesa, R. A., Gotlib, J. R., Levy, R. S., Gupta, V., DiPersio, J. F., Catalano, j., Deininger, M., Miller, C. B., Silver, R. T., Talpaz, M., Winton, E. F., Harvey, J. H., Vaddi, K., Erickson-Viitanen, S. K., Koumenis, I., Sun, W., Sandor, V., Kantarjian, H., on behalf of all COMFORT-I investigators (2011). Results of COMFORT-I, a randomized double-blind phase III trial of JAK 1/2 inhibitor INCB18424 (424) versus placebo (PB) for patients with myelofibrosis (MF). *Journal of Clinical Oncology*, 29:15s.

Volasertib FDA Approval for CLL Drug, Orphan Drug Status for AML Therapy. (2014) *Oncology Times* May 10, 2014 oncology-times.com.

von Tresckow, J., Cramer, P., Bahlo, J., et al. (2019). CLL2-BIG: sequential treatment with bendamustine, ibrutinib and Obinutuzumab (GA101) in chronic lymphocytic leukemia. *Leukemia*, 33(5): 1161–1172.

Walker, A. J., Wedam, S., Amiri-Kordestani, L., Bloomquist, E., Tang, S., Sridhara, R., Chen, W., Palmby, T. R., Fourie Zirkelbach, J., Fu, W., Liu, Q., Tilley, A., Kim, G., Kluetz, P. G., McKee, A. E., & Pazdur, R. (2016a). FDA Approval of Palbociclib in Combination with Fulvestrant for the Treatment of Hormone Receptor-Positive, HER2-Negative Metastatic Breast Cancer. *Clinical Cancer Research: an Official Journal of the American Association for Cancer Research*, 22(20), 4968–4972.

Walker, A. R., Bhatnagar, B., Marcondes, A. M. Q., DiPaolo, J., Vasu, S., Mims, A. S., Klisovic, R. B., Walsh, K. J., Canning, R., Behbehani, G. K., Garzon, R., Blachly, J. S., Johnson, A. J., Abella-Dominicis, E., Byrd, J. C., and Blum, W. (2016b). Interim Results of a Phase 1b/2 Study of Entospletinib (GS-9973) Monotherapy and in Combination with Chemotherapy in Patients with Acute Myeloid Leukemia. *Blood*, 128 (22): 2831-2831.

Walker, A. R., Byrd, J. C., Blum, W., Lin, T., Crosswell, H. E., Zhang, D., Gao, J., Rao, A. V., Minden, M. D., & Stock, W. (2018). High response rates with entospletinib in patients with (v;11q23.3); KMT2A rearranged acute myeloid leukemia and acute lymphoblastic leukemia. *Cancer Research*, 78(13 Supplement): 819.

Wang, F., Li, H., Yan, X. G., Zhou, Z. W., Yi, Z. G., He, Z. X., Pan, S. T., Yang, Y. X., Wang, Z. Z., Zhang, X., Yang, T., Qiu, J. X., &Zhou, S. F. (2015). Alisertib induces cell cycle arrest and autophagy and suppresses Epithelial-to-Mesenchymal Transition involving PI3K/Akt/mTOR and sirtuin 1-mediated signaling pathways in human pancreatic cancer cells. *Drug Design, Development and Therapy*, 9: 575-601.

Wang, G., Jiang, Q., & Zhang, C. (2014). The role of mitotic kinases in coupling the centrosome cycle with the assembly of the mitotic spindle. *Journal of Cell Science*, 127(Pt 19), 4111–4122.

Wang, J. X., Zhang, L., Huang, Z. W., Zhang, X. N., Jiang, Y. Y., Liu, F. J., Long, L., Xue, M. J., Lu, G., Liu, Q., & Long, Z. J. (2020). Aurora Kinase Inhibitor restrains STAT5-activated leukemic cell proliferation by inducing mitochondrial impairment. *Journal of Cellular Physiology*, doi: 10.1002/jcp.29680.

Wang, J., Yang, S., Zhang, H., Song, Y., Zhang, X., Qian, H., Han, X., & Shi Y. (2011). Aurora-A as an independent molecular prognostic marker in gastric cancer. *Oncology Reports*, 26 (1): 23-32.

Wang, M. L., Blum, K. A., Martin, P., Goy, A., Auer, R., Kahl, B. S., Jurczak, W., Advani, R. H., Romaguera, J. E., Williams, M. E., Barrientos, J. C., Chmielowska, E., Radford, J., Stilgenbauer, S., Dreyling, M., Jedrzejczak, W. W., Johnson, P., Spurgeon, S. E., Zhang, L., Baher, L., … Rule, S. (2015). Long-term follow-up of MCL patients treated with single-agent ibrutinib: updated safety and efficacy results. *Blood*, 126(6), 739–745.

Wang, M. L., Lee, H., Chuang, H., Wagner-Bartak, N., Hagemeister, F., Westin, J., Fayad, L., Samaniego, F., Turturro, F., Oki, Y., Chen, W., Badillo, M., Nomie, K., DeLa Rosa, M., Zhao, D., Lam, L., Addison, A., Zhang, H., Young, K. H., Li, S., … Zhang, L. (2016). Ibrutinib in combination with rituximab in relapsed or refractory mantle cell lymphoma: a single-centre, open-label, phase 2 trial. *The Lancet. Oncology*, 17(1), 48–56.

Wang, M. L., Lee, H., Thirumurthi, S., Chuang, H., Chuang, H., Hagemeister, F., Westin, J., Fayad, L., Samaniego, F., Turturro, F., Chen, W., Oriabure, O., Feng, L., Zhou, S., Huang, S., Li, S., Zhang, L.,

Badillo, M., Wu, L., Ahmed, M., Yan, F., Nomie, K., Lam, L., Addison, A., Romaguera, J. (2017). Ibrutinib-Rituximab followed by reduced chemo-immunotherapy consolidation in young, newly diagnosed mantle cell lymphoma patients: a window of opportunity to reduce chemo. *Hematological Oncology*, 35(S2): 142–143.

Wang, M. L., Rule, S., Martin, P., Goy, A., Auer, R., Kahl, B. S., Jurczak, W., Advani, R. H., Romaguera, J. E., Williams, M. E., Barrientos, J. C., Chmielowska, E., Radford, J., Stilgenbauer, S., Dreyling, M., Jedrzejczak, W. W., Johnson, P., Spurgeon, S. E., Li, L., Zhang, L., … Blum, K. A. (2013). Targeting BTK with ibrutinib in relapsed or refractory mantle-cell lymphoma. *The New England Journal of Medicine*, 369(6), 507–516.

Wang, M., Lee, H. J., Thirumurthi, S., Chuang, H. H., Hagemeister, F. B., Westin, J. R., Fayad, L. E., Samaniego, F., Turturro, F., Chen, W., Oriabure, O., Huang, S. Y., Li, S., Zhang, L., Badillo, M., Hartig, K. H., Ahmed, M., Nomie, K., Lam, L. T., Addison, A. A., Romaguera, J. E. (2016). Chemotherapy-Free Induction with Ibrutinib-Rituximab Followed By Shortened Cycles of Chemo-Immunotherapy Consolidation in Young, Newly Diagnosed Mantle Cell Lymphoma Patients: A Phase II Clinical Trial. *Blood*, 128(22): 147.

Wang, M., Rule, S., Zinzani, P. L., Goy, A., Casasnovas, O., Smith, S. D., Damaj, G., Doorduijn, J., Lamy, T., Morschhauser, F., Panizo, C., Shah, B., Davies, A., Eek, R., Dupuis, J., Jacobsen, E., Kater, A. P., Le Gouill, S., Oberic, L., Robak, T., … Jurczak, W. (2018). Acalabrutinib in relapsed or refractory mantle cell lymphoma (ACE-LY-004): a single-arm, multicentre, phase 2 trial. *Lancet (London, England),* 391(10121), 659–667.

Wang, M., Rule, S., Zinzani, P. L., Goy, A., Casasnovas, O., Smith, S. D., Damaj, G, Doorduijn, J. K., Lamy, T., Morschhauser, F., Panizo, C., Shah, B. D., Davies, A.,Eek, R., Dupuis, J., Jacobsen, E., Kater, A. P., Gouill, S. L. E., Oberic, L., Robak, T., Dua, R., Frigault, M. M., Izumi, R., Nguyen, D., Patel, P., Yin, M., Jurczak, W. (2018). Long-term follow-up of acalabrutinib monotherapy in patients with relapsed/refractory mantle cell lymphoma. *Blood,* 132 (Supplement 1): 2876.

Wang, X., Ding, J., & Meng, L. H. (2015). PI3K isoform-selective inhibitors: next-generation targeted cancer therapies. *Acta Pharmacologica Sinica*, 36(10): 1170–1176.

Wang, X., Li, B., Ciotkowska, A., Rutz, B., Erlander, M. G., Ridinger, M., Wang, R., Tamalunas, A., Waidelich, R., Stief, C. G., & Hennenberg, M. (2020). Onvansertib, a Polo-like Kinase 1 inhibitor, inhibits prostate stromal cell growth and prostate smooth muscle contraction, which is additive to inhibition by α 1-blockers. *European Journal of Pharmacology*, 873: 172985.

Weichert, W., Denkert, C., Schmidt, M., Gekeler, V., Wolf, G., Köbel, M., Dietel, M., & Hauptmann, S. (2004). Polo-like kinase isoform expression is a prognostic factor in ovarian carcinoma. *British Journal Cancer*, 90 (4): 815-21.

Weinblatt, M. E., Kavanaugh, A., Burgos-Vargas, R., Dikranian, A. H., Medrano-Ramirez, G., Morales-Torres, J. L., Murphy, F. T., Musser, T. K., Straniero, N., Vicente-Gonzales, A. V., and Grossbard, E. (2008). Treatment of rheumatoid arthritis with a syk kinase inhibitor: A twelve-week, randomized, placebo-controlled trial. *Arthritis & Rheumatism*, 58 (11): 3309-3318.

Weiß, L., & Efferth, T. (2012). Polo-like kinase 1 as target for cancer therapy. *Experimental Hematology and Oncology*, 1 (1): 38.

Wells, S. A., Jr, Robinson, B. G., Gagel, R. F., Dralle, H., Fagin, J. A., Santoro, M., Baudin, E., Elisei, R., Jarzab, B., Vasselli, J. R., Read, J., Langmuir, P., Ryan, A. J., & Schlumberger, M. J. (2012). Vandetanib in patients with locally advanced or metastatic medullary thyroid cancer: a randomized, double-blind phase III trial. *Journal of Clinical Oncology: Official Journal of the American Society of Clinical Oncology*, 30(2), 134–141.

Westerweel, P. E., te Boekhorst, P. A. W., Levin, M.-D., & Cornelissen, J. J. (2019). New Approaches and Treatment Combinations for the Management of Chronic Myeloid Leukemia. *Frontiers in Oncology*, 9 (665).

White, D. L., Saunders, V. A., Dang, P., Engler, J., Venables, A., Zrim, S., Zannettino, A., Lynch, K., Manley, P. W., & Hughes, T. (2007). Most CML patients who have a suboptimal response to Imatinib have low OCT-1 activity: higher doses of Imatinib may overcome the negative impact of low OCT-1 activity. *Blood*, 110 (12): 4064-4072.

Wilkinson, R. W., Odedra, R., Heaton, S. P., Wedge, S. R., Keen, N. J., Crafter, C., Foster, J. R., Brady, M. C., Bigley, A., Brown, E., Byth, K. F., Barrass, N. C., Mundt, K. E., Foote, K. M., Heron, N. M., Jung, F. H., Mortlock, Boyle, F. T., & Green, S. (2007). AZD1152, a selective inhibitor of aurora B kinase, inhibits human tumor xenograft growth by inducing apoptosis. *Clinical Cancer Research*, 13 (12): 3682-8.

Winkles, J. A., & Alberts, G. F. (2005). Differential regulation of polo-like kinase 1, 2, 3, and 4 gene expression in mammalian cells and tissues. *Oncogene*, 24 (2): 260-6.

Wirth L. J., Kohno T., Udagawa H., Matsumoto S., Ishii G., Ebata K., Tuch, B. B., Zhu, E. Y., Nguyen, M., Smith, S., Hanson, L. M., Burkard, M. R., Cable, L., Blake, J. F., Condroski, K. R., Brandhuber, B. J., Andrews, S., Rothenberg, S. M., & Goto, K. (2019). Emergence and Targeting of Acquired and Hereditary Resistance to Multikinase RET Inhibition in Patients With RET-Altered Cancer. *JCO Precision Oncology*, 11;(3):1–7.

Woyach, J. A., Ruppert, A. S., Heerema, N. A., Zhao, W., Booth, A. M., Ding, W., Bartlett, N. L., Brander, D. M., Barr, P. M., Rogers, K. A., Parikh, S. A., Coutre, S., Hurria, A., Brown, J. R., Lozanski, G., Blachly, J. S., Ozer, H. G., Major-Elechi, B., Fruth, B., Nattam, S., … Byrd, J. C. (2018). Ibrutinib Regimens versus Chemoimmunotherapy in Older Patients with Untreated CLL. *The New England Journal of Medicine*, 379(26), 2517–2528.

Wu J., Liu C., Tsui S. T. and Liu D (2016). Second-generation inhibitors of Bruton tyrosine kinase. *Journal of Hematololy and Oncology*, 9(1):80-87.

Wylie, A. A., Schoepfer, J., Jahnke, W., Cowan-Jacob, S. W., Loo, A., Furet, P., Marzinzik, A. L., Pelle, X., Donovan, J., Zhu, W., Buonamici, S., Hassan, A. Q., Lombardo, F., Iyer, V., Palmer, M., Berellini, G., Dodd,

S., Thohan, S., Bitter, H., … Sellers, W. R. (2017). The allosteric inhibitor ABL001 enables dual targeting of BCR–ABL1. *Nature*, 543 (7647): 733-737.

Xie, Y. H., Chen, Y. X., & Fang, J. Y. (2020). Comprehensive review of targeted therapy for colorectal cancer. *Signal transduction and targeted therapy*, 5(1), 22.

Xu, F., He, Q., Li, X., Chang, C.-K., Wu, L.-Y., Zhang, Z., Liu, L., Shi, W.-H., Zhu, Y., Zhao, Y.-S., Gu, S.-C., Fei, C.-M., Guo, J., Wu, D., & Zhou, L. (2014). Rigosertib as a selective anti-tumor agent can ameliorate multiple dysregulated signaling transduction pathways in high-grade Myelodysplastic Syndrome. *Scientific Reports*, 4: 7310.

Xu. W., Yang, S., Zhou, K., Pan, L., Li, Z., Zhou, J., Gao, S., Zhou, D., Hu, J., Feng, R., Huang, H., Ji, M., Guo, H., Huang, J., Novotny, W., Feng, S., Li, J. (2019). Zanubrutinib for patients with relapsed or refractory chronic lymphocytic leukemia. *Hematological Oncology*, 37(Suppl 2): 87–8.

Yamaguchi, T., Kakefuda, R., Tajima, N., Sowa, Y., & Sakai, T. (2011). Antitumor activities of JTP-74057 (GSK1120212), a novel MEK1/2 inhibitor, on colorectal cancer cell lines in vitro and in vivo. *International Journal of Oncology*, 39 (1): 23-31.

Yamaguchi, T., Kakefuda, R., Tajima, N., Sowa, Y., & Sakai, T. (2011). Antitumor activities of JTP-74057 (GSK1120212), a novel MEK1/2 inhibitor, on colorectal cancer cell lines in vitro and in vivo. *International Journal of Oncology*, 39(1), 23–31.

Yamaoka, K., Saharinen, P., Pesu, M., Holt, V. E., 3rd, Silvennoinen, O., & O'Shea, J. J. (2004). The Janus kinases (Jaks). *Genome Biology*, 5(12): 253.

Yamaoka, T., Kusumoto, S., Ando, K., Ohba, M., & Ohmori, T. (2018). Receptor Tyrosine Kinase-Targeted Cancer Therapy. *International journal of molecular sciences,* 19(11), 3491.

Yamaoka, T., Kusumoto, S., Ando, K., Ohba, M., & Ohmori, T. (2018). Receptor Tyrosine Kinase-Targeted Cancer Therapy. *International Journal of Molecular Sciences,* 19(11), 3491.

Yan, C., Huang, M., Li, X., Wang, T., & Ling, R. (2019). Relationship between BRAF V600E and clinical features in papillary thyroid carcinoma. *Endocrine connections*, 8(7), 988–996.

Yang, J., Ikezoe, T., Nishioka, C., Tasaka, T., Taniguchi, A., Kuwayama, Y., Komatsu, N., Bandobashi, K., Togitani, K., Koeffler, H. P., Taguchi, H., and Yokoyama, A. (2007). AZD1152, a novel and selective aurora B kinase inhibitor, induces growth arrest, apoptosis, and sensitization for tubulin depolymerizing agent or topoisomerase II inhibitor in human acute leukemia cells in vitro and in vivo. *Blood*, 110 (6): 2034-2040.

Yang, J., Nie, J., Ma, X., Wei, Y., Peng, Y., & Wei, X. (2019). Targeting PI3K in cancer: mechanisms and advances in clinical trials. *Molecular Cancer*, 18(1), 26.

Yang, K., & Fu, L.-w. (2015). Mechanisms of resistance to BCR–ABL TKIs and the therapeutic strategies: A review. *Critical Reviews in Oncology/Hematology*, 93 (3): 277-292.

Yang, N., Deng, W., Sun, Q., Liang, J., Wang, L., Fan, S., Tang, R., Yu, Y., Sun, J., Zhou, F., Dai, G., Qing, W., Su, W., and Ren, Y. (2016). HMPL-523, a Novel SYK Inhibitor Showed Anti-Tumor Activities In Vitro and In Vivo. *Blood,* 128 (22): 3970-3970.

Yang, X., Pan, X., Cheng, X., Kuang, Y., & Cheng, Y. (2018). Risk of Gastrointestinal Events during Lapatinib Therapy: A Meta-Analysis From 12,402 Patients With Cancer. *American Journal of Therapeutics*, 25(4), e412–e422.

Yang, Y., Ding, l., Zhou, Q., Fen, L., Cao, Y., Sun, J., Zhou, X., & Liu, A. (2020). Silencing of AURKA augments the antitumor efficacy of the AURKA inhibitor MLN8237 on neuroblastoma cells. *Cancer Cell International*, 20: 9.

Yarden, Y., & Pines, G. (2012). The ERBB network: at last, cancer therapy meets systems biology. *Nature reviews. Cancer*, 12(8), 553–563.

Yoh, K., Seto, T., Satouchi, M., Nishio, M., Yamamoto, N., Murakami, H., Nogami, N., Matsumoto, S., Kohno, T., Tsuta, K., Tsuchihara, K., Ishii, G., Nomura, S., Sato, A., Ohtsu, A., Ohe, Y., & Goto, K. (2017). Vandetanib in patients with previously treated RET-rearranged advanced non-small-cell lung cancer (LURET): an open-label, multicentre phase 2 trial. *The Lancet. Respiratory Medicine*, 5(1), 42–50.

Young, R. M., Hardy, I. R., Clarke, R. L., Lundy, N., Pine, P., Turner, B. C., Potter, T. A., and Refaeli, Y. (2009). Mouse models of non-Hodgkin lymphoma reveal Syk as an important therapeutic target. *Blood*, 113 (11): 2508-16.

Yu, Z., Liu, Y., & Li, Z. (2012). Structure-function Relationship of the Polo-like Kinase in Trypanosoma Brucei. *Journal of Cell Sciences*, 125 (Pt 6): 1519-30.

Yuan, C.-X., Zhou, Z.-W., Yang, Y.-X., He, Z.-X., Zhang, X., Wang, D., Yang, T., Wang, N.-J., Zhao, R. J., & Zhou, S.-F. (2015). Inhibition of mitotic aurora kinase A by alisertib induces apoptosis and autophagy of human gastric cancer AGS and NCI-N78 cells. *Drug Design, Development and Therapy*, 9: 487-508.

Yuan, J., Sanhaji, M., Krämer, A., Reindl, W., Hofmann, M., Kreis, N.-N., Zimmer, B., Berg, T., & Strebhardt K. (2011). Polo-box domain inhibitor poloxin activates the spindle assembly checkpoint and inhibits tumor growth *in vivo*. *American Journal of Pathology*, 179 (4): 2091-9.

Zabriskie, M. S., Eide, C. A., Tantravahi, S. K., Vellore, N. A., Estrada, J., Nicolini, F. E., Khoury, H. J., Larson, R. A., Konopleva, M., Cortes, J. E., Kantarjian, H., Jabbour, E. J., Kornblau, S. M., Lipton, J. H., Rea, D., Stenke, L., Barbany, G., Lange, T., Hernández-Boluda, J. C., Ossenkoppele, G. J., … O'Hare, T. (2014). BCR-ABL1 compound mutations combining key kinase domain positions confer clinical resistance to ponatinib in Ph chromosome-positive leukemia. *Cancer Cell*, 26(3), 428–442.

Zeidan, A. M., Schiller, G. I., Lin, T. L., Becker, P. S., Patel, P. A., Wang, E. S., Spira, A. I., Tsai, M. L., Ridinger, M., Croucher, P. J., Erlander, M., & Silberman, S. L. (2019) Safety, Efficacy and Biomarker Analysis of a Phase 1b/2 Study of Onvansertib (ONV), a Polo-like Kinase 1 (PLK1) Inhibitor, in Combination with Low-Dose Cytarabine (LDAC) or Decitabine (DEC) in Patients (pts) with Relapsed/Refractory Acute Myeloid Leukemia (R/R AML). *Blood,* 134 (Supplement_1): 230

Zeidan, A. M., Becker, P., Spira, A. I., Patel, P. A., Schiller, G. J., Tsai, M. L., Lin, T. L., Ridinger, M., Erlander, M., Silberman, S. L., & Cortes, J. E. (2019). Phase Ib safety, preliminary anti-leukemic activity and biomarker analysis of the polo-like kinase 1 (PLK1) inhibitor, onvansertib, in combination with low-dose cytarabine or decitabine in patients with relapsed or refractory acute myeloid leukemia. *Cancer Research*, 79 (13 Supplement): CT102.

Zelenetz, A. D., Barrientos, J. C., Brown, J. R., Coiffier, B., Delgado, J., Egyed, M., Ghia, P., Illés, Á., Jurczak, W., Marlton, P., Montillo, M., Morschhauser, F., Pristupa, A. S., Robak, T., Sharman, J. P., Simpson, D., Smolej, L., Tausch, E., Adewoye, A. H., Dreiling, L. K., … Hillmen, P. (2017). Idelalisib or placebo in combination with bendamustine and rituximab in patients with relapsed or refractory chronic lymphocytic leukaemia: interim results from a phase 3, randomised, double-blind, placebo-controlled trial. *The Lancet. Oncology*, 18(3), 297–311.

Zhan, J. Y., Ma, J., & Zheng, Q. C. (2019). Molecular dynamics investigation on the Asciminib resistance mechanism of I502L and V468F mutations in BCR-ABL. *Journal of Molecular Graphics and Modelling*, 89: 242-249.

Zhang, G., Scarborough, H., Kim, J., Rozhok, A. I., Chen, Y. A., Zhang, X., Song, L., Bai, Y., Fang, B., Liu, R. Z., Koomen, J., Tan, A. C., Degregori, J., & Haura, E. B. (2016). Coupling an EML4-ALK-centric interactome with RNA interference identifies sensitizers to ALK inhibitors. *Science signaling,* 9(450), rs12.

Zhang, G., Zhou, X., & Lin, C. (2015). Efficacy of chemotherapy plus bevacizumab as first-line therapy in patients with metastatic colorectal cancer: a meta-analysis and up-date. *International journal of clinical and experimental medicine,* 8(1), 1434–1445.

Zhang, J., Yang, P. L., & Gray, N. S. (2009). Targeting cancer with small molecule kinase inhibitors. *Nature reviews. Cancer*, 9(1), 28–39.

Zhang, S. Q., Smith, S. M., Zhang, S. Y., & Lynn Wang, Y. (2015). Mechanisms of ibrutinib resistance in chronic lymphocytic leukaemia and non-Hodgkin lymphoma. *British Journal of Haematology*, 170(4): 445–456.

Zhou, C., Wu, Y. L., Chen, G., Feng, J., Liu, X. Q., Wang, C., Zhang, S., Wang, J., Zhou, S., Ren, S., Lu, S., Zhang, L., Hu, C., Hu, C., Luo, Y., Chen, L., Ye, M., Huang, J., Zhi, X., Zhang, Y., ... You, C. (2011). Erlotinib versus chemotherapy as first-line treatment for patients with advanced EGFR mutation-positive non-small-cell lung cancer (OPTIMAL, CTONG-0802): a multicentre, open-label, randomised, phase 3 study. *The Lancet. Oncology*, 12(8), 735–742.

Zhou, Y., Fu, C., Kong, Y., Pan, D., Wang, Y., Huang, S., Li, Z., Ning, Z., Lu, X., Shan, S., & Xin, L. (2016). Antitumor and immunomodulatory effects of a novel multitarget inhibitor, CS2164, in mouse hepatocellular carcinoma models. *Anticancer Drugs*, 30 (9): 909-916.

Zhou, Y., Shan, S., Li, Z. B., Xin, L. J., Pan, D. S., Yang, Q. J., Liu, Y. P., Yue, X. P., Liu, X. R., Gao, J. Z., Zhang, J. W., Ning, Z. Q., & Lu, X. P. (2017). CS2164, a novel multi-target inhibitor against tumor angiogenesis, mitosis and chronic inflammation with anti-tumor potency. *Cancer Science*, 108 (3): 469-477.

Zhu, J., Cao, J., Qiu, L., Qi, J., Song, Y., Tu, M., Ji, D., Shen, W., Sun, M., Hua, Y., Yang, C., Yu, C., Wang, J., Dai, G., and Su, W. (2018). Preliminary Results from a Phase 1 Study of HMPL-523, a Highly Selective Syk Inhibitor, in Chinese Patients with Mature B-Cell Lymphomas. *Blood*, 132 (Supplement 1): 5324-5324.

Zirlik, K., &Veelken H. 2018. "Small Molecules in Hematology," Part of the *Recent Results in Cancer Research book series* (RECENT CANCER, volume 212), edited by U. M. Martens (ed.), 243-264, Springer International Publishing AG, part of Springer Nature.

In: An Introduction to Cancer Therapy
Editor: Neville Charron
ISBN: 978-1-53618-450-1

Chapter 3

CURRENT STRATEGIES IN CANCER GENE THERAPY

Betül Bozdoğan*[1], *PhD, Göknur Kara*[2], *PhD and Emir Baki Denkbaş*[3,*], *PhD
[1]Chemistry Department, Aksaray University, Aksaray, Turkey
[2]Chemistry Department, Ordu University, Ordu, Turkey
[3]Biomedical Engineering Department, Başkent University, Ankara, Turkey

ABSTRACT

Cancer ranks second among the causes of death in developed countries. It is stated that 9.6 million people died in 2018 due to cancer. The clinical failure of conventional cancer treatments like chemotherapy, radiotherapy, and surgery necessitates novel therapeutic strategies that minimize the side effects and enhance long-term patient survival. In the past two decades, there have been dramatic scientific and technological advances in cancer genomic research, and consequently, gene therapy has emerged as a promising approach for cancer treatment. Since gene therapy is developed, 60% of research is focused on cancer. In its most general definition, gene therapy can be described the correction of a genetic

[*] Corresponding Author's E-mail: ebdenkbas@baskent.edu.tr, emirbaki@gmail.com.

deficiency by inserting a wild type version of a defective or missing gene into the somatic cells, by silencing the gene that causes a disease, or by inserting new genes to overcome a disease thereby treating a disorder or disease. There are several prospective strategies for gene therapy of cancer. These are suicide gene therapy, anti-angiogenic gene therapy, immunomodulatory gene therapy, chemoprotection approach, RNA interference therapy, and pro-apoptotic gene therapy. In this chapter, the currently employed gene therapy strategies, obstacles, and challenges in cancer gene therapy were presented. The theme was focused on the latest nanotechnological advancements in this field including gene transfer methods, vectors, and their current successful applications in cancer gene therapy.

Keywords: gene therapy, cancer, suicide gene therapy, anti-angiogenic gene therapy, immunomodulatory gene therapy, chemoprotection, RNA interference, pro-apoptotic gene therapy

1. Introduction

Cancer, the second leading cause of death worldwide, is one of the most complex diseases with its great number of cellular abnormalities and various genetic disorders. According to the data of the World Health Organization (WHO), it is estimated that approximately 10 million people die from cancer by 2020 [1]. The unsatisfactory efficacy and undesirable systemic toxicity of chemotherapy and radiotherapy, which are traditional cancer treatments, pose a serious threat to human health. In particular, the rapid development of cell resistance against chemotherapeutic agents, or even the presence of drug resistance before treatment, causes chemotherapy to have a low therapeutic rate for many tumors. Both radiotherapy and surgery are limited due to tumor invasion and the spread to external areas where the treatment is directly accessible. For these reasons, new treatment forms need to be developed urgently to ensure long-term survival, especially for patients with poor prognosis [2, 3].

Significant advances have been made in cancer research and genomics over the past two decades, with two independent draft versions of the human genome sequence and approximately 30,000 genes identified and published in 2001. This revolutionary development has shed light on extensive investigations in molecular genetics about gene function and biological processes that cause genetic deviation and malignant transformation [4]. With the emergence of genetic information about cancer, therapeutic approaches, called gene therapy, have been developed, based on the transfer of genetic material (DNA or RNA) into damaged cells and to fix the underlying defect or eliminate the neoplastic cell [5].

To date, there are many gene therapy strategies developed against cancer that has proven success *in vitro*, *in vivo*, and even clinically, and are highly promising for cancer patients. In the suicide gene therapy, cell suicide-inducing transgenes encoding an enzyme such as herpes simplex thymidine kinase (HSV-TK) or bacterial cytosine deaminase (CD) are introduced into tumor cells. Following, the prodrug, which is converted into a cytotoxic metabolite by the enzyme, is administrated [6]. Another strategy is anti-angiogenic gene therapy in which a therapeutic gene is transferred to cancer cells to down-regulation of proangiogenic factors (e.g.: vascular endothelial growth factor, fibroblast growth factor, and platelet-derived growth factor) and up-regulation of angiogenesis inhibitor factors (e.g.: endostatin, and angiostatin) [7]. In the immunomodulatory gene therapy, the patient's immune response can be stimulated with the tumor-specific expression of immunostimulators and the antitumor immune response may be augmented for the selective destruction of cancer cells [8]. Treating cancer with chemotherapy not only affects malignant cells but also damages non-cancerous cells. Chemoprotection cancer gene therapy is an interesting approach to protect normal cells from drug toxicity during chemotherapy and to increase the effectiveness of chemotherapy. There are many successful results in which genes such as multidrug resistance (MDR), O^6-Methylguanine methyltransferase (MGMT), and dihydrofolate reductase (DHFR) are given to normal cells, protecting those cells from the toxic side effects of MDR drugs, alkylating agents, and antifolates, respectively. This strategy, therefore, has the potential to be used in combination with higher dosages of chemotherapy drugs for the treatment of several malignancies [9]. In RNAi-based cancer gene therapy, non-encoded RNA molecules inhibit the expression of mRNAs encoding pathogenic factors and the formation of the related protein. This strategy has drawn great attention in particular for several therapeutic oncogene targets that have proven to be undruggable [10, 11]. It is important to target the apoptotic machinery in cancer gene therapy, as imbalances or mutations in the expression of pro-apoptotic genes in tumors cause erroneous apoptotic signaling. Therefore, pro-apoptotic cancer gene therapy has emerged as a powerful strategy that aims to the introduction of genes that trigger apoptosis [12].

2. Cancer Gene Therapy

2.1. Suicide Gene Therapy

Among cancer gene therapies, suicide gene therapy has gained considerable attention. Suicide gene therapy, gene-directed enzyme prodrug therapy (GDEPT), consists of two steps: (i) vector-mediated delivery of a prodrug activator suicide genes into target cancer cells and (ii) subsequent activation of the suicide mechanism by the administration of a specific prodrug. The inactive prodrugs were converted into cytotoxic metabolites (chemotherapeutic agents) by the suicide enzyme. This treatment can also be considered as "intracellular chemotherapy".

The concept of suicide gene therapy was first introduced as "tumor chemosensitivity" in 1986. The anti-herpes drug acyclovir exhibits minimal toxicity to cells lacking herpes simplex virus thymidine kinase (HSV-TK) gene but exhibits selective toxicity to cells expressing the HSV-TK gene. It is converted to toxic form by HSV-TK activity and inhibits DNA synthesis of the infected cells [13]. The viral thymidine kinase converts 9-([2-hydroxy-1-(hydroxymethyl)ethoxy]methyl) guanine, called "ganciclovir", which is a better substrate for HSV-TK than acyclovir, into ganciclovir monophosphate, and then this product is diphosphotylated into ganciclovir triphosphate by cellular enzymes. Ganciclovir triphosphate incorporates into DNA and triggers the apoptotic signals. Introduction of HSV-TK gene into the cancer cells and followed by treatment with acyclovir, ganciclovir, or brivudin caused the regression of the tumors, systemic side effects are minimized, and therapy is localized to the gene transfection site. This gene therapy approach opened the field of suicide gene therapy [14]. This HSV-TK/ganciclovir system, the most widely used suicide gene therapy, pioneered other enzyme-encoding suicide gene/prodrug combinations including cytosine deaminase/5-fluorocytosine, horseradish peroxidase/ indole-3-acetic acid, carboxypeptidase G2/ N,N-[(2-chloroethyl) (2-mesyloxy-ethyl) amino] benzoyl-L-glutamic acid, and purine nucleoside phosphorylase/6-methylpurine deoxyriboside.

The enzyme cytosine deaminase from *Escherichia coli* can deaminate nontoxic prodrug 5-fluorocytosine to the toxic molecule 5-fluorouracil to achieve the suicide gene therapy [15]. The purine nucleoside phosphorylase (PNP) enzyme system of *Escherichia coli*, which catalyzed the conversion of nontoxic deoxyadenosine analogs and purine nucleosides like (6-methylpurine-20-deoxyriboside or arabinofuranosyl-2-fluoroadenine monophosphate) to toxic adenine analogs, was utilized in the treatment of human malignant tumors [16]. Human phase I clinical trial (NCT 01310179; IND 14271) was conducted to evaluate efficacy and safety of adenoviral vector expressing E. coli purine nucleoside phosphorylase in combination with intravenous fludarabine monophosphate that is a clinically approved chemotherapeutic for the treatment of solid tumors [17]. The process disrupts RNA and protein synthesis, furthermore, fluoroadenine has the unique bystander killing, which is the ability to kill neighboring cells. Another enzyme/prodrug combination is horseradish peroxidase and plant hormone indole-3-acetic acid (auxin) which is converted by this enzyme into the toxic product, 3-methylene-2-oxindole [18]. Other suicide gene therapy systems are the cytochrome P450 reductase/cyclophosphamide and ifosfamide, *E. coli* nitroreductase /5-(aziridin-1-yl)-2,4-dinitrobenzamide, linamarase/linamarin, beta-lactamase/Cephalosporin doxorubicin and 7-(4-carboxybutanamido)-cephalosporin mustard, carboxypeptidase A/ methotrexate-a-peptides, and human carboxylesterase gene/irinotecan. All of them were patented [19, 20]. Every year, several new or modified enzyme/prodrug systems are discovered and only some of them moved towards preclinical and clinical studies.

2.1.1. Delivery Systems for Suicide Gene Therapy

Although more than 100 clinical trials on suicide gene therapy have been performed globally, the clinical translations of these systems have been largely failed due to limitations such as low cancer specificity, poor therapeutic outcome, and the high dose required for prodrug administration. Consequently, the need to develop new strategies especially carrier systems for suicide genes has emerged. These carrier systems should deliver the suicide gene and prodrug targeted and simultaneously to the tumor at appropriate doses. The suicide gene therapy should be combined with other treatment modalities for maximum synergistic efficacy. The monitoring of carrier and evaluation of the therapeutic performance can improve the outcome of the treatment of cancer.

With the advent of nanotechnology, numerous nanomaterials had been promising carriers in suicide gene therapy. These nanoparticles can be targeted to tumors by active targeting with tumor-specific antibodies or peptides and passive targeting due to Enhanced Permeation and Retention (EPR) effect. The viral or non-viral vectors are developed to transfect tumor cells with a gene encoding a specific exogenous enzyme. One of the current strategies of suicide gene therapy is the development of effective non-viral gene delivery vectors for penetration of genes through tumor cells, endosomal escape to the cytosol, efficient cancer cell uptake, and biodegradability. Multifunctional polymeric, organic, and inorganic nanoparticles could be employed as non-viral suicide gene carriers. An ideal gene carrier should have some critical features like (i) low toxicity, (ii) non-immunogenicity, (iii) improving genetic material stability, (iv) increasing the transfection efficacy, and (v) specific targeting [21].

The favorite candidate materials for gene vector are cationic lipids and polymers. Because, genes can be easily loaded by electrostatic interactions between positively charged groups of cationic polymers (e.g., polylysine or polyethyleneimine) and the negatively-charged phosphate backbone of nucleic acids [21]. Cationic lipids are the most used non-viral carrier used in 4.5% of clinical trials performed so far [22]. Salvioni and coworkers developed a novel delivery system based on cationic lipid-protamine nanoparticles for a suicide plasmid gene encoding saporin (SAP). SAP plasmid is higher cytotoxic for triple negative breast cancer cells. Protamine is a polycation and a condensing agent which improve the lipofection efficacy. The transfection of cancer cells with lipid-protamine-plasmid DNA nanotherapeutic resulted in tumor mass reduction without systemic toxicity and organ damage [23].

A research group developed nanoparticles as effective non-viral HSV-TK vectors from cationic poly(beta-amino ester)s (PBAE) polymers, poly(ethylene glycol)-modified PBAEs, and end-modified PBAEs by electrostatic interaction with nucleic acids [24, 25]. These PBAEs vectors are promising for the suicide gene therapy of human brain cancers. Sukumar and coworkers synthesized nanoparticles from poly(D-L-lactic-co-glycolic acid), poly(ethylene glycol), and polyethyleneimine (PLGA-PEG-PEI) triblock copolymers. The nanoparticles were used to deliver a thymidine kinase-p53-nitroreductase triple therapeutic gene (TK-p53-NTR) for synergistic therapy against hepatocellular carcinoma. The developed nanoparticles showed high loading efficiency for triple gene and markedly bettered suicide gene therapy with the simultaneous co-expression of p53 and subsequent administration of prodrugs. Resulting, a superior therapeutic outcome was established [26]. As an efficient gene delivery system, graphene oxide-hydroxyapatite (GO-Hap) nanocomposites were developed. The transfection cells with these nanocomposites resulted in inhibited proliferation, induced cell apoptosis, and minimum toxicity in human breast cancer cells. The GO-HAp nanocomposites have a significant capability as a gene delivery vector [27]. Magnetic nanoparticles (MNPs) can be a potential candidate for suicide gene carrier systems. According to the results of the research carried out by Wang and coworkers, rod-like mesoporous silica nanoparticles exhibited faster prodrug release behavior, better hyperthermia properties, and higher gene loading capacity. Magnetically-targeted, magnetic resonance imaging (MRI)-guided, hyperthermia-enhanced, and therapeutic outcome-monitored suicide gene therapy with rod-like mesoporous silica nanoparticles have provided highly effective therapy for cancer *in vivo* [28]. Yuan et al. developed magnetic nanoparticles for combining suicide gene therapy, magnetic hyperthermia, and imaging probe for simultaneous treatment and diagnosis of cancer, namely theragnosis of cancer [29]. Chitosan stabilized quantum dots and fluorescent emitting gold nanoclusters were also used as a nanocarrier for delivery of cytosine deaminase-uracilphosphoribosyl transferase suicide gene and real-time monitoring of gene delivery [30, 31]. In a study of Malik and coworkers, polylysine-modified polyethylenimine copolymer was used as a non-viral transfection agent for the delivery of the suicidal gene (HSV-TK) and tumor necrosis factor-related apoptosis-inducing ligand (TRAIL) gene in mesenchymal stem cells. The TRAIL protein encoded by the TRAIL gene can specifically induce apoptosis and enhance the activity of HSV-TK/GCV. These transfected mesenchymal stem cells provided combinational, cost-effective, tumor-targeted, and low immunogenic therapy for glioblastoma treatment [32]. Biocompatible and low immunogenic serum cationic albumin can form a stable polyplex with plasmid DNA and be also used as a gene delivery vehicle by conjugated with polyethyleneimine [33].

One of the challenges in this pHSV-TK/ganciclovir combination suicide gene therapy is short plasma half-life (~2–6 h), and the very low oral bioavailability (~5%) of ganciclovir. Ganciclovir has to be injected (5 mg/kg) daily to maintain the therapeutic plasma concentration. Therefore, a carrier that can efficiently deliver both suicide genes and prodrug can further the efficacy of this suicide gene therapy. The cationic, amphiphilic copolymer-based nanoparticles from poly (lactide-co-glycolide) -graft-polyethyleneimine (PgP) demonstrated effective suicide gene/drug carrier properties in both rat glioma (C6) cells *in vitro* and T5 SCT animal model *in vivo*. The PgP/pHSV-TK with ganciclovir treatment increases apoptosis of tumor cells and consequently reduces tumor size in a rat model [34].

Another non-viral approach to suicide gene delivery is cell-based delivery systems like mesenchymal stem cells (MSCs). MSCs are the most suitable cells as the delivery agent due to hypo-immunogenicity, ease of isolation, expansion, the capability of self-renewal, and genetic manipulation. In a study, plasmids containing both the firefly luciferase and the yeast cytosine deaminase uracil phosphoribosyl transferase (CDUPRT) genes were loaded in murine MSCs as vehicles of suicide gene therapy. The fusion with the uracil phosphoribosyl transferase gene improves the cytosine deaminase system by sensitizing 5-FU-resistant tumor cells to low concentrations of 5-FU. *In vitro* bioluminescence imaging showed that luciferase can be used as an *in vitro* reporter system for monitoring the cytotoxic effect of the suicide gene [35]. In another study, MSCs were transfected with HSVTK- and murine interferon-gamma-expressing plasmid vectors. IFN-gamma has a high antitumor activity and a higher therapeutic effect. The MSCs that were sensitive to ganciclovir and released IFN-gamma significantly suppressed the proliferation of murine adenocarcinoma cell lines *in vitro* and *in vivo* [36].

Viruses have the ability to introduce their genetic material in host cells. Due to their ability, they are widely used as gene vectors. Adenoviruses, herpes viruses, retroviruses, poxviruses, adeno-associated viruses (parvoviruses), lentiviruses, vaccinia virus, Epstein-Barr virus, and human cytomegalovirus can be used viral vectors. Retroviral replicating vectors (RRVs) are the inability to infect non-dividing cells but show inherent specificity for mitotically active cells. Because of this reason, they can achieve tumor-selective transduction. RRVs are non-cytolytic in contrast to other viruses utilized in gene delivery [37]. RRVs can be engineered to carry prodrug activator genes that highly efficiently kill a wide variety of cancer cells upon prodrug administration, *in vitro* and *in vivo* [38-40]. Phase I clinical trials for RRV-mediated prodrug activator gene therapy resulted in long-term survival and T cells-mediated systemic antitumor immunity inpatient with recurrent glioblastoma [41]. RRVs are currently evaluated in an international phase III trial for recurrent high-grade glioma.

Oncolytic viruses are anti-tumor agents and can kill cancer cells. In 2015, the US Food and Drug Administration (FDA) approved first oncolytic viruses for the treatment of melanoma, genetically engineered herpes simplex virus. The growing trend is the combining of oncolytic viruses with other cancer treatments, such as gene therapies and chemotherapies. Vaccinia virus-thymidine kinase deleted oncolytic vaccinia viruses containing a mutant HSV-TK transgene reduced the replication in tumors by >50% and demonstrated tumor selectivity and sensitivity to GCV [42].

2.1.2. Combination with other Therapeutic Strategies

Cancer cells can transform resistant to any chemotherapeutic agent. Therefore, combination regimes by additive or synergetic effects are essential for reducing the risk of resistance and enhancing the antitumor effect. The combination of the prodrug activator genes herpes simplex virus thymidine kinase and cytosine deaminase in the presence of the respective prodrugs ganciclovir and 5-fluorocytosine produced synergistic cytocidal effects [43]. The phenomenon, in which toxic drug and its metabolites diffuse into the surrounding non-recipient cells and kills them, is named the "bystander effect". Toxic ganciclovir molecules diffuse into surrounding cells via connexin-based Gap junctions. It is known that resveratrol induces the upregulation of connexin in hepatocellular carcinoma cells (HCC). According to the results of a study planned based on this fact, the killing effect of the HSV-TK suicide gene on HCC cells is boosted by the promotion of resveratrol to the bystander effect [44].

The current strategies for enhancing the therapeutic effect of suicide mechanisms are combinatorial approaches. In combination therapy, two or more enzyme/prodrugs couples with a similar or different mode of action combined with chemotherapy, radiation therapy, or ultrasound to realize synergistic anticancer therapeutic potentials. The combination of radiofrequency hyperthermia with green fluorescent protein (GFP)/herpes simplex virus thymidine kinase (HSV-TK)/ganciclovir (GCV) gene therapy was evaluated for the treatment of cholangiocarcinoma, which is a most lethal malignancy resistant to chemotherapy. The combination of suicide gene therapy with radiofrequency hyperthermia significantly decreased tumor volumes compared to individual effects. On the other hand, this research provided monitoring of the therapeutic outcome by bioluminescent optical imaging [45]. The success of molecular image-guided, intratumoral radiofrequency hyperthermia–enhanced herpes simplex virus thymidine kinase/ganciclovir gene therapy in the treatment of non–small-cell lung cancer and ovarian cancer has also been demonstrated [46, 47]. It is known that the utilization of tissue- or cell-specific promoters elevates the expression of HSV-TK genes. The heat shock protein (HSP) synthesis, which is low under normal conditions, increases in the presence of extreme temperatures. The image-guided delivery of suicide gene and intratumoral radiofrequency hyperthermia increased the targeted expression of HSP promoter-mediated HSV-TK gene and curative effect of HSV-TK/ganciclovir suicide gene therapy system [48].

Another combination approach for suicide gene therapy is focused on ultrasound-induced microbubble cavitation for reversibly and locally opening blood-brain barrier (BBB) for enhancing suicide gene delivery in glioma. By focused ultrasound-induced BBB opening, adenoviral-mediated HSV-TK gene can be effectively delivered and overexpressed in the brain tumor. In *in vivo* experiments, the stronger anti-tumor effect and longer survival time were observed after the administration of ganciclovir [49]. Ultrasound and microbubble mediated sonoporation were also used for effective suicide gene delivery vehicle, which was polyethylene glycol (PEG)ylated-poly(lactic-co-glycolic acid)/polyethyleneimine nanoparticles (PLGA/PEI NPs) [50].

2.2. Anti-Angiogenic Gene Therapy

Angiogenesis in which novel capillary blood vessels form is a normal physiological process. It only occurs at the embryonic development, bone repair, wound repair, and the female reproductive cycle in normal conditions. It is a key element in tissue engineering and regenerative medicine applications [51]. Angiogenesis is a complex process. It is induced by degradation of the basement membrane glycoproteins and extracellular matrix components; endothelial cells activate, migrate, and proliferate; endothelial cells transform into tubular structures; form capillary vessels; and develop novel basement membrane. Anomalous increasing angiogenesis is a marker of solid tumor development and growth. The association between angiogenesis and tumorigenesis was explained by Folkman in 1971. He hypothesized anti-angiogenesis therapy to treat cancer [52]. Microvasculature network supplies the nutrient, oxygen, and drainage the metabolites to the tumor.

The angiogenesis mediated signaling pathways during pathogenesis and carcinogenesis activate the angiogenesis and lead to the development of impaired pathological neovascularization. Some proangiogenic regulators including vascular endothelial growth factor (VEGF), epidermal growth factor, transforming growth factor-α and -β (TGF-α and -β), placental-derived growth factor, basic fibroblast growth factor, platelet-derived growth factor, and angiopoietin 1 and 2 underpin abnormal tumor vasculatures or tumor angiogenesis mechanisms. Genetic mutations (loss of tumor-suppressor genes or activation of oncogenes), metabolic stress (low pH, hypoxia, or hypoglycemia), and the immune/inflammatory response trigger the angiogenic signaling. Tumor angiogenesis is a target for anti-angiogenic cancer therapy. Antiangiogenic drugs such as monoclonal antibodies, receptor tyrosine kinase inhibitors, or various protein inhibitors of VEGF are administered to treat cancer. They have the disadvantages of high cost, short half-life, and tendency to interference by endogenous substances. Using VEGF inhibitors alone or in combination with other chemotherapeutics caused the resistance of the therapy in patients [8]. Compared with monoclonal antibodies and pharmaceutical proteins used in anti-angiogenic therapies, gene therapy presents sustained and localized expression of the anti-angiogenic gene product, fewer side effects, lower cost. In 2015, more than 2,200 clinical trials had been conducted on gene therapy. Over 60% of them were on cancer gene therapy. Anti-angiogenic gene therapy is one of the most studied gene therapy strategies for cancer treatment. Current anti-angiogenic gene therapies are based on two principles. In (i) gene augmentation, the expression of exogenous anti-angiogenic genes introduced stop tumor angiogenesis. In (ii) gene blockade, exogenous anti-angiogenic genes inhibit the excessive expression of pro-angiogenic genes. The genes of interest are pro-angiogenic genes for gene blockade and anti-angiogenic genes for gene augmentation [8].

2.2.1. Interleukin-12 (IL-12)

IL-12 is a pro-inflammatory cytokine with immunoregulatory functions. IL-12 exhibits an anti-tumor effect due to its ability to stimulate immunity and inhibit tumor angiogenesis. Phase 1 clinical study on intratumoral electroporation of plasmid IL-12 provided long-term overall survival in patients with malignant melanoma [53]. The phase 2 study of IL-12 electroporation therapy in melanoma results that tumor responses in 31% of patients were induced, and no severe systemic or local side effect was observed [54]. The current strategies in IL-12 anti-angiogenic gene therapy are the development of different delivery systems with high specificity, low toxicity, and sustained local expression of the gene. Viral vectors for IL-12 such as herpes simplex virus mutants, Semliki Forest virus, and adenoviruses provided effective gene delivery for some cancer like malignant melanoma [55], metastatic breast cancer [56], and pancreatic cancer [57]. Other current strategies for IL-12 anti-angiogenic gene therapy were combining with the suicide gene therapy approach [58], chemotherapeutics such as bleomycin, and electroporation [59].

2.2.2. Angiostatin

Plasminogen is an angiogenesis inhibitor and has an anti-tumor effect. Angiostatin is one of the four domains of a proteolytic fragment of plasminogen. Angiostatin and other plasminogen derivatives show anticancer activities. Angiostatin exhibits a limited therapeutic activity due to its short half-life [60]. To overcome this limitation, various delivery agents were developed. Viruses especially herpes simplex virus, oncolytic measles virus, adenovirus, adeno-associated virus, vaccinia virus, and lentivirus can be used as viral vectors. Herpes simplex virus, which has a potential for the targeting to cancer stem cells, can be used as a vector for angiostatin gene. Zhang and coworkers engineered a herpes simplex virus expressing an endostatin–angiostatin fusion gene for targeting of glioblastoma stem cells. It expressed an endostatin–angiostatin fusion gene and exhibited antitumor effect by limiting tumor microvasculature development [61]. Angiostatin gene is often co-transfected with endostatin gene or other genes in combination for a synergistically anti-tumor effect. Medulloblastomas are the most common pediatric brain tumors. Medulloblastomas are highly vascularized and can be efficiently treated with angiogenesis inhibitors. Hutzen et al. developed a virotherapy approach by oncolytic measles virus expressing a fusion protein of two endogenous angiogenesis inhibitors: endostatin and angiostatin. The oncolytic measles viruses expressing anti-angiogenic fusion gene inhibited the formation of tumor-associated angiogenesis [62]. In anti-angiogenic therapy, targeting endothelial cells is more practical than targeting tumor cells. The inhibition of EC proliferation, migration, and EC apoptosis may damage the viability of numerous tumor cells. Another viral vector, lentivirus was used as an anti-angiogenic gene carrier including angiostatin, endostatin, and vascular endothelial growth factor receptor 2 (sFlk1) genes. Lentivirus mediated combinatorial anti-angiogenic gene therapy targeting different endothelial growth factor signaling pathways inhibited endothelial cell proliferation in malignant mesothelioma cells [63]. As an application of non-viral vectors, cationic liposomes have been examined in the co-transfection of IL-12 gene with anti-angiogenic endostatin, saxatilin, and angiostatin genes. This liposome-mediated co-transfection strategy synergistically inhibited melanoma growth [64].

2.2.3. Endostatin

Endostatin, a fragment of type XVIII collagen, is an endogenous angiogenesis inhibitor [65]. Endostatin gene therapy studies primarily focused on (i) combining endostatin with other gene therapy strategies [66, 67] or other techniques like chemotherapy or radiotherapy [68]; (ii) and developing a more effective gene delivery system. Among the recent researches on gene delivery systems, Liang and coworkers' work attracts attention because they constructed a bacterial vector. Salmonella typhimurium are Gram-negative facultative anaerobic bacteria. They attenuate their virulence and enhance their tumor-targeting and immunostimulatory ability by designing a mutant, which delivers endostatin plasmid. The results showed that Salmonella colonization and endostatin expression increase the apoptosis and suppress the tumor angiogenesis within cancerous tissues [69]. Zhuo et al. developed a novel liposomal delivery system with dual functions. The liposome exhibits anti-angiogenesis gene delivery and targeted tumor imaging functions. Loaded liposomes have spherical shape and diameter of 122 ± 11 nm. It is targeted to tumor-derived endothelial cells. Endostatin-loaded liposomes enhanced tumor targeting, imaging, and gene transfer; and suppressed tumor growth by 71% [70]. A research group encapsulated recombinant plasmids co-expressing endostatin and DESI2, which is a novel pro-apoptotic gene and induces apoptosis, within DOTAP/Cholesterol cationic liposome as a delivery agent. Combination of endostatin with DESI2 inhibited proliferation of colon carcinoma and lung cancer cells via inducing apoptosis and suppressing angiogenesis *in vitro* and *in vivo*. The combined gene therapy importantly inhibited tumor growth and prolonged survival [66]. Folate-decorated and endostatin loaded nanoparticles were used in the anti-angiogenic gene delivery application. Positively charged nanoparticles exhibited pH-responsive endostatin release and anti-proliferative effect [71].

2.2.4. Tumstatin

Tumstatin, a cleavage fragment of type IV collagen, is an alternative endogenous angiogenesis inhibitor. Its anti-angiogenic activity is 10-fold higher than endostatin. Its anti-angiogenesis is through the inhibition of cell proliferation and tube formation in endothelial cells and induction of endothelial cells apoptosis [72]. The use of bacteria for cancer treatment has a long history. Anaerobic intestinal probiotics E. coli Nissle 1917 (EcN) have been licensed as a pharmaceutical for the treatment of diarrhea and colitis ulcerosa. Moreover, EcN colonizes and replicates in the necrotic tumor tissue. It is also used as a Tum-5 carrier in gene therapy. Tum-5 is an anti-angiogenic active fragment of tumstatin. The expression of Tum-5 in the EcN, which infects the tumor tissue, restrained B16 melanoma tumor growth [73]. Nonpathogenic and anaerobic Bifidobacterium longum (BL) selectively localize and grow in the hypoxia region within tumor tissue. A vector expressing tumstatin was built and transformed into BL. Tum-transformed BL can be represented as an effective gene delivery system for cancer treatment [74].

2.2.5. Anti-Angiogenic Metargidin Peptide (AMEP)

AMEP is a novel anticancer agent. It binds to $\alpha5\beta1$ and $\alpha V\beta3$ integrins via its Arg-Gly-Asp (RGD) integrin-binding sequence [75]. Electroporation-mediated gene therapy with AMEP-coding plasmids was evaluated on low and highly metastatic B16 melanoma variants. The study resulted in attenuation of angiogenesis; inhibition of proliferation, invasion, and migration of melanoma cells; and reduction of metastasis [76]. AMEP plasmids can be delivered via electrotransfer, the use of electric pulses to transfer genes. In phase 1 clinical study, treatment with electrotransfer-mediated AMEP plasmid delivery applications is effective, safe, and tolerable in patients [77, 78].

2.2.6. NK4

NK4 is a novel bifunctional anti-tumor agent. NK4 exhibits anti-angiogenic activity via indirectly inhibiting VEGF expression and directly affecting endothelial cells. Mesenchymal stem cells (MSCs) selectively migrate toward the tumor tissue and is one of the most preferred delivery vehicles for cancer targeting. The anti-angiogenic effect of human placenta-derived MSCs expressing NK4 was examined in patients with glioblastoma multiforme. The proliferation of GBM cells and the growth of tumor were inhibited by the induction of apoptosis after coculture with MSCs expressing NK4 *in vitro* [79]. Cai and coworkers combined MSCs with an adenovirus vector to deliver the NK4 gene in order not to induce the immunological rejection. MSCs significantly migrated to high metastasis liver carcinoma cells. Co-culture with NK4-modified MSCs significantly suppressed the proliferation and migration of cancer cells *in vitro.* In animal studies, angiogenesis and tumor growth were significantly restrained [80].

2.2.7. Endoglin

Endoglin is a TGF-β co-receptor and activates a complex signaling pathway concerning the proliferation, adhesion, and migration of endothelial cells. Increased expression of endoglin in the endothelial cells of tumor vascular is a predictive factor for prognosis. In the anti-angiogenic gene therapy, the silencing endoglin gene by RNA interference strategy demonstrated good anti-angiogenic and antitumor efficacy. Intratumoral gene electrotransfer (GET) of plasmids encoding shRNA against endoglin has been explored for antitumor efficacy in a study. GET-mediated silencing of endoglin with irradiation. The combined treatment significantly decreased the number of blood vessels and proliferating, and increased necrosis, apoptosis, and hypoxia [81]. Transfection properties of polyplexes of modular peptide carrier L1 and siRNAs for silencing VEGFA, VEGFR1, and endoglin genes were studied in endothelial cells EA.Hy926 and breast cancer cells MDA-MB-231. Anti-angiogenic treatment of cancer was synergistically improved via down-regulation of proliferation and migration of endothelial cells by anti-VEGFA, -VEGFR1, and -endoglin siRNAs [82].

2.3. Immunomodulatory Gene Therapy

Immunotherapy emerged as a novel strategy for cancer therapy. The immunotherapy utilizes the inherent immune system and its components and induces the anticancer immune response to exterminate cancer. Two main components of the immune system to combat foreign antigens are B-cells and T-cells. B-cells secrete antibodies that circulate in the blood to bind their antigens. T-cells don't secrete antibodies, interact directly with their antigens, and mediate multiple immune reactions. All cancer cells express tumor-specific antigens, namely tumor-associated antigens (TAAs), and are immunogenic. The objective of immunotherapy is to enhance the recognition and presentation of TAAs. The most important challenge in cancer immunotherapy is the strongly immunosuppressive micro-environment of the tumor. Also, cancer cells can escape from the immune system by secreting immunosuppressive factors and downregulating antigen expression. Immunotherapy may employ one or more of the below approaches for fighting against cancer. In active immunotherapy (vaccine therapy), the patient's immune response is stimulated by cytokines and gene vaccines. In the case of passive immunotherapy, cytokines and antibodies are administrated to directly affect the cancer cells. In adoptive immunotherapy, the patient's T-cells or dendritic cells are manipulated *ex vivo* and then inoculated back to enhance antitumor response. Lastly, immune enhancement therapy augments immune stimulatory molecules or deactivates immune inhibitory molecules [3, 4].

The genetic immunotherapy strategies comprise the transfer of genes encoding immune-stimulating molecules, cytokines. Cytokines can modulate tumor growth by inducing and activating the innate immune response. In recent years, IL-4, IL-6, IL-7, IL-12, IL-15, IL-18, IL-21, and IL-2 are explored in clinical trials for immunomodulatory cancer therapy [83]. Another genetic immunotherapy strategy is the manipulation of antigen-presenting cells. Genetically engineered dendritic cells expressing antigens that are the most powerful antigen-presenting cells can provoke a strong immune reaction against cancer cells (cell vaccines). Either, the desired immune reaction can be induced by direct antigen-encoding genes vaccination [84].

2.3.1. Interleukin-2 (IL-2)

IL-2 is a key cytokine that induces the proliferation of T-cells and cytotoxic T lymphocytes (CTLs) immune response. IL-2 is a strong immunostimulator. FDA approved IL-2 for the treatment of renal cell carcinoma in 1992 and for metastatic melanoma in 1998. The systemic IL-2 treatment caused toxicity affecting almost all organs and the protein of IL-2 had a short half-life. For the solution to this obstacle, local IL-2 delivery was employed [83]. Nonreplicating adenoviral vectors encoding human IL-2 complementary DNA were constructed. Direct intratumoral administration of IL-2 vectors was effective in tumor growth inhibition [85]. Huang et al. proposed a dual-targeted immunogene therapy. They utilize the synergistic effect of plasmid DNA encoding IL-2 for promoting antitumor immunity and siRNA against the immune checkpoint PD-L1 for silencing immunosuppressive factors. To overcome short half-life, inefficient intracellular release and lack of specificity of siRNA/pDNA, they designed unique dendrimer-calcium phosphate nanoparticles containing an-HCC-targeting peptide (SP94) and thymine-capped polyamidoamine dendrimer. This nanoparticle exhibits efficient intracellular delivery of genes by targeting, the pH-responsive release of genes by CaP core, enhanced endosomal escape and nuclear entry of genes by thymine-capped polyamidoamine dendrimer, and promoted cellular immunity by stimulating interferon genes. Nanoparticles-mediated and tumor-targeted delivery of immunomodulatory genes ensure tumor-specific expression of immunostimulators and downregulation of immunosuppressors [86].

2.3.2. Interleukin-12 (IL-12)

IL-12 is a pivotal cytokine that activates both innate and adaptive immunities. Pathogen-associated molecular pattern recognition trigger IL-12 which causes the secretion of interferon-γ by T-cells, dendritic cells, and natural killer cells. This secretion causes additional IL-12 production. IL-12 gene therapy is the most used technique of immunomodulatory gene therapy. Liu et al. developed a methoxy poly(ethylene glycol)-poly(lactide) (MPEG-PLA) and 1,2-dioleoyl-3-trimethylammonium-propan(DOTAP) based delivery system for IL-12 via self-assembly method. Treatment with proposed therapeutic inhibited tumor growth *in vivo* by inhibiting angiogenesis, activating immunity, reducing proliferation, and promoting apoptosis [87]. Men and coworkers synthesized monomethoxy poly(ethylene glycol)poly(epsilon-caprolactone) with the DOTAP lipid-based cationic micelles for delivery of IL-12 for cancer immunogene therapy. The micelles showed strong inhibition of cancer cell growth *in vitro*. Local and systemic administration of micelles demonstrated multiple anti-cancer activities including TNF- α secretion, angiogenesis inhibition, T-cell infiltration, and apoptosis induction *in vivo* [88]. Polyamidoamine (PAMAM) is a more largely investigated gene carrier. PAMAM was modified with cholesteryl chloroformate and alkyl-PEG and loaded with plasmid encoding IL-12 gene for colon cancer immunogene therapy. This non-viral immunogene delivery agent provided an efficient and safe alternative for delivering genes [89]. Nissim et al. constructed an RNA-based gene circuit platform for tumor-specific expression of immunostimulators. Their circuit includes novel synthetic cancer-specific promoters and RNA-based AND gate which generates combinatorial outputs only when both promoters are decidedly and mutually active. While input promoter 1 modulates an auto-inhibitory mRNA encoding the output protein, input promoter 2 modulates an RNA molecule that attenuates the auto-inhibition and increases the production of outputs. The circuit produces immunomodulatory outputs including an immunogenic cell surface antigen

(STE), a chemokine, which provokes T-cells delivery to tumor areas (CCL21), a cytokine that activates and regulates T-cell function (IL-12), and a checkpoint inhibitor antibody (anti-PD1). The circuit selectively triggered the T-cell mediated killing of cancerous cells, *in vitro*. Lentiviral mediated delivery of circuit significantly diminished the tumor and prolonged survival time in ovarian cancer model. This circuit design reduced off-target immunogenic effects [90]. Combination approaches of immunogenic therapy with physical methods such as electropermeabilization-based treatments show promising results. In a study, a peritumoral plasmid IL-12 electrotransfer was combined with partial-irreversible electropermeabilization treatment of melanoma to kill cancer cells and release of tumor antigens, which are able to activate immune cells. This two-step combined treatment delayed the tumor growth and restrained a second tumor by activation of the immune system [91]. The phase II clinical trial of electroporated tavokinogene telseplasmid IL-12 was recently conducted in advanced melanoma patients. The treatment drove changes in immune responses with minimal local or systemic toxicity. This in situ tumor vaccination can be a safe and effective treatment for cancer [92].

2.3.3. Bispecific T-cell Engager Antibodies (BiTEs)

BITEs possess two specific single-chains for connection to the surface antigen on cancer cells and ligand on T-cells and play a linking role. It promotes the immune synapse on the cancer cells and T-cells. A research team discovered stearic acid grafted polyethyleneimine (stPEI) and calcium phosphate (CaP) based delivery system to carry minicircle DNA expressing BiTE antibodies. This delivery system with high transfection efficiency, low cytotoxicity, and long-term effects promoted the production of BiTEs and showed a high T cell-directed cytotoxicity on HCC [93].

2.3.4. Interferons (INFs)

INFs are other well-established cytokines in cancer immunotherapy. The IFNs are proteins and glycoproteins with antiproliferative, immunomodulatory, and antiviral effects. Their secretion augments cytotoxic T lymphocytes, natural killer cells, and macrophages activity.

Interferon-β is a potent antiangiogenic and antimetastatic molecule. Interferon-α induces apoptosis of tumor cells and inhibits angiogenesis. Type I interferon (IFN-I) has an anti-tumor effect against urothelial carcinoma by stimulating the immune response. Phase 1 clinical trials with adenoviral interferon-α resulted in increased expression of T-cells and IL-6-mediated antitumor response [94]. MSCs expressing IFN-β were administrated to the tumor-bearing mice and observed reduction in tumor size and weight in prostate cancer [95] and bladder cancer [96].

2.4. Chemoprotection Gene Therapy

The primary principle of medicine, "primum non nocere" or in other words "first, do no harm" is not all the time coherent with the oncological interventions, such as chemotherapy, targeted therapy, and radiotherapy, as they often cause remarkable toxicities [97]. Although the term "Medical Machiavellianism" describes the paradigm of "first, do harm to do good" for oncological treatment approaches in which toxicity and benefit are inseparably linked, anti-Medical Machiavellianism takes place as the toxicity goes beyond the benefit [98].

Systemic chemotherapy is currently one of the most widely used forms of treatment in many types of cancer. To date, numerous chemotherapeutic agents either alone or in combination have been developed that can kill tumor cells [99]. Chemotherapy has been successful in treating most patients with Hodgkin's disease, testicular cancer, and pediatric acute lymphocytic leukemia. However, for several other types of cancers like adult carcinomas, chemotherapy only had marginal impacts [100]. One of the reasons for this problem is that tumor cells can develop MDR [101, 102]. The other reason of the problem is that anticancer drugs do not have specificity for tumor cells, that is, they affect not only the malignancies, but also cause serious damage to healthy cells and tissues [100]. Chemotherapeutic agents have side effects including alopecia, immunosuppression, stomatitis, vomiting, nausea, and anorexia which lead to decreased functional competence and quality of life in cancer patients [103, 104]. As a result of these toxicities, a reduction in chemotherapy dose and frequency of administration, or discontinuation of treatment in extreme cases may be required. Limitations in the agent doses used result in insufficient tumor cell killing and failure to achieve disease-free remission [99].

Chemotherapy drugs exhibit significant toxicity in especially rapidly proliferating cells, such as those in the gastrointestinal tract and the blood-forming hematopoietic system. In particular, hematological toxicity prevents the administration of chemotherapy on time and thus the therapeutic success by causing severe infectious complications, thrombocytopenia, and myelosuppression. In this regard, to protect hematopoietic cells from the negative influences of chemotherapy drugs, researchers have developed a number of gene therapy approaches. The basic idea behind this approach is to transfer appropriate drug resistance genes to hematopoietic stem cells (HSCs) to prevent myelosuppression and preserve blood formation during chemotherapy thus to reduce the toxic side effects of anticancer agents [4, 100]. Overexpression or transgene expression of drug resistance genes in HSCs and/or progenitor cells is also called chemoprotection or myeloprotection gene therapy and has emerged as a potential approach to overcome this issue [105, 106].

The proposed clinical procedure for the insertion of the drug-resistance gene into HSCs is accomplished by autologous transplantation. With this strategy, HSCs are obtained from the patient's own bone marrow or peripheral blood of patients treated with stem-cell mobilization procedures. By using one of the known phenotypic markers like the CD34 antigen, stem cells are enriched [100, 107, 108]. Moreover, the stem cells are *ex vivo* transduced with a viral vector containing the chemotherapy resistance gene. The patient then receives chemotherapy not only to destroy cancer cells but also to facilitate engraftment of the genetically modified stem cells that will be afterward infused. After CD34+ stem cell transplantation, chemotherapy drugs are administered in a sequential dose-intense manner with the expectation that the genetically modified stem cells will avoid otherwise inadmissible toxicity [100, 108]. Reducing toxic side effects, in particular in myelosuppression after chemotherapy, may provide using overdose intensive drug combinations to ultimately obviate tumor resistance [108].

A number of drug resistance genes have been identified and studied for their chemoprotective characteristics from cytotoxic drugs mediated toxicities.

2.4.1. Multidrug-Resistance 1 Gene (MDR1)

There are multiple mechanisms that regulate the formation of drug resistance in the cells. One of the major causes of MDR is the overexpression of ATP binding cassette (ABC) transport protein, P-glycoprotein (P-gp). P-gp is the product of MDR gene ABCB1 (ABC transporter family B member 1, also known as MDR-1) [102, 109, 110] and functions as a drug efflux pump by excreting various compounds including chemotherapeutic drugs including actinomycin D, epipodophyllotoxins, anthracyclines, vinca alkaloids, taxol and taxotere out of cells in an ATP-dependent-manner [3]. P-gp is highly expressed in normal human cells to hinder drug accumulation while in erythroid and myeloid bone marrow cells its expression is too reduced to act as a protective factor. Therefore, these cells become vulnerable to cytotoxic chemotherapy [107]. A large number of studies using MDR1 transgenic mice have successfully demonstrated that hematopoietic cells can be protected from chemotherapy drugs.

A previous study reported that the transplantation of MDR1 gene transduced human placenta mesenchymal stem cells (MSCs) in nude mice resulted in the protection of bone marrow toxicity arising through chemotherapeutic agent paclitaxel [111]. As a result of MDR1-MSCs transplantation, the survival rate of mice drastically increased after receiving paclitaxel indicating the transplantation might improve resistance to chemotherapeutic toxicity.

Gene transfer targeting HSCs was also studied using more than one protective genes [106]. In the context of myelodysplasia and acute myeloid leukemia, the researchers investigated *in vitro* combined overexpression of MDR1 and cytidine deaminase (CDA) to protect the lymphohematopoietic system against the side effects of combination chemotherapy that includes cytosine arabinoside (Ara-C) and anthracyclines. For this purpose, myeloid 32D cells, and primary lineage marker negative (lin−) murine bone marrow cells were transduced with 3rd generation, self-inactivating (SIN) lentiviral vectors. MDR1 and CDA transduced cells exhibited successful resistance against Ara-C and anthracycline application at concentrations 5–20 times the LD50 of non-transduced control cells. In addition, it has been also revealed that the transduced cells significantly enriched following Ara-C/anthracycline administration.

2.4.2. O^6-Methylguanine Methyltransferase (MGMT)

MGMT is a protein that hampers the DNA damage caused by bischloroethylnitrosourea (BCNU), temozolomide (TMZ), and chloroethylnitrosourea (CCNU), that are frequently used alkylating agents in solid malignancies in particular brain tumors, by directly removing the alkyl residue [112]. The high expression level of MGMT in primary brain tumors is related to drug resistance and failure of the treatment [113]. O^6-benzylguanine (O^{6}BG) is a substrate analog that eliminates drug resistance in tumor cells by depleting MGMT. However, the combination of O^{6}BG with alkylating agents is limited in clinical use as it causes severe hematopoietic toxicity [114].

Adair et al. conducted clinical trials with glioblastoma patients using chemoprotective HSC gene therapy approaches. In their study conducted in 2012, mutant MGMT (P140K) gene-modified HSCs were transplanted into patients to remove hematopoietic toxicity arising from O^{6}BG/TMZ combination therapy in glioblastoma patients with high MGMT levels. Thus, the safety and feasibility of this strategy were proved based on the results of the first three patients participating in this trial [115]. As a continuation of this study, this time, 7 patients in total were treated to achieve enhanced chemotherapy tolerance and improved outcome results [116]. Glioblastoma patients with high MGMT tumors were given BCNU and then received autologous gene-modified HSCs. Patients underwent O^{6}BG/TMZ chemotherapy in 28-day cycles following hematopoietic recovery. The results of gene therapy indicated that a marked increase in the mean number of tolerated O^{6}BG/TMZ cycles in comparison to historical controls without gene therapy was observed. In addition, it has been also revealed that there is a significantly delayed tumor growth at low cumulative

TMZ dosages in patients in comparison to the patients receiving standard TMZ regimens without O^6BG.

2.4.3. Cytidine Deaminase

Human cytidine deaminase (hCDA, EC 3.5.4.5) is an important enzyme in the nucleotide salvage pathway, and it deaminates cytidine (CR) and deoxycytidine (CdR) into uridine and deoxyuridine, respectively [117]. hCDA also catalyzes the deamination of various cytidine nucleoside analogs used in cancer treatment such as Ara-C, azacytidine, decitabine, gemcitabine, and turn them into inactive metabolites lacking antineoplastic properties [9, 118].

In a previous work, the *in vivo* myeloprotection capability of lentiviral vectors mediated Dox-induced hCDA overexpression was investigated using a murine transplant model. The research revealed that the hematopoietic system of mice was protected and dramatically avoided from Ara-C toxicity with the accelerated recovery of platelets and granulocytes [119]. In 2015, Lachmann et al. presented a promising *in vitro* hCDD-based myeloprotective gene therapy strategy with minimal background activity. They developed doxycycline (Dox)-inducible 'all-in-one' self-inactivating (SIN) lentiviral vector using a pTET-T11 (TII) minimal-promoter and a reverse transactivator protein (rtTA2S-M2) driven by the phosphoglycerate kinase promoter to be used for tight regulation of transgene expression (Lv.TII vectors) in human hematopoietic cells. The vector was modified with the CDA gene, and rapid and dose-dependent transgene expression onset was detected in K562 and primary human CD34+ hematopoietic cells after Dox administration. In Lv.TII.CDA-transduced K562 cells, Dox-inducible hCDA expression provided a 10-fold increase in resistance against Ara-C. Additionally, it was observed that Lv.TII.CDD-transduced CD34+ myeloid cells were durable up to 300 nM Ara-C while control cells were influenced by 50 nM [120].

2.4.4. Dihydrofolate Reductase (DHFR)

DHFR reduces folate to dihydrofolate, and dihydrofolate to tetrahydrofolate in an NADPH-dependent manner in mammalians cells

[121]. A variant of the DHFR gene was used in the first drug resistance vector, where its capability to protect bone marrow cells against chemotherapeutics *in vivo* was studied [122]. The DHFR enzyme has been reported to contain several amino acid substitutions that confer resistance to an antifolate drug, methotrexate (MTX), toxicity in drug-sensitive normal cells [121, 123]. MTX is a clinically potent chemotherapeutic agent used in the treatment of many cancer types such as osteosarcoma, non-Hodgkin's lymphoma, and acute lymphoblastic leukemia [124]. Hematopoietic cells can be protected from both *in vitro* and *in vivo* antifolate effects by the retroviral vectors expressing these variants [125].

A non-viral transposon system that is called sleeping beauty (SB) and has the ability to introduce new sequences into the chromosomes of vertebrate cells was used by Hyland et al. In the study, hematopoietic progenitor cells (HPCs) were modified by SB transposon system for DHFR-tyr22 expression thus the cells can resist to high amounts of MTX indicating a selective and chemoprotective approach [123].

2.4.5. Challenges of Chemoprotection Gene Therapy

With this approach, gastrointestinal cells cannot be preserved. There is also the risk that drug resistance genes can transfer to the cancer cells and make them insensitive to chemotherapeutic drugs. In addition, with the incorporation of a new gene to a host stem cell's genome may allow other oncogenes to develop malign characteristics and change other adjacent genes to create other diseases [4]. These challenges should be taken into consideration to maintain the performance of chemoprotection cancer gene therapy.

2.5. RNAi Based Gene Therapy

Cancer is a genetic disease characterized by a high level of both intra- and inter-tumoral heterogeneity and as well as intra- and inter-patient heterogeneity. This molecular heterogeneity plays a great role in distinctly varied responses to standard therapeutic applications. Therefore, to identify the molecular profile of each patient and develop personalized treatment programs in line with this information remain very important [126]. The currently used cancer treatments have disadvantages such as being non-selective, leading side effects responsible for long-term and costly recovery, and causing relapse at later time points. In this regard, targeted therapies can offer more effective and less harmful approaches [1, 127]. RNA interference (RNAi) is a rapidly emerging strategy that has a wide potential as personalized gene therapy for cancer, due to its target specificity, wide targeting capacity, and adaptability [10, 126].

2.5.1. RNAi Mechanism

RNAi is a conserved and naturally occurring process that regulates gene expression and prevents the conversion of genes into protein. It is also used in cells as a defense mechanism against foreign nucleic acids from bacteria and viruses [128, 129]. RNAi was first discovered by Fire and Mello in 1998 and described as a sequence-specific post-transcriptional gene silencing by double-stranded RNA (dsRNA) molecules. In this cellular mechanism, long non-coding RNA transcripts are diced into short dsRNA fragments by Dicer enzyme, and these dsRNAs interact with the RNA-induced silencing complex (RISC) that contains several proteins, including Argonaute and transactivation response RNA-binding protein. Within the activation of the RISC complex, one of the strands which is called "passenger or sense strand" is discarded and the other strand which is called "guide or antisense strand" complementarily pairs and binds with the homologous target mRNA sequence. Hereby, the mRNA and subsequently its expression is degraded namely silenced by induction of RNAse-mediated cleavage [130-132].

In mammalian cells, usually long dsRNAs cannot cleave into small interfering RNA (siRNA), and long dsRNA injection triggers an interferon response. Elbashir et al. first demonstrated that 21 nucleotide-long RNAs can mediate RNAi machinery to silence gene expression in mammalian cells [133]. This paved the way for the researchers to transfer synthetic short dsRNAs to mammalian cells for gene silencing approaches.

siRNAs (exogenous, synthetic double-stranded molecules) and microRNAs (miRNAs, endogenous, inherent, genome-origin single-stranded molecules) are the key molecules that trigger RNAi mechanism [134]. The mechanism of action of siRNAs and miRNAs is pretty similar in terms of post-transcriptional gene silencing [135]. The difference in the mode of action between the miRNA and siRNA is that a single miRNA can target a number of mRNAs whereas siRNA can target only one specific mRNA [134]. In addition, miRNAs often use eight nucleotides from 5' end to recognize their target mRNA sequences and use their inhibitory functions in the translation process. However, siRNAs use almost their full length to identify target sequences and mediate cleavage of the target mRNA [136, 137]. This chapter will focus on siRNA-based RNAi applications and challenges in cancer treatment.

RNAi holds great promise in oncology for the design and development of new molecular therapeutic drugs against the cancer-causing or -related genes, In particular, RNAi technology is groundbreaking with its new generation treatment approach for the genes that encode so-called "non-druggable" targets and are not amenable to traditional treatments [10, 138].

2.5.2. Challenges of siRNA-Based RNAi Therapy

There are early-phase trials reporting successful clinical responses to RNAi therapies in cancer patients however, improvements in RNAi-based therapeutics are required in various areas [10]. In order for siRNA-based therapeutic approaches to move from the bench to the clinic, several challenges such as efficient *in vivo* delivery of siRNAs, long-term serum stability of siRNA, biological safety and, off-target effects need to be overcome [139].

The major biological barrier faced by siRNA administered *in vivo* is the nucleases in plasma and tissues. siRNAs can be easily degraded by nucleases in the systemic circulation and filtered out by the renal system, resulting in a short half-life *in vivo* [140]. It was previously reported that the half-life of naked or free (unmodified) siRNA in serum ranges between several minutes and 1 h [141]. Another barrier to the effective *in vivo* administration of siRNA is that it is uptaken by the reticuloendothelial system (RES), which consists of macrophages and monocytes responsible for removing cellular debris and foreign pathogens [142]. Additionally, cellular uptake of siRNA is also poor due to the fact that hydrophilic and anionic siRNA cannot efficaciously pass through the biological membranes [126].

Artificial siRNAs have been demonstrated as potent promoters of the innate immune response inducing inflammatory cytokines in vitro and *in vivo* [143]. siRNA therapeutics-based toxicity may occur because of inappropriate target recognition of exogenously introduced RNA. Inappropriate target recognition may be caused by the RISC choosing the passenger strand instead of the guide strand, or by poor annealing of guide to the target mRNA [144, 145]. Besides, partial homology between siRNA and off-target mRNA transcripts can cause undesired gene silencing. The main determinant of off-target silencing is the part called the seed region where contains bases 2-7 from 5′ ends of the guide strand, and the possibility of cross homology of this region should be considered during the siRNA drug design for clinical use [146, 147].

Chemically modification (like phosphorothioate (PS) modification and cholesterol/ligand conjugation) and vector-based encapsulation of siRNA have demonstrated protection and maintained effective dosage and stability in the site of action. However, caution is required when chemically modifying siRNAs because some modifications prevent the siRNA from integrating properly into the RISC complex, leading to loss of mRNA targeting [1, 129]. Although viral vectors are highly effective with respect to *in vivo* siRNA applications, safety-related problems limit their use. For this reason, nanotechnology-based non-viral vectors became promising for improved *in vivo* siRNA delivery with their overall biocompatibility [127].

2.5.3. Current Clinical Trials of siRNA-Based Therapies for Various Cancer Types

The therapeutic potential of siRNA therapies has been broadly shown in preclinical studies. Despite the challenges, some of the siRNA therapeutics have been investigated in clinical trials for the treatment of several diseases including cancer. A variety of siRNA carriers have been increasingly developed to overcome the problems and maintain clinically appropriate siRNA-based drugs. These carriers are typically cationic cell-penetrating peptide, polymer, or lipid-based nanoparticle systems that provide siRNA encapsulation and delivery [148]. Table 1. shows the nanocarrier system integrated siRNA-based cancer drugs such as siRNA-EphA2-DOPC, TKM-080301, siG12D-LODER, Atu027, and DCR-MYC, which have recently entered phase I/II of human clinical trials.

2.5.3.1. siRNA-EphA2-DOPC

The researchers in MD Anderson Cancer Center formulated siRNA-EphA2-DOPC drug containing neutral DOPC nanoliposomes encapsulated with EphA2 siRNAs that knockdown EphA2. EphA2 is a cell surface receptor tyrosine kinase and responsible for neuronal cell migration. It was reported that overexpression of EphA2 is related to cancer, tumor growth, and poor clinical outcome [149]. Preclinical results demonstrated that DOPC mediated silencing of EphA2 led to reduced tumorigenicity in breast and pancreatic cancers. Inhibition of EphA2 suppressed the tumor growth in ovarian cancer model in mice and enhanced anti-tumor activity when using in combination with chemotherapeutics [150]. In addition, preclinical trials carried out with non-human primates indicated that siRNA-EphA2-DOPC drug was well tolerated and there is no dose-dependent side effect. Currently, the siRNA-EphA2-DOPC drug is recruited in MD Anderson Cancer Center under Phase I clinical trials. In the trial, 40 patients with advanced solid tumors are intravenously administered with EphA2 encapsulated DOPC liposomes twice a week (clinicaltrials.gov identifier NCT01591356).

2.5.3.2. TKM-080301

A siRNA drug called TKM-PLK1 or TKM-080301 that targets PLK1 was developed by Arbutus Biopharma Corporation to treat the patients who have HCC, Gastrointestinal Neuroendocrine Tumors (GI-NET) and Adrenocortical carcinoma (ACC) [151]. The PLK1 is excessively expressed in cancer cells and involved in tumor cell growth. The clinical trials focused on patients with HCC were completed using LNPs as a transfection agent to deliver siRNA against PLK1. TKM-PLK1 was administered to 43 patients as a four-week cycle, containing three weeks injection and then a rest week. The data obtained from Phase I/II clinical trials indicated that the drug reduced the tumor density up to 59% (clinicaltrials.gov identifier NCT02191878).

2.5.3.3. siG12D-LODER

Silenseed manufactured the product called KRAS-LODER or siG12D-LODER to treat human pancreatic cancers, which is a poly(lactic-co-glycolic) acid (PLGA) complex releasing a G12D-mutated KRAS-targeted siRNA in a sustained manner for four months [152]. Since more than 90% of pancreatic ductal adenocarcinomas (PDAC) involves G12D mutation in the KRAS oncogene, silencing this gene has emerged as a promising antitumor strategy. During Phase I clinical trials, siG12D-LODER was administered into the patients with non-operable, locally advanced pancreatic cancer (LAPC) via an EUS biopsy needle in a dose escalation design. Patients were also received standard-of-care chemotherapy, mostly Gemcitabine, and in a number of instances FOLFIRINOX. The data obtained from 13 patients showed that no drug-related adverse side effects were observed considering the drug as safe and well-tolerated. While 9 patients treated with a single dose of LODER and Gemcitabine exhibited a median overall survival of 12.0 months, 3 patients treated with a LODER + modified FOLFIRINOX exhibited a median overall survival of 28.3 months (clinicaltrials.gov identifier NCT01188785). Currently, siG12D-LODER has proceeded to Phase II/III trials along with chemotherapy (gemcitabine+nab-paclitaxel) (clinicaltrials.gov identifier NCT01676259).

2.5.3.4. ATU-027

Silence therapeutics conducted clinical trials of Atu-027, which targets and silences PKN3 using lipoplex. PKN3 was reported to carry a crucial role in tumor growth and metastasis [155]. The lipoplex consists of positively charged lipid nanoparticles and negatively charges siRNAs [156]. Atu-027 was investigated under Phase II clinical trial in combination with gemcitabine for the treatment of patients with advanced or metastatic pancreatic adenocarcinoma (clinicaltrials.gov identifier: NCT01808638).

Table 1. siRNA therapeutics in clinical trials

Therapeutic Name	Target	Cancer Type	Delivery Vehicle	Route of Administ.	Phase	Sponsor	Recruitment Status	ClinicalTrials.gov identifier	Related Article
siRNA-EphA2-DOPC	EphA2	Advanced solid tumors	DOPC liposomes	IV	I	MD Anderson Cancer Center	Recruiting	NCT01591356	[150]
TKM-080301	PLK1	Advanced HCC	LNP	IV	I/II	Arbutus Biopharma Corporation	Completed/2015	NCT02191878	[153]
siG12D-LODER	KRAS G12D	Advanced pancreatic cancer	Biodegradable polymeric matrix	EUS biopsy needle	II	Silenceed Ltd	Recruiting	NCT01676259	[154]
Atu027	PKN3	Advanced or Metastatic Pancreatic Cancer	Liposomal particles	IV	I/II	Silence therapeutics	Completed/2016	NCT01808638	[155]

EphA2: ephrin type-A receptor 2.
DOPC: 1,2-dioleoyl-sn-glycero-3-phosphatidylcholine.
PLK1: polo-like kinase.
LNP: Lipid nanoparticles.
PKN3: protein kinase N3.
HCC: Hepatocellular carcinoma.
LODER: Local drug eluter.
EUS: endoscope ultrasound.

Clinical trials were carried out in two separate arms, in which two different doses of Atu-027 were used. Patients in arm 2 were exposed to 33% more Atu-027 than those in arm 1. Atu-027 was revealed to well-tolerated with the combined application with gemcitabine for pancreatic cancer patients. Using a higher dose of Atu-027 in the test arm 2 provided the patients to have higher overall survival and long-term of progression-free survival (PFS) rate than the patients in the test arm 1 [157].

2.6. Pro-Apoptotic Gene Therapy

Apoptosis is programmed cell death, which is described by a number of morphological and biochemical changes that include a number of regulated molecular interactions or signaling cascades [158]. While traditional cancer therapy approaches such as chemotherapy and radiation therapy cause a great deal of apoptosis in tumor cells, they unfortunately induce indistinguishable killing of normal cells as well [159]. Therefore, the development of pro-apoptotic drugs that target only the tumor and induce apoptosis without causing serious deterioration in the normal organism has provided new approaches to cancer treatment [160].

One of the common features observed in tumors is that they often exhibit abnormalities in programmed cell death pathways including apoptosis. Defective apoptotic signaling caused by mutations or imbalances in the expression of pro-apoptotic genes in malignant cells leads to targeting the apoptotic machine in cancer gene therapy. Triggering apoptosis by integrating genes encoding apoptosis inducer, mediator, or executioner into cells is one of the most frequently used gene therapy approaches [12].

To date, several pro-apoptotic molecules have been identified in tumors that are active in the apoptotic pathway and control the apoptotic threshold. One of the most important of these is p53, a tumor suppressor that has the ability to activate apoptosis [161]. Tumor necrosis factor-related apoptosis-inducing ligand (TRAIL) is another promising molecule used in cancer therapy by triggering apoptosis and killing tumor cells with high specificity [162]. However, due to the short serum half-life of the genes and the lack of effective *in vivo* administration approaches, the clinical use of therapeutically active pro-apoptotic genes has largely hindered. A great number of studies using nanoparticle systems as carriers are currently available that illuminate new ways to gene therapy approach for the treatment of several types of human malignancies.

2.6.1. p53

The TP53 that encodes p53 is the most commonly mutated gene in several human tumors such as ovarian cancer (96%), small cell lung cancer (85%), pancreatic cancer (75%), head and neck cancer (60%) and breast cancer (54%). In addition, TP53 mutations were reported to be associated with worse prognosis in various cancer types [163]. p53 has an important role in a variety of biological processes like cell cycle, apoptosis, angiogenesis, immune response, DNA metabolism, and cellular differentiation [164]. Besides, it acts as a tumor suppressor that promotes apoptosis by directly acting on the intrinsic apoptotic pathway or attenuating growth signals. When DNA damage occurs, p53 is phosphorylated and stabilized by the activation of DNA checkpoint proteins, and the gene transcription of other pro-apoptotic genes like Bax and Bid or tumor suppressors such as phosphatase and tensin homolog (PTEN) that lead to apoptosis, initiates [159].

The *in vitro* and *in vivo* therapeutic potential of p53 gene therapy in breast cancer was investigated in 2016 [165]. Transferrin modified silica nanoparticles (SiNPs) were prepared and used as a cationic non-viral gene delivery tool. Transferrin receptor-expressing breast carcinoma cells, MCF-7 were treated with transferrin-SiNPs-p53 complex and the transfected cells exhibited growth inhibition of 60.7% and apoptosis induction of 20.5%. Wild-type p53 expression and increased Bax expression were also obtained after transferrin-SiNPs-p53 treatment *in vitro* and *in vivo*. *In vivo* introduction of transferrin-SiNPs-p53 remarkably reduced tumor growth in the MCF-7 tumor model in nude mice suggesting that this inhibitory effect is due to the induction of apoptosis via p53 expression.

Li and colleagues co-encapsulated p53 gene and doxorubicin (DOX) in star-shaped polymeric micelles to reveal a combined anticancer effect.

Promising *in vitro* stability, biocompatibility, and gene transfection efficiency of the produced polyplexes were achieved in serum circumstances. It was observed that the polyplex system enables co-delivery of p53 and DOX, resulting in the enhanced apoptotic rate of tumor cells both *in vitro* and *in vivo.* The results also demonstrated not only a strong antitumor efficacy but also few side effects [166].

2.6.2. Tumor Necrosis Factor-Related Apoptosis-Inducing Ligand (TRAIL)

TRAIL (also known as APO2L or TNFSF10) is a type II membrane protein and a member of the TNF receptor superfamily. It is a promising anticancer death ligand that has attracted great interest due to its capability to trigger apoptosis in several cancer cells without killing non-cancerous cells. Therefore, TRAIL has emerged as a safe pro-apoptotic drug target and rapidly excited its entry into clinical trials [167]. TRAIL interacts with the death receptors (DR4 and DR5) which are preferentially expressed in malignant cells whereas in non-cancerous cells their expression is not significant. Together with Fas-associated death domain protein (FADD) and procaspase-8/10, death-inducing signaling complex (DISC) forms. With the formation of DISC, caspase 8 and cleaved caspase 8 are activated, and cell apoptosis is directly induced by activation of the downstream substrates of the apoptosis pathway [168].

Wang et al. studied a nanoparticle (NP) mediated targeted pro-apoptotic gene transfection for the treatment of glioblastoma (GBM). For this purpose, they designed chlorotoxin (CTX) conjugated chitosan–polyethylene glycol (PEG)-grafted polyethyleneimine (PEI) copolymer (CP-PEI) coated iron oxide nanoparticles (NPs) for effectively delivery TRAIL encoding plasmid DNA *in vitro* and *in vivo*. NP–TRAIL–CTX treatment-induced apoptosis threefold in T98G GBM cells in comparison to the control DNA bound NPs. More importantly, near-zero tumor growth and markedly induced apoptosis were obtained after systemic administration of NP–TRAIL–CTX to mice bearing T98G xenografts [169].

References

[1] Mahmoodi Chalbatani, G., Dana, H., Gharagouzloo, E., Grijalvo, S., Eritja, R., Logsdon, C. D., Memari, F., Miri, S. R., Rad, M. R., and Marmari, V. 2019. "Small interfering RNAs (siRNAs) in cancer therapy: a nano-based approach." *International journal of nanomedicine* 14: 3111-3128.

[2] McCormick, F. 2001. "Cancer gene therapy: fringe or cutting edge?" *Nature Reviews Cancer* 1 (2): 130-141.

[3] Ortiz, R., Melguizo, C., Prados, J., Álvarez, P.J., Caba, O., Rodríguez-Serrano, F., Hita, F., and Aránega, A. 2012. "New gene therapy strategies for cancer treatment: a review of recent patents." *Recent Pat Anticancer Drug Discov* 7 (3): 297-312.

[4] Amer, M. H. 2014. "Gene therapy for cancer: present status and future perspective." *Molecular and cellular therapies* 2: 27-27.

[5] Prados, J., Melguizo, C., Boulaiz, H., Marchal, J. A., and Aránega, A. 2005. "Cancer gene therapy: strategies and clinical trials." *Cell Mol Biol (Noisy-le-grand)* 51:1: 23-36.

[6] Zarogoulidis, P., Darwiche, K., Sakkas, A., Yarmus, L., Huang, H., Li, Q., Freitag, L., Zarogoulidis, K., and Malecki, M. 2013. "Suicide Gene Therapy for Cancer - Current Strategies." *J Genet Syndr Gene Ther* 4: 16849.

[7] Gatson, N. N., Chiocca, E. A., and Kaur, B. 2012. "Anti-angiogenic gene therapy in the treatment of malignant gliomas." *Neuroscience letters* 527 (2): 62-70.

[8] Li, T., Kang, G., Wang, T., and Huang, H. 2018. "Tumor angiogenesis and anti-angiogenic gene therapy for cancer (Review)." *Oncology Letters* 16 (1): 687-702.

[9] Beauséjour, C. M., Eliopoulos, N., Momparler, L., Le, N. L., and Momparler, R. L. 2001. "Selection of drug-resistant transduced cells with cytosine nucleoside analogs using the human cytidine deaminase gene." *Cancer Gene Ther* 8 (9): 669-76.

[10] Wu, S. Y., Lopez-Berestein, G., Calin, G. A., and Sood, A. K. 2014. "RNAi Therapies: Drugging the Undruggable." *Science Translational Medicine* 6: 240.

[11] Zhong, X., Zhang, D., Xiong, M., and Zhang, L. 2016. "Noncoding RNA for Cancer Gene Therapy." *Recent Results Cancer Res* 209: 51-60.

[12] Das, S. K., Menezes, M. E., Bhatia, S., Wang, X. Y., Emdad, L., Sarkar, D., and Fisher, P. B. 2015. "Gene Therapies for Cancer: Strategies, Challenges and Successes." *Journal of cellular physiology* 230 (2): 259-271.

[13] Field, A. K., Davies, M. E., DeWitt, C., Perry, H. C., Liou, R., Germershausen, J., Karkas, J. D., Ashton, W. T., Johnston, D. B., and Tolman, R. L. 1983. "9-([2-hydroxy-1-(hydroxymethyl) ethoxy]methyl)guanine: a selective inhibitor of herpes group virus replication." *Proc Natl Acad Sci USA* 80 (13): 4139-43.

[14] Moolten, F. L. 1986. "Tumor chemosensitivity conferred by inserted herpes thymidine kinase genes: paradigm for a prospective cancer control strategy." *Cancer Res* 46 (10): 5276-81.

[15] Austin, E. A. and Huber, B. E. 1993. "A first step in the development of gene therapy for colorectal carcinoma: cloning, sequencing, and expression of Escherichia coli cytosine deaminase." *Mol Pharmacol* 43 (3): 380-7.

[16] Sorscher, E. J., Peng, S., Bebok, Z., Allan, P. W., Bennett, L. L., Jr., and Parker, W. B. 1994. "Tumor cell bystander killing in colonic carcinoma utilizing the Escherichia coli DeoD gene to generate toxic purines." *Gene Ther* 1 (4): 233-8.

[17] Rosenthal, E. L., Chung, T. K., Parker, W. B., Allan, P. W., Clemons, L., Lowman, D., Hong, J., Hunt, F. R., Richman, J., Conry, R. M., Mannion, K., Carroll, W. R., Nabell, L., and Sorscher, E. J. 2015. "Phase I dose-escalating trial of *Escherichia coli* purine nucleoside phosphorylase and fludarabine gene therapy for advanced solid tumors." *Ann Oncol* 26 (7): 1481-7.

[18] Tupper, J., Stratford, M. R., Hill, S., Tozer, G. M., and Dachs, G. U. 2010. "*In vivo* characterization of horseradish peroxidase with indole-

3-acetic acid and 5-bromoindole-3-acetic acid for gene therapy of cancer." *Cancer Gene Ther* 17 (6): 420-8.

[19] Düzgüneş, N. 2019. "Origins of Suicide Gene Therapy." In *Suicide Gene Therapy: Methods and Protocols*, edited by N. Düzgüneş, 1-9. New York, NY: Springer New York.

[20] Navarro, S. A., Carrillo, E., Griñán-Lisón, C., Martín, A., Perán, M., Marchal, J. A., and Boulaiz, H. 2016. "Cancer suicide gene therapy: a patent review." *Expert Opinion on Therapeutic Patents* 26 (9): 1095-1104.

[21] Vago, R., Collico, V., Zuppone, S., Prosperi, D., and Colombo, M. 2016. "Nanoparticle-mediated delivery of suicide genes in cancer therapy." *Pharmacological Research* 111: 619-641.

[22] Ginn, S. L., Amaya, A. K., Alexander, I. E., Edelstein, M., and Abedi, M. R. 2018. "Gene therapy clinical trials worldwide to 2017: An update." *The Journal of Gene Medicine* 20 (5): 3015.

[23] Salvioni, L., Zuppone, S., Andreata, F., Monieri, M., Mazzucchelli, S., Di Carlo, C., Morelli, L., Cordiglieri, C., Donnici, L., De Francesco, R., Corsi, F., Prosperi, D., Vago, R., and Colombo, M. 2020. "Nanoparticle-Mediated Suicide Gene Therapy for Triple Negative Breast Cancer Treatment." *Advanced Therapeutics*: 2000007.

[24] Kim, J., Mondal, S. K., Tzeng, S. Y., Rui, Y., Al-Kharboosh, R., Kozielski, K. K., Bhargav, A. G., Garcia, C. A., Quiñones-Hinojosa, A., and Green, J. J. 2020. "Poly(ethylene glycol)–Poly(beta-amino ester)-Based Nanoparticles for Suicide Gene Therapy Enhance Brain Penetration and Extend Survival in a Preclinical Human Glioblastoma Orthotopic Xenograft Model." *ACS Biomaterials Science & Engineering* 6 (5): 2943-2955.

[25] Mangraviti, A., Tzeng, S. Y., Kozielski, K. L., Wang, Y., Jin, Y., Gullotti, D., Pedone, M., Buaron, N., Liu, A., Wilson, D. R., Hansen, S. K., Rodriguez, F. J., Gao, G.-D., DiMeco, F., Brem, H., Olivi, A., Tyler, B., and Green, J. J. 2015. "Polymeric Nanoparticles for Nonviral Gene Therapy Extend Brain Tumor Survival *in Vivo*." *ACS Nano* 9 (2): 1236-1249.

[26] Sukumar, U. K., Rajendran, J. C. B., Gambhir, S. S., Massoud, T. F., and Paulmurugan, R. 2020. "SP94-Targeted Triblock Copolymer Nanoparticle Delivers Thymidine Kinase-p53-Nitroreductase Triple Therapeutic Gene and Restores Anticancer Function against Hepatocellular Carcinoma *in Vivo*." *Acs Applied Materials & Interfaces* 12 (10): 11307-11319.

[27] Cheang, T. Y., Lei, Y. Y., Zhang, Z. Q., Zhou, H. Y., Ye, R. Y., Lin, Y., and Wang, S. 2018. "Graphene oxide-hydroxyapatite nanocomposites effectively deliver HSV-TK suicide gene to inhibit human breast cancer growth." *J Biomater Appl* 33 (2): 216-226.

[28] Wang, Z., Chang, Z., Lu, M., Shao, D., Yue, J., Yang, D., Zheng, X., Li, M., He, K., Zhang, M., Chen, L., and Dong, W.-f. 2018. "Shape-controlled magnetic mesoporous silica nanoparticles for magnetically-mediated suicide gene therapy of hepatocellular carcinoma." *Biomaterials* 154: 147-157.

[29] Yuan, C., An, Y., Zhang, J., Li, H., Zhang, H., Wang, L., and Zhang, D. 2014. "Magnetic nanoparticles for targeted therapeutic gene delivery and magnetic-inducing heating on hepatoma." *Nanotechnology* 25 (34): 345101.

[30] Sahoo, A. K., Banerjee, S., Ghosh, S. S., and Chattopadhyay, A. 2014. "Simultaneous RGB emitting Au nanoclusters in chitosan nanoparticles for anticancer gene theranostics." *ACS Appl Mater Interfaces* 6 (1): 712-24.

[31] Shao, D., Li, J., Pan, Y., Zhang, X., Zheng, X., Wang, Z., Zhang, M., Zhang, H., and Chen, L. 2015. "Noninvasive theranostic imaging of HSV-TK/GCV suicide gene therapy in liver cancer by folate-targeted quantum dot-based liposomes." *Biomater Sci* 3 (6): 833-41.

[32] Malik, Y. S., Sheikh, M. A., Xing, Z., Guo, Z., Zhu, X., Tian, H., and Chen, X. 2018. "Polylysine-modified polyethylenimine polymer can generate genetically engineered mesenchymal stem cells for combinational suicidal gene therapy in glioblastoma." *Acta Biomaterialia* 80: 144-153.

[33] Kumar, S. U. and Gopinath, P. 2016. "Nanotechnology- A Promising Approach for Suicide Gene Therapy." *Austin J Nanomed Nanotechnol* 4 (1): 1042.

[34] Gwak, S. J. and Lee, J. S. 2019. "Suicide Gene Therapy By Amphiphilic Copolymer Nanocarrier for Spinal Cord Tumor." *Nanomaterials* 9 (4): 573.

[35] Gerace, D., Martiniello-Wilks, R., Habib, R., and Simpson, A. M. 2019. "Luciferase-based reporting of suicide gene activity in murine mesenchymal stem cells." *PLOS ONE* 14 (7): 0220013.

[36] Tsujimura, M., Kusamori, K., Katsumi, H., Sakane, T., Yamamoto, A., and Nishikawa, M. 2019. "Cell-based interferon gene therapy using proliferation-controllable, interferon-releasing mesenchymal stem cells." *Scientific Reports* 9:1.

[37] Dalba, C., Klatzmann, D., Logg, C. R., and Kasahara, N. 2005. "Beyond oncolytic virotherapy: replication-competent retrovirus vectors for selective and stable transduction of tumors." *Curr Gene Ther* 5 (6): 655-67.

[38] Tai, C. K., Wang, W. J., Chen, T. C., and Kasahara, N. 2005. "Single-shot, multicycle suicide gene therapy by replication-competent retrovirus vectors achieves long-term survival benefit in experimental glioma." *Mol Ther* 12 (5): 842-51.

[39] Huang, T. T., Parab, S., Burnett, R., Diago, O., Ostertag, D., Hofman, F. M., Espinoza, F. L., Martin, B., Ibañez, C. E., Kasahara, N., Gruber, H. E., Pertschuk, D., Jolly, D. J., and Robbins, J. M. 2015. "Intravenous administration of retroviral replicating vector, Toca 511, demonstrates therapeutic efficacy in orthotopic immune-competent mouse glioma model." *Hum Gene Ther* 26 (2): 82-93.

[40] Kawasaki, Y., Tamamoto, A., Takagi-Kimura, M., Maeyama, Y., Yamaoka, N., Terada, N., Okamura, H., Kasahara, N., and Kubo, S. 2011. "Replication-competent retrovirus vector-mediated prodrug activator gene therapy in experimental models of human malignant mesothelioma." *Cancer Gene Therapy* 18 (8): 571-578.

[41] Cloughesy, T. F., Landolfi, J., Hogan, D. J., Bloomfield, S., Carter, B., Chen, C. C., Elder, J. B., Kalkanis, S. N., Kesari, S., Lai, A., Lee,

I. Y., Liau, L. M., Mikkelsen, T., Nghiemphu, P. L., Piccioni, D., Walbert, T., Chu, A., Das, A., Diago, O. R., Gammon, D., Gruber, H. E., Hanna, M., Jolly, D. J., Kasahara, N., McCarthy, D., Mitchell, L., Ostertag, D., Robbins, J. M., Rodriguez-Aguirre, M., and Vogelbaum, M. A. 2016. "Phase 1 trial of vocimagene amiretrorepvec and 5-fluorocytosine for recurrent high-grade glioma." *Sci Transl Med* 8:341: 341ra75.

[42] Islam, S. M. B. U., Lee, B., Jiang, F., Kim, E.-K., Ahn, S. C., and Hwang, T.-H. 2020. "Engineering and Characterization of Oncolytic Vaccinia Virus Expressing Truncated Herpes Simplex Virus Thymidine Kinase." *Cancers* 12 (1): 228.

[43] Kubo, S., Takagi-Kimura, M., Tagawa, M., and Kasahara, N. 2019. "Dual-vector prodrug activator gene therapy using retroviral replicating vectors." *Cancer Gene Therapy* 26: 128-135.

[44] Xiao, J., Wang, X., Wu, Y., Zhao, Q., Liu, X., Zhang, G., Zhao, Z., Ning, Y., Wang, K., Tan, Y., and Du, B. 2019. "Synergistic effect of resveratrol and HSV-TK/GCV therapy on murine hepatoma cells." *Cancer Biology & Therapy* 20 (2): 183-191.

[45] Jin, Y., Gao, J., Weng, Q., Xiong, F., Gu, S., Shivaram, G., Zhang, F., and Yang, X. 2018. "Cholangiocarcinoma: molecular imaging-guided radiofrequency hyperthermia-enhanced intratumoral herpes simplex virus thymidine kinase gene therapy." *Am J Cancer Res* 8 (3): 502-513.

[46] Ji, J., Weng, Q., Zhang, F., Xiong, F., Jin, Y., Hui, J., Song, J., Gao, J., Chen, M., Li, Q., Shin, D., and Yang, X. 2018. "Non–Small-Cell Lung Cancer: Feasibility of Intratumoral Radiofrequency Hyperthermia–enhanced Herpes Simplex Virus Thymidine Kinase Gene Therapy." *Radiology* 288 (2): 612-620.

[47] Li, Y., Zhao, S., Zhang, F., Jin, G., Zhou, Y., Li, P., Shin, D., and Yang, X. 2020. "Molecular imaging-monitored radiofrequency hyperthermia-enhanced intratumoral herpes simplex virus-thymidine kinase gene therapy for rat orthotopic ovarian cancer." *Int J Hyperthermia* 37 (1): 101-109.

[48] Luo, J., Zhou, J., Xie, F., Zhu, Y., Zhou, F., Zhang, S., Jiang, S., He, J., Liu, J., Wu, X., Zhang, Y., Sun, J., and Yang, X. 2018. "Combined treatment of cholangiocarcinoma with interventional radiofrequency hyperthermia and heat shock protein promoter-mediated HSV-TK gene therapy." *Am J Cancer Res* 8 (8): 1595-1603.

[49] Pan, M., Zhang, Y., Deng, Z., Yan, F., and Hong, G. 2018. "Noninvasive and Local Delivery of Adenoviral-Mediated Herpes Simplex Virus Thymidine Kinase to Treat Glioma Through Focused Ultrasound-Induced Blood-Brain Barrier Opening in Rats." *J Biomed Nanotechnol* 14 (12): 2031-2041.

[50] Devulapally, R., Lee, T., Barghava-Shah, A., Sekar, T. V., Foygel, K., Bachawal, S. V., Willmann, J. K., and Paulmurugan, R. 2018. "Ultrasound-guided delivery of thymidine kinase-nitroreductase dual therapeutic genes by PEGylated-PLGA/PIE nanoparticles for enhanced triple negative breast cancer therapy." *Nanomedicine (Lond)* 13 (9): 1051-1066.

[51] Teleanu, R. I., Chircov, C., Grumezescu, A. M., and Teleanu, D. M. 2020. "Tumor Angiogenesis and Anti-Angiogenic Strategies for Cancer Treatment." *J. Clin. Med.* 9: 84.

[52] Folkman, J. 1971. "Tumor angiogenesis: therapeutic implications." *N Engl J Med* 285 (21): 1182-6.

[53] Daud, A., Takamura, K. T., Diep, T., Heller, R., and Pierce, R. H. 2015. "Long-term overall survival from a phase I trial using intratumoral plasmid interleukin-12 with electroporation in patients with melanoma." *Journal of Translational Medicine* 13: O3.

[54] Daud, A., Algazi, A., Ashworth, M., Buljan, M., Takamura, K. T., Diep, T., Pierce, R. H., and Bhatia, S. 2015. "Intratumoral electroporation of plasmid interleukin-12: efficacy and biomarker analyses from a phase 2 study in melanoma (OMS-I100)." *Journal of Translational Medicine* 13: O11.

[55] Markert, J. M., Cody, J. J., Parker, J. N., Coleman, J. M., Price, K. H., Kern, E. R., Quenelle, D. C., Lakeman, A. D., Schoeb, T. R., Palmer, C. A., Cartner, S. C., Gillespie, G. Y., and Whitley, R. J. 2012.

"Preclinical evaluation of a genetically engineered herpes simplex virus expressing interleukin-12." *J Virol* 86 (9): 5304-13.

[56] Kramer, M. G., Masner, M., Casales, E., Moreno, M., Smerdou, C., and Chabalgoity, J. A. 2015. "Neoadjuvant administration of Semliki Forest virus expressing interleukin-12 combined with attenuated Salmonella eradicates breast cancer metastasis and achieves long-term survival in immunocompetent mice." *BMC Cancer* 15: 620.

[57] Poutou, J., Bunuales, M., Gonzalez-Aparicio, M., Garcia-Aragoncillo, E., Quetglas, J. I., Casado, R., Bravo-Perez, C., Alzuguren, P., and Hernandez-Alcoceba, R. 2015. "Safety and antitumor effect of oncolytic and helper-dependent adenoviruses expressing interleukin-12 variants in a hamster pancreatic cancer model." *Gene Ther* 22 (9): 696-706.

[58] Freytag, S. O., Zhang, Y., and Siddiqui, F. 2015. "Preclinical toxicology of oncolytic adenovirus-mediated cytotoxic and interleukin-12 gene therapy for prostate cancer." *Mol Ther Oncolytics* 2: 15006.

[59] Cutrera, J., King, G., Jones, P., Kicenuik, K., Gumpel, E., Xia, X., and Li, S. 2015. "Safe and effective treatment of spontaneous neoplasms with interleukin 12 electro-chemo-gene therapy." *J Cell Mol Med* 19 (3): 664-75.

[60] Wahl, M. L., Moser, T. L., and Pizzo, S. V. 2004. "Angiostatin and anti-angiogenic therapy in human disease." *Recent Prog Horm Res* 59: 73-104.

[61] Zhang, G., Jin, G., Nie, X., Mi, R., Zhu, G., Jia, W., and Liu, F. 2014. "Enhanced antitumor efficacy of an oncolytic herpes simplex virus expressing an endostatin-angiostatin fusion gene in human glioblastoma stem cell xenografts." *PLoS One* 9 (4): e95872.

[62] Hutzen, B., Bid, H. K., Houghton, P. J., Pierson, C. R., Powell, K., Bratasz, A., Raffel, C., and Studebaker, A. W. 2014. "Treatment of medulloblastoma with oncolytic measles viruses expressing the angiogenesis inhibitors endostatin and angiostatin." *BMC Cancer* 14: 206.

[63] Kubo, S., Takagi-Kimura, M., and Kasahara, N. 2015. "Combinatorial anti-angiogenic gene therapy in a human malignant mesothelioma model." *Oncol Rep* 34 (2): 633-8.

[64] Kim, H. S., Jeong, H. Y., Lee, Y. K., Kim, K. S., and Park, Y. S. 2013. "Synergistic antitumoral effect of IL-12 gene cotransfected with antiangiogenic genes for angiostatin, endostatin, and saxatilin." *Oncol Res* 21 (4): 209-16.

[65] Sasaki, T., Fukai, N., Mann, K., Göhring, W., Olsen, B. R., and Timpl, R. 1998. "Structure, function and tissue forms of the C-terminal globular domain of collagen XVIII containing the angiogenesis inhibitor endostatin." *Embo j* 17 (15): 4249-56.

[66] Yan, H., Guo, W., Li, K., Tang, M., Zhao, X., Lei, Y., Nie, C.-l., and Yuan, Z. 2018. "Combination of DESI2 and endostatin gene therapy significantly improves antitumor efficacy by accumulating DNA lesions, inducing apoptosis and inhibiting angiogenesis." *Experimental Cell Research* 371 (1): 50-62.

[67] Zhang, Y. L., Zhou, T. Y., Ai, J., Chen, S. Q., Chen, F., Nie, C. H., Chen, X. H., Zhou, G. H., Wang, H. L., Zhu, T. Y., Wang, B. Q., Yu, Z. N., Jing, L., Wu, L. M., Zheng, S. S., and Sun, J. H. 2020. "Gene Therapy with Cytosine Deaminase and Endostatin Fusion Gene Mediated by Endothelial Progenitor Cells in Hepatomas." *Cancer management and research* 12: 3023-3031.

[68] Huiqi, G., Jing, Z., Peng, F., Yong, L., and Baozhong, S. 2015. "*In vivo* study of the effect of combining endostatin gene therapy with 32P-colloid on hepatocarcinoma and its functioning mechanism." *J buon* 20 (4): 1042-7.

[69] Liang, K., Liu, Q., Li, P., Han, Y., Bian, X., Tang, Y., and Kong, Q. 2018. "Endostatin gene therapy delivered by attenuated Salmonella typhimurium in murine tumor models." *Cancer Gene Ther* 25 (7-8): 167-183.

[70] Zhuo, H., Zheng, B., Liu, J., Huang, Y., Wang, H., Zheng, D., Mao, N., Meng, J., Zhou, S., Zhong, L., and Zhao, Y. 2018. "Efficient targeted tumor imaging and secreted endostatin gene delivery by anti-

CD105 immunoliposomes." *Journal of Experimental & Clinical Cancer Research* 37 (1): 42.

[71] Adeyemi, S. A., Choonara, Y. E., Kumar, P., du Toit, L. C., Marimuthu, T., Kondiah, P. P. D., and Pillay, V. 2019. "Folate-decorated, endostatin-loaded, nanoparticles for anti-proliferative chemotherapy in esophaegeal squamous cell carcinoma." *Biomedicine & Pharmacotherapy* 119: 109450.

[72] Maeshima, Y., Colorado, P. C., Torre, A., Holthaus, K. A., Grunkemeyer, J. A., Ericksen, M. B., Hopfer, H., Xiao, Y., Stillman, I. E., and Kalluri, R. 2000. "Distinct antitumor properties of a type IV collagen domain derived from basement membrane." *J Biol Chem* 275 (28): 21340-8.

[73] He, L., Yang, H. J., Liu, F., Chen, Y. Y., Tang, S. J., Ji, W., Tang, J. L., Liu, Z. D., Sun, Y. J., Hu, S. B. A., Zhang, Y. M., Liu, X., Huang, W. T., Ding, X. Z., and Xia, L. Q. 2017. "Escherichia coli Nissle 1917 engineered to express Tum-5 can restrain murine melanoma growth." *Oncotarget* 8 (49): 85772-85782.

[74] Wei, C., Xun, A. Y., Wei, X. X., Yao, J., Wang, J. Y., Shi, R. Y., Yang, G. H., Li, Y. X., Xu, Z. L., Lai, M. G., Zhang, R., Wang, L. S., and Zeng, W. S. 2016. "Bifidobacteria Expressing Tumstatin Protein for Antitumor Therapy in Tumor-Bearing Mice." *Technology in Cancer Research & Treatment* 15 (3): 498-508.

[75] Trochon-Joseph, V., Martel-Renoir, D., Mir, L. M., Thomaïdis, A., Opolon, P., Connault, E., Li, H., Grenet, C., Fauvel-Lafève, F., Soria, J., Legrand, C., Soria, C., Perricaudet, M., and Lu, H. 2004. "Evidence of antiangiogenic and antimetastatic activities of the recombinant disintegrin domain of metargidin." *Cancer Res* 64 (6): 2062-9.

[76] Bosnjak, M., Dolinsek, T., Cemazar, M., Kranjc, S., Blagus, T., Markelc, B., Stimac, M., Zavrsnik, J., Kamensek, U., Heller, L., Bouquet, C., Turk, B., and Sersa, G. 2015. "Gene electrotransfer of plasmid AMEP, an integrin-targeted therapy, has antitumor and antiangiogenic action in murine B16 melanoma." *Gene Therapy* 22 (7): 578-590.

[77] Spanggaard, I., Dahlstroem, K., Laessoee, L., Hansen, R. H., Johannesen, H. H., Hendel, H. W., Bouquet, C., Attali, P., and Gehl, J. 2017. "Gene therapy for patients with advanced solid tumors: a phase I study using gene electrotransfer to muscle with the integrin inhibitor plasmid AMEP." *Acta Oncologica* 56 (7): 909-916.

[78] Spanggaard, I. and Gehl, J. 2015. "Antiangiogenic Metargidin Peptide (AMEP) Gene Therapy in Disseminated Melanoma." *Methods Mol Biol* 1317: 359-64.

[79] Jabbarpour, Z., Kiani, J., Keshtkar, S., Saidijam, M., Ghahremani, M. H., and Ahmadbeigi, N. 2020. "Effects of human placenta-derived mesenchymal stem cells with NK4 gene expression on glioblastoma multiforme cell lines." *Journal of Cellular Biochemistry* 121 (2): 1362-1373.

[80] Cai, C., Hou, L., Zhang, J., Zhao, D., Wang, Z., Hu, H., He, J., Guan, W., and Ma, Y. 2017. "The Inhibitory Effect of Mesenchymal Stem Cells with rAd-NK4 on Liver Cancer." *Applied Biochemistry and Biotechnology* 183 (1): 444-459.

[81] Stimac, M., Kamensek, U., Cemazar, M., Kranjc, S., Coer, A., and Sersa, G. 2016. "Tumor radiosensitization by gene therapy against endoglin." *Cancer Gene Therapy* 23 (7): 214-220.

[82] Egorova, A. A., Shtykalova, S. V., Maretina, M. A., Sokolov, D. I., Selkov, S. A., Baranov, V. S., and Kiselev, A. V. 2019. "Synergistic Anti-Angiogenic Effects Using Peptide-Based Combinatorial Delivery of siRNAs Targeting VEGFA, VEGFR1, and Endoglin Genes." *Pharmaceutics* 11: 261.

[83] Mosallaei, M., Simonian, M., Ehtesham, N., Karimzadeh, M. R., Vatandoost, N., Negahdari, B., and Salehi, R. 2020. "Genetically engineered mesenchymal stem cells: targeted delivery of immunomodulatory agents for tumor eradication." *Cancer Gene Therapy*.

[84] El-Aneed, A. 2004. "Current strategies in cancer gene therapy." *Eur J Pharmacol* 498 (1-3): 1-8.

[85] Chaurasiya, S., Hew, P., Crosley, P., Sharon, D., Potts, K., Agopsowicz, K., Long, M., Shi, C., and Hitt, M. M. 2016. "Breast

cancer gene therapy using an adenovirus encoding human IL-2 under control of mammaglobin promoter/enhancer sequences." *Cancer Gene Ther* 23 (6): 178-87.

[86] Huang, K. W., Hsu, F. F., Qiu, J. T., Chern, G. J., Lee, Y. A., Chang, C. C., Huang, Y. T., Sung, Y. C., Chiang, C. C., Huang, R. L., Lin, C. C., Dinh, T. K., Huang, H. C., Shih, Y. C., Alson, D., Lin, C. Y., Lin, Y. C., Chang, P. C., Lin, S. Y., and Chen, Y. 2020. "Highly efficient and tumor-selective nanoparticles for dual-targeted immunogene therapy against cancer." *Science Advances* 6 (3): eaax5032.

[87] Liu, X., Gao, X., Zheng, S., Wang, B., Li, Y., Zhao, C., Muftuoglu, Y., Chen, S., Li, Y., Yao, H., Sun, H., Mao, Q., You, C., Guo, G., and Wei, Y. 2017. "Modified nanoparticle mediated IL-12 immunogene therapy for colon cancer." *Nanomedicine: Nanotechnology, Biology and Medicine* 13 (6): 1993-2004.

[88] Men, K., Huang, R., Zhang, X. Y., Zhang, R., Zhang, Y. F., He, M. X., Tong, R. S., Yang, L., Wei, Y. Q., and Duan, X. M. 2018. "Local and Systemic Delivery of Interleukin-12 Gene by Cationic Micelles for Cancer Immunogene Therapy." *Journal of Biomedical Nanotechnology* 14 (10): 1719-1730.

[89] Pishavar, E., Oroojalian, F., Ramezani, M., and Hashemi, M. 2020. "Cholesterol-conjugated PEGylated PAMAM as an efficient nanocarrier for plasmid encoding interleukin-12 immunogene delivery toward colon cancer cells." *Biotechnol Prog* 36 (3): e2952.

[90] Nissim, L., Wu, M.-R., Pery, E., Binder-Nissim, A., Suzuki, H. I., Stupp, D., Wehrspaun, C., Tabach, Y., Sharp, P.A ., and Lu, T. K. 2017. "Synthetic RNA-Based Immunomodulatory Gene Circuits for Cancer Immunotherapy." *Cell* 171 (5): 1138-1150.e15.

[91] Pasquet, L., Bellard, E., Chabot, S., Markelc, B., Rols, M. P., Teissie, J., and Golzio, M. 2019. "Pre-clinical investigation of the synergy effect of interleukin-12 gene-electro-transfer during partially irreversible electropermeabilization against melanoma." *J Immunother Cancer* 7 (1): 161.

[92] Algazi, A., Bhatia, S., Agarwala, S., Molina, M., Lewis, K., Faries, M., Fong, L., Levine, L. P., Franco, M., Oglesby, A., Ballesteros-

Merino, C., Bifulco, C. B., Fox, B. A., Bannavong, D., Talia, R., Browning, E., Le, M. H., Pierce, R. H., Gargosky, S., Tsai, K. K., Twitty, C., and Daud, A. I. 2020. "Intratumoral delivery of tavokinogene telseplasmid yields systemic immune responses in metastatic melanoma patients." *Annals of Oncology* 31 (4): 532-540.

[93] Chen, P., Liu, Y., Zhao, J., Pang, X., Zhang, P., Hou, X., Chen, P., He, C.-Y., Wang, Z., and Chen, Z.-Y. 2018. "The synthesis of amphiphilic polyethyleneimine/calcium phosphate composites for bispecific T-cell engager based immunogene therapy." *Biomaterials Science* 6 (3): 633-641.

[94] Plote, D., Choi, W., Mokkapati, S., Sundi, D., Ferguson, J. E., Duplisea, J., Parker, N. R., Yla-Herttuala, S., Committee, S. U. O. C. T. C. B., McConkey, D., Schluns, K. S., and Dinney, C. P. 2019. "Inhibition of urothelial carcinoma through targeted type I interferon-mediated immune activation." *OncoImmunology* 8 (5): e1577125.

[95] Wang, G. X., Zhan, Y. A., Hu, H. L., Wang, Y., and Fu, B. 2012. "Mesenchymal stem cells modified to express interferon-β inhibit the growth of prostate cancer in a mouse model." *J Int Med Res* 40 (1): 317-27.

[96] Bitsika, V., Roubelakis, M. G., Zagoura, D., Trohatou, O., Makridakis, M., Pappa, K. I., Marini, F. C., Vlahou, A., and Anagnou, N. P. 2012. "Human amniotic fluid-derived mesenchymal stem cells as therapeutic vehicles: a novel approach for the treatment of bladder cancer." *Stem Cells Dev* 21 (7): 1097-111.

[97] Oronsky, B., Goyal, S., Kim, M. M., Cabrales, P., Lybeck, M., Caroen, S., Oronsky, N., Burbano, E., Carter, C., and Oronsky, A. 2018. "A Review of Clinical Radioprotection and Chemoprotection for Oral Mucositis." *Transl Oncol* 11 (3): 771-778.

[98] Oronsky, B., Carter, C., Scicinska, A., Oronsky, A., Oronsky, N., Lybeck, M., and Scicinski, J. 2016. "Medical Machiavellianism: the tradeoff between benefit and harm with targeted chemotherapy." *Oncotarget* 7 (8): 9041-5.

[99] Rafferty, J. A., Hickson, I., Chinnasamy, N., Lashford, L. S., Margison, G. P., Dexter, T. M., and Fairbairn, L. J. 1996.

"Chemoprotection of normal tissues by transfer of drug resistance genes." *Cancer and Metastasis Reviews* 15 (3): 365-383.

[100] Sorrentino, B. P. 2002. "Gene therapy to protect haematopoietic cells from cytotoxic cancer drugs." *Nat Rev Cancer* 2:6: 431-41.

[101] Gottesman, M. M. 2002. "Mechanisms of cancer drug resistance." *Annu Rev Med* 53: 615-27.

[102] Gottesman, M. M., Fojo, T., and Bates, S. E. 2002. "Multidrug resistance in cancer: role of ATP-dependent transporters." *Nat Rev Cancer* 2 (1): 48-58.

[103] Groopman, J. E. and Itri, L. M. 1999. "Chemotherapy-induced anemia in adults: incidence and treatment." *J Natl Cancer Inst* 91 (19): 1616-34.

[104] Wang, Y., Probin, V., and Zhou, D. 2006. "Cancer therapy-induced residual bone marrow injury-Mechanisms of induction and implication for therapy." *Curr Cancer Ther Rev* 2 (3): 271-279.

[105] Moritz, T. and Williams, D. A. 2001. "Marrow protection - transduction of hematopoietic cells with drug resistance genes." *Cytotherapy* 3 (2): 67-84.

[106] Brennig, S., Lachmann, N., Buchegger, T., Hetzel, M., Schambach, A., and Moritz, T. 2015. "Chemoprotection of murine hematopoietic cells by combined gene transfer of cytidine deaminase (CDD) and multidrug resistance 1 gene (MDR1)." *J Exp Clin Cancer Res* 34: 148.

[107] Guo, C.-B., Li, Y.-C., and Jin, X.-Q. 2006. "Chemoprotection effect of retroviral vector encoding multidrug resistance 1 gene to allow intensified chemotherapy *in vivo*." *Cancer Chemotherapy and Pharmacology* 58 (1): 40-49.

[108] Maier, P., Spier, I., Laufs, S., Veldwijk, M. R., Fruehauf, S., Wenz, F., and Zeller, W. J. 2010. "Chemoprotection of human hematopoietic stem cells by simultaneous lentiviral overexpression of multidrug resistance 1 and O(6)-methylguanine-DNA methyltransferase (P140K)." *Gene Ther* 17 (3): 389-99.

[109] Yang, X., Yang, P., Shen, J., Osaka, E., Choy, E., Cote, G., Harmon, D., Zhang, Z., Mankin, H., Hornicek, F. J., and Duan, Z. 2014.

"Prevention of multidrug resistance (MDR) in osteosarcoma by NSC23925." *British journal of cancer* 110 (12): 2896-2904.

[110] Higgins, C. F. 2007. "Multiple molecular mechanisms for multidrug resistance transporters." *Nature* 446 (7137): 749-57.

[111] Han, L. Y., Li, Y. P., Ye, M. Z., Wang, B. W., Wang, Q., Zhao, S. H., and Li, H. L. 2012. "Transduction of mesenchymal stem cells with multidrug resistance gene provides protection for bone marrow toxicity after being transplanted into a nude mice model." *Chin Med J (Engl)* 125 (18): 3246-50.

[112] Brent, T. P., Dolan, M. E., Fraenkel-Conrat, H., Hall, J., Karran, P., Laval, L., Margison, G. P., Montesano, R., Pegg, A. E., Potter, P. M., and et al. 1988. "Repair of O-alkylpyrimidines in mammalian cells: a present consensus." *Proceedings of the National Academy of Sciences of the United States of America* 85 (6): 1759-1762.

[113] Middlemas, D. S., Stewart, C. F., Kirstein, M. N., Poquette, C., Friedman, H. S., Houghton, P. J., and Brent, T. P. 2000. "Biochemical correlates of temozolomide sensitivity in pediatric solid tumor xenograft models." *Clin Cancer Res* 6 (3): 998-1007.

[114] Quinn, J. A., Jiang, S. X., Reardon, D. A., Desjardins, A., Vredenburgh, J. J., Rich, J. N., Gururangan, S., Friedman, A. H., Bigner, D. D., Sampson, J. H., McLendon, R. E., Herndon, J. E., 2nd, Walker, A., and Friedman, H. S. 2009. "Phase II trial of temozolomide plus o6-benzylguanine in adults with recurrent, temozolomide-resistant malignant glioma." *J Clin Oncol* 27 (8): 1262-7.

[115] Adair, J. E., Beard, B. C., Trobridge, G. D., Neff, T., Rockhill, J. K., Silbergeld, D. L., Mrugala, M. M., and Kiem, H. P. 2012. "Extended survival of glioblastoma patients after chemoprotective HSC gene therapy." *Sci Transl Med* 4 (133): 133ra57.

[116] Adair, J. E., Johnston, S. K., Mrugala, M. M., Beard, B. C., Guyman, L. A., Baldock, A. L., Bridge, C. A., Hawkins-Daarud, A., Gori, J. L., Born, D. E., Gonzalez-Cuyar, L. F., Silbergeld, D. L., Rockne, R. C., Storer, B. E., Rockhill, J. K., Swanson, K. R., and Kiem, H. P. 2014.

"Gene therapy enhances chemotherapy tolerance and efficacy in glioblastoma patients." *J Clin Invest* 124 (9): 4082-92.

[117] Ruan, H., Qiu, S., Beard, B. C., and Black, M. E. 2016. "Creation of zebularine-resistant human cytidine deaminase mutants to enhance the chemoprotection of hematopoietic stem cells." *Protein Engineering, Design and Selection* 29 (12): 573-582.

[118] Bouffard, D. Y., Laliberté, J., and Momparler, R. L. 1993. "Kinetic studies on 2',2'-difluorodeoxycytidine (Gemcitabine) with purified human deoxycytidine kinase and cytidine deaminase." *Biochem Pharmacol* 45 (9): 1857-61.

[119] Lachmann, N., Brennig, S., Phaltane, R., Flasshove, M., Dilloo, D., and Moritz, T. 2013. "Myeloprotection by cytidine deaminase gene transfer in antileukemic therapy." *Neoplasia (New York, N.Y.)* 15 (3): 239-248.

[120] Lachmann, N., Brennig, S., Hillje, R., Schermeier, H., Phaltane, R., Dahlmann, J., Gruh, I., Heinz, N., Schiedlmeier, B., Baum, C., and Moritz, T. 2015. "Tightly regulated 'all-in-one' lentiviral vectors for protection of human hematopoietic cells from anticancer chemotherapy." *Gene Ther* 22 (11): 883-92.

[121] Gori, J. L., Beard, B. C., Williams, N. P., Ironside, C., Swanson, D., Scott McIvor, R., and Kiem, H. P. 2013. "*In vivo* protection of activated Tyr22-dihydrofolate reductase gene-modified canine T lymphocytes from methotrexate." *J Gene Med* 15 (6-7): 233-41.

[122] Williams, D. A., Hsieh, K., DeSilva, A., and Mulligan, R. C. 1987. "Protection of bone marrow transplant recipients from lethal doses of methotrexate by the generation of methotrexate-resistant bone marrow." *J Exp Med* 166 (1): 210-8.

[123] Hyland, K. A., Olson, E. R., and McIvor, R. S. 2015. "Sleeping Beauty-Mediated Drug Resistance Gene Transfer in Human Hematopoietic Progenitor Cells." *Hum Gene Ther* 26 (10): 657-63.

[124] Bertino, J.R. 1993. "Karnofsky memorial lecture. Ode to methotrexate." *Journal of clinical oncology: official journal of the American Society of Clinical Oncology* 11 (1): 5-14.

[125] Blakley, R. L. and Sorrentino, B. P. 1998. "*In vitro* mutations in dihydrofolate reductase that confer resistance to methotrexate: potential for clinical application." *Hum Mutat* 11 (4): 259-63.

[126] Wang, Z., Rao, D. D., Senzer, N., and Nemunaitis, J. 2011. "RNA interference and cancer therapy." *Pharm Res* 28 (12): 2983-95.

[127] Saxena, V. 2014. "RNAi-based Cancer Therapeutics: Are we there yet?" *Journal of Pharmacovigilance* 02.

[128] Ozcan, G., Ozpolat, B., Coleman, R. L., Sood, A. K., and Lopez-Berestein, G. 2015. "Preclinical and clinical development of siRNA-based therapeutics." *Adv Drug Deliv Rev* 87: 108-19.

[129] Chery, J. 2016. "RNA therapeutics: RNAi and antisense mechanisms and clinical applications*."* *Postdoc J* 4 (7): 35-50.

[130] Bora, R. S., Gupta, D., Mukkur, T. K., and Saini, K. S. 2012. "RNA interference therapeutics for cancer: challenges and opportunities (review)." *Mol Med Rep* 6 (1): 9-15.

[131] Kole, R., Krainer, A. R., and Altman, S. 2012. "RNA therapeutics: beyond RNA interference and antisense oligonucleotides*." Nature reviews. Drug discovery* 11 (2): 125-140.

[132] Bobbin, M. L. and Rossi, J. J. 2016. "RNA Interference (RNAi)-Based Therapeutics: Delivering on the Promise?" *Annu Rev Pharmacol Toxicol* 56: 103-22.

[133] Elbashir, S. M., Harborth, J., Lendeckel, W., Yalcin, A., Weber, K., and Tuschl, T. 2001. "Duplexes of 21-nucleotide RNAs mediate RNA interference in cultured mammalian cells." *Nature* 411 (6836): 494-498.

[134] Lam, J. K. W., Chow, M. Y. T., Zhang, Y., and Leung, S. W. S. 2015. "siRNA Versus miRNA as Therapeutics for Gene Silencing." *Molecular therapy. Nucleic acids* 4 (9): e252.

[135] Kim, V. N., Han, J., and Siomi, M. C. 2009. "Biogenesis of small RNAs in animals." *Nat Rev Mol Cell Biol* 10:2: 126-39.

[136] Wang, J., Lu, Z., Wientjes, M. G., and Au, J. L. 2010. "Delivery of siRNA therapeutics: barriers and carriers." *Aaps j* 12 (4): 492-503.

[137] Chakraborty, C., Sharma, A. R., Sharma, G., Doss, C. G. P., and Lee, S. S. 2017. "Therapeutic miRNA and siRNA: Moving from Bench to

Clinic as Next Generation Medicine." *Mol Ther Nucleic Acids* 8: 132-143.

[138] Xin, Y., Huang, M., Guo, W. W., Huang, Q., Zhang, L. Z., and Jiang, G. 2017. "Nano-based delivery of RNAi in cancer therapy." *Molecular Cancer* 16 (1): 134.

[139] Guzman-Villanueva, D., El-Sherbiny, I. M., Herrera-Ruiz, D., Vlassov, A. V., and Smyth, H. D. 2012. "Formulation approaches to short interfering RNA and MicroRNA: challenges and implications." *J Pharm Sci* 101 (11): 4046-66.

[140] Sullenger, B. A. and Nair, S. 2016. "From the RNA world to the clinic." *Science* 352 (6292): 1417.

[141] Layzer, J. M., McCaffrey, A. P., Tanner, A. K., Huang, Z., Kay, M. A., and Sullenger, B. A. 2004. "*In vivo* activity of nuclease-resistant siRNAs." *RNA (New York, N.Y.)* 10 (5): 766-771.

[142] Xu, C.-f. and Wang, J. 2015. "Delivery systems for siRNA drug development in cancer therapy." *Asian Journal of Pharmaceutical Sciences* 10 (1): 1-12.

[143] Marques, J. T. and Williams, B. R. G. 2005. "Activation of the mammalian immune system by siRNAs." *Nature Biotechnology* 23 (11): 1399-1405.

[144] Foged, C. 2012. "siRNA delivery with lipid-based systems: promises and pitfalls." *Curr Top Med Chem* 12 (2): 97-107.

[145] Noland, C. L. and Doudna, J. A. 2013. "Multiple sensors ensure guide strand selection in human RNAi pathways." *RNA (New York, N.Y.)* 19 (5): 639-648.

[146] Birmingham, A., Anderson, E. M., Reynolds, A., Ilsley-Tyree, D., Leake, D., Fedorov, Y., Baskerville, S., Maksimova, E., Robinson, K., Karpilow, J., Marshall, W. S., and Khvorova, A. 2006. "3′ UTR seed matches, but not overall identity, are associated with RNAi off-targets." *Nature Methods* 3 (3): 199-204.

[147] Jackson, A. L., Burchard, J., Schelter, J., Chau, B. N., Cleary, M., Lim, L., and Linsley, P. S. 2006. "Widespread siRNA "off-target" transcript silencing mediated by seed region sequence complementarity." *RNA* 12 (7): 1179-87.

[148] Barata, P., Sood, A. K., and Hong, D. S. 2016. "RNA-targeted therapeutics in cancer clinical trials: Current status and future directions." *Cancer Treat Rev* 50: 35-47.

[149] Shen, H., Rodriguez-Aguayo, C., Xu, R., Gonzalez-Villasana, V., Mai, J., Huang, Y., Zhang, G., Guo, X., Bai, L., Qin, G., Deng, X., Li, Q., Erm, D. R., Aslan, B., Liu, X., Sakamoto, J., Chavez-Reyes, A., Han, H. D., Sood, A. K., Ferrari, M., and Lopez-Berestein, G. 2013. "Enhancing chemotherapy response with sustained EphA2 silencing using multistage vector delivery." *Clin Cancer Res* 19 (7): 1806-15.

[150] Wagner, M. J., Mitra, R., McArthur, M. J., Baze, W., Barnhart, K., Wu, S. Y., Rodriguez-Aguayo, C., Zhang, X., Coleman, R. L., Lopez-Berestein, G., and Sood, A. K. 2017. "Preclinical Mammalian Safety Studies of EPHARNA (DOPC Nanoliposomal EphA2-Targeted siRNA)." *Mol Cancer Ther* 16 (6): 1114-1123.

[151] Arbutus Biopharma. *TKM-PLK1 clinical trials*. 2020 [Access date: 15 June 2020]; Available from: http://arbutusbio.com/portfolio/tkm-plk1.php.

[152] Silenseed, *Kras-Loder for Pancreatic Cancer*, Phase 2 Clinical Trials, 2020 [Access date: 15 June 2020]; Available from: https://www.silenseed.com/kras-loder-for-pancreatic-cancer/

[153] El Dika, I., Lim, H. Y., Yong, W. P., Lin, C. C., Yoon, J. H., Modiano, M., Freilich, B., Choi, H. J., Chao, T. Y., Kelley, R. K., Brown, J., Knox, J., Ryoo, B. Y., Yau, T., and Abou-Alfa, G. K. 2019. "An Open-Label, Multicenter, Phase I, Dose Escalation Study with Phase II Expansion Cohort to Determine the Safety, Pharmacokinetics, and Preliminary Antitumor Activity of Intravenous TKM-080301 in Subjects with Advanced Hepatocellular Carcinoma." *Oncologist* 24 (6): 747-e218.

[154] Golan, T., Khvalevsky, E. Z., Hubert, A., Gabai, R. M., Hen, N., Segal, A., Domb, A., Harari, G., David, E. B., Raskin, S., Goldes, Y., Goldin, E., Eliakim, R., Lahav, M., Kopleman, Y., Dancour, A., Shemi, A., and Galun, E. 2015. "RNAi therapy targeting KRAS in

combination with chemotherapy for locally advanced pancreatic cancer patients." *Oncotarget* 6 (27): 24560-24570.

[155] Schultheis, B., Strumberg, D., Santel, A., Vank, C., Gebhardt, F., Keil, O., Lange, C., Giese, K., Kaufmann, J., Khan, M., and Drevs, J. 2014. "First-in-human phase I study of the liposomal RNA interference therapeutic Atu027 in patients with advanced solid tumors." *J Clin Oncol* 32 (36): 4141-8.

[156] Santel, A., Aleku, M., Keil, O., Endruschat, J., Esche, V., Fisch, G., Dames, S., Löffler, K., Fechtner, M., Arnold, W., Giese, K., Klippel, A., and Kaufmann, J. 2006. "A novel siRNA-lipoplex technology for RNA interference in the mouse vascular endothelium." *Gene Therapy* 13 (16): 1222-1234.

[157] Titze-de-Almeida, R., David, C., and Titze-de-Almeida, S. S. 2017. "The Race of 10 Synthetic RNAi-Based Drugs to the Pharmaceutical Market." *Pharm Res* 34 (7): 1339-1363.

[158] Portt, L., Norman, G., Clapp, C., Greenwood, M., and Greenwood, M. T. 2011. "Anti-apoptosis and cell survival: a review." *Biochim Biophys Acta* 1813 (1): 238-59.

[159] Jia, L. T., Chen, S. Y., and Yang, A. G. 2012. "Cancer gene therapy targeting cellular apoptosis machinery." *Cancer Treat Rev* 38 (7): 868-76.

[160] Wong, R. S. Y. 2011. "Apoptosis in cancer: from pathogenesis to treatment." *Journal of Experimental & Clinical Cancer Research* 30 (1): 87.

[161] Leonard, C. J., Canman, C. E., and Kastan, M. B. 1995. "The role of p53 in cell-cycle control and apoptosis: implications for cancer." *Important Adv Oncol*: 33-42.

[162] Pietro, R. D. and Zauli, G. 2004. "Emerging non-apoptotic functions of tumor necrosis factor-related apoptosis-inducing ligand (TRAIL)/Apo2L." *Journal of Cellular Physiology* 201 (3): 331-340.

[163] Blandino, G. and Di Agostino, S. 2018. "New therapeutic strategies to treat human cancers expressing mutant p53 proteins." *Journal of experimental & clinical cancer research: CR* 37 (1): 30.

[164] Suzuki, K. and Matsubara, H. 2011. "Recent advances in p53 research and cancer treatment." *J Biomed Biotechnol* 2011: 978312.

[165] Rejeeth, C. and Kannan, S. 2016. "p53 gene therapy of human breast carcinoma: using a transferrin-modified silica nanoparticle." *Breast Cancer* 23 (1): 101-110.

[166] Li, Y., Xu, B., Bai, T., and Liu, W. 2015. "Co-delivery of doxorubicin and tumor-suppressing p53 gene using a POSS-based star-shaped polymer for cancer therapy." *Biomaterials* 55: 12-23.

[167] Farooqi, A. A., Gadaleta, C. D., Ranieri, G., Fayyaz, S., and Marech, I. 2016. "New Frontiers in Promoting TRAIL-Mediated Cell Death: Focus on Natural Sensitizers, miRNAs, and Nanotechnological Advancements." *Cell Biochemistry and Biophysics* 74 (1): 3-10.

[168] Wang, S., Shao, M., Zhong, Z., Wang, A., Cao, J., Lu, Y., Wang, Y., and Zhang, J. 2017. "Co-delivery of gambogic acid and TRAIL plasmid by hyaluronic acid grafted PEI-PLGA nanoparticles for the treatment of triple negative breast cancer." *Drug Deliv* 24 (1): 1791-1800.

[169] Wang, K., Kievit, F. M., Jeon, M., Silber, J. R., Ellenbogen, R. G., and Zhang, M. 2015. "Nanoparticle-Mediated Target Delivery of TRAIL as Gene Therapy for Glioblastoma." *Adv Healthc Mater* 4 (17): 2719-26.

In: An Introduction to Cancer Therapy
Editor: Neville Charron
ISBN: 978-1-53618-450-1

Chapter 4

SULFONAMIDES: A VALUABLE WEAPON AGAINST CANCER WITH SULFAMETHOXAZOLE AS A POTENTIAL REPURPOSED LEAD MOLECULE

Avirup Malla[1,2], Suvroma Gupta[1,*] and Runa Sur[2,†]
[1]Department of Biotechnology, Haldia Institute of Technology, Haldia, Purba Medinipur, West Bengal
[2]Department of Biophysics, Molecular Biology and Bioinformatics, University of Calcutta, West Bengal

ABSTRACT

Drug development in the field of oncology is facing an acute 'productivity crisis,' where the success rate for new drugs from Phase I trial to US Food and Drug Administration (FDA) approval in the period 2003 to 2011 was around 6.7%. A figure that is about half the rate for non-oncological drugs. This apparent slow pace of new oncology drug production is occurring against two challenges, one of increased cancer incidence across the globe, and the other of existing significant therapeutic

[*] Corresponding Author's E-mail: suvroma.gupta@gmail.com.
[†] Corresponding Author's E-mail: runasur2013@gmail.com.

resistance in many types of malignant disease. To overcome these hurdles, the Repurposing Drugs in Oncology (ReDO) project is focussed to find existing and widely-used non-cancer drugs with hidden attributes of anticancer potential. In contrast to the de novo development of new molecules, drug repurposing begins with known pharmaceutical agents with a prehistory of clinical use. In this regard, Sulfamethoxazole (SMX) has long been known for combating several microbial infections. It affects folic acid biosynthesis inhibiting dihydropteroate synthetase. Although some toxic effects of SMX and its derivatives have been reported in patients, specific target of SMX or its derivatives in eukaryotic system has not been identified precisely. Earlier some sulfonamide group of compounds like E-7010 and many others were found to selectively inhibit microtubule assembly by binding to tubulin at the colchicine site. A wealth of information exists regarding inhibitory activity of sulfonamides against a panel of human cancer cell lines. Because the sulfonamide moiety (O=S=O) is common to many anticancer sulphur group drugs, it is tempting to explore SMX for its anticancer potential. Binding interaction of SMX with microtubule and lactate dehydrogenase is indicative of additional mode of action of SMX along with the cytotoxicity exhibited by the drug against Hela cancer cell lines.

Keywords: repurposing, cytotoxicity, microtubule, sulfonamide

1. INTRODUCTION

1.1. Sulfonamides: A Valuable Weapon against Cancer

Drug development in the field of oncology is facing an acute ‘productivity crisis.’ The success rate for new drugs considering Phase I trial to US Food and Drug Administration (FDA) approval, during the period 2003 to 2011 was around 6.7%. This figure is about half the rate for the development of non-oncological drugs (Hay et al., 2014). This apparent slowdown of new oncology drug production is confronting two challenges namely one of increased cancer incidence across the globe, and the other of existing significant therapeutic resistance in many types of malignant disease (Pantziarka et al., 2014). The global distribution of cancer incidence is also continuously changing. It is predicted that by 2030 cancer incidence in the low to medium human development index (HDI) countries will represent 52% of the global total, or 10.6 million cases (Bray et al., 2012). To overcome these hurdles, the Repurposing Drugs in Oncology (ReDO) project, finds that existing and widely used non-cancer drugs may represent a relatively untapped source of novel therapies for cancer. In contrast to the development of new molecules, drug repurposing initiates with known pharmaceutical agents with a prehistory of clinical use. Because repurposing builds upon previous research and development efforts, these drugs could be ready for clinical trials quickly, speeding their timeframe for review, approval and integration into health care (Pantziarka et al., 2014).

Cancer is a broad term. It is an uncontrolled growth and division of cells that forms different types of malignant tumors. Some varieties of cancer cause fast cell growth whereas in some other cancers cells grow and divide at a slower rate. Most of the cancers have been classified into three main groups like carcinomas, sarcomas and leukaemia or lymphomas. Carcinomas comprise around 90% of human cancers and arises from epithelial tissue. Sarcomas cover solid tumors of connective tissues, like muscle, bone, animal tissue and plant tissue whereas leukaemia and lymphomas arise from the blood-forming cells and from cells of the system.

Sulfamethoxazole (SMX)	**Sulfapyridine**	**Sulfadiazine**
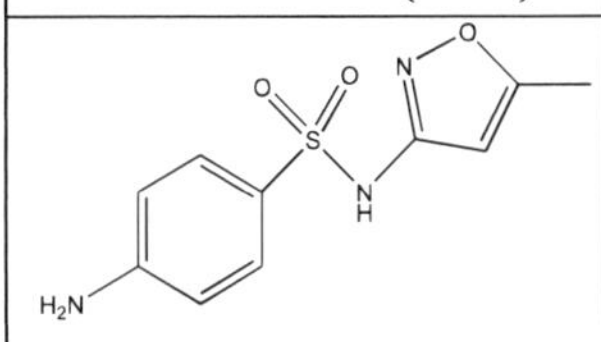	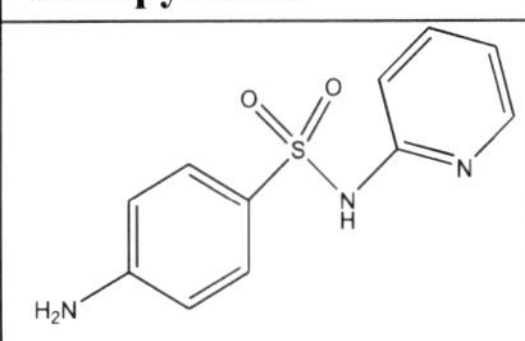	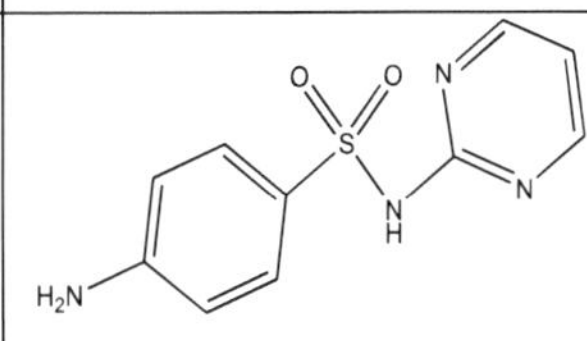

Figure 1. Structure of different sulfonamide group of drugs.

1.2. Drug Repurposing: A Newly Emerging Concept

Repurposing of so called "old" drugs is evolving to treat numerous diseases because of low costs, de-risks (their pharmacokinetics and toxicity have already been established) and short development timelines (Pushpakom et al., 2019). Various so called "old" drugs have now been treated to cure numerous diseases like diabetes, inflammation, many viral and bacterial infections as well as cancers. However, some technological challenges exist in the administration of these drugs which still needs to be addressed. Different types of diseases are emerging day by day and newly developed chemotherapeutic agents do not successfully combat many critical cancers albeit a huge advancement of technology in the field of drug discovery. The success level of these cancer drugs in human context is surprisingly low. Thus, there exists an increasing requirement for the development of new potent drugs, however pharmaceutical industries are facing various kinds of challenges that include high attrition rates, longer time frames to produce new drugs and huge costs. Inspite of efforts spent on new drug discovery by various Research and Development projects (R&D) of many countries, satisfactory results are not visible yet. This justifies Drug Repurposing.

Drug repurposing indicates the strategy of finding new aspects of various "old" drugs outside the scope of their original medicinal indications. There are many advantages of repurposing old drugs to treat many critical diseases. First, in the use of these old drugs chances of failure is lower because their activity has been found to be safe and well established in various pre-clinical models and in humans. Second, the period of drug development pattern is reduced as there are many novel drugs showing significant results in various pre-clinical models albeit having failed in human trials which is a major drawback in drug designing and development industries. Third, drug repurposing reduces financial investments because a huge amount of money was invested in pre-clinical and clinical trials on the drugs. These low risks, already established clinical implications, limited toxicity levels, less time and lower financial investment selects drug repurposing as a new and emerging topic to counter numerous diseases.

Drug repurposing project shows promising success to treat various types of diseases in clinical trials that immediately suggests that derivatives of these old drugs might have better potency to cure many diseases. These following examples illustrate some successful outcomes of drug repurposing schemes.

Table 1. Successful outcomes of drug ReDO project

Name of Drugs	Original Indication	New Indication
Adenosine	Conversion to rhythm of paroxysmal supraventricular tachycardia, including that associated with accessory bypass tracts (Wolff-Parkinson-White Syndrome).	For use in conjunction with BCNU in the treatment of brain tumors.
Amiloride HCl Solution for Inhalation	As adjunctive treatment with thiazide diuretics or other kaliuretic-diuretic agents in congestive heart failure or hypertension to: help restore normal serum potassium levels in patients who develop hypokalaemia on the kaliuretic diuretic; prevent development of hypokalaemia in patients who would be exposed to particular risk if hypokalaemia were to develop, digitalized patients or patients with significant cardiac arrhythmias.	Treatment of cystic fibrosis.
Alitretinoin	Topical treatment of cutaneous lesions in patients with AIDS-related Kaposi's sarcoma.	Treatment of acute promyelocytic leukemia.
Bacitracin	The use of intramuscular bacitracin should be limited to the treatment of infants with pneumonia and empyema caused by staphylococci shown to be susceptible to the drug.	Treatment of antibiotic-associated pseudomembranous enterocolitis caused by toxins A and B elaborated by Clostridium difficile.
Bupivacaine	Indicated for the production of local or regional anaesthesia or analgesia for surgery, dental and oral surgery procedures, diagnostic and therapeutic procedures, and for obstetrical procedures.	Relief of persistent pain associated with postherpetic neuralgia.
Celecoxib	Osteoarthritis and adult rheumatoid arthritis	Familial adenomatous polyposis.
Difluprednat	Difluprednate ophthalmic emulsion 0.05%, a topical corticosteroid, is indicated for the treatment of inflammation and pain associated with ocular surgery.	Treatment of endogenous and traumatic anterior uveitis and panuveitis.
Eculizumab	Treatment of paroxysmal nocturnal hemoglobinuria to reduce hemolysis	Treatment of dermatomyositis.
Finasteride	Benign prostatic hyperplasia	Hair loss.
Galantamine	Polio, paralysis and anaesthesia.	Alzheimer s disease
Histamine	Positive Skin Test Control - Histamine is indicated as an adjunct in allergy skin test for diagnosis, as a positive control to test wheal-flare response of skin for evaluation of skin test response to allergenic extracts.	For use as an adjunct to cytokine therapy in the treatment of malignant melanoma.
Idoxuridine	Treatment of keratitis caused by the virus of herpes simplex.	Treatment of nonparenchymatous sarcomas

Table 1. (Continued)

Name of Drugs	Original Indication	New Indication
Mannitol	Mannitol Injection is indicated for: Promotion of diuresis, in the prevention and/or treatment of the oliguric phase of acute renal failure before irreversible renal failure becomes established. Reduction of intracranial pressure and treatment of cerebral edema by reducing brain mass. Reduction of elevated intraocular pressure when the pressure cannot be lowered by other means. Promotion of urinary excretion of toxins.	For use to facilitate clearance of mucus in patients with bronchiectasis and in patients with cystic fibrosis at risk for bronchiectasis.
Nitazoxanide	Treatment of diarrhoea caused by Cryptosporidium parvum and Giardia lamblia.	Treatment for intestinal amebiasis.
Nevirapine	Use in combination with other antiretroviral agents for the treatment of HIV-1 infection.	Prevention of HIV infection in pediatric patients under the age of 16 years.
Oxaliplatin	Used in combination with infusional 5-FU/LV, it is indicated for adjuvant treatment of stage III colon cancer in patients who have undergone complete resection of the primary tumor. It is used for treatment of advanced colorectal cancer.	Treatment of ovarian cancer.
Pazopanib	Treatment of patients with advanced renal cell carcinoma	Treatment of soft tissue sarcomas
Paclitaxel	Cancer	Restenosis
Rituximab	Treatment of patients with Non-Hodgkin s Lymphoma and Chronic Lymphocytic Leukemia.	Treatment of immune thrombocytopenic purpura.
Rifabutin	Prevention of disseminated Mycobacterium avium complex disease in patients with advanced HIV infections.	Treatment of disseminated Mycobacterium avium complex disease.
Ropinirole	Hypertension.	Restless leg syndrome.
Somatropin	For long-term treatment of children who have growth failure due to a lack of adequate endogenous growth hormone secretion.	Adjunct for the induction of ovulation in women with infertility due to hypogonadotropic hypogonadism or bilateral tubal occlusion or unexplained infertility, who are undergoing in vivo or in vitro fertilization procedures.

Name of Drugs	Original Indication	New Indication
Sermorelin Acetate	Treatment of idiopathic or organic growth hormone deficiency in children with growth failure	Adjunct to gonadotropin therapy in the induction of ovulation in women with anovulatory or oligo-ovulatory infertility who fail to ovulate in response to adequate treatment with clomiphene citrate alone and gonadotropin therapy alone.
Sibutramine	Depression.	Obesity.
Tadalafil	Inflammation and cardiovascular disease.	Male erectile dysfunction.
Tiotropium Bromide	Tiotropium bromide inhalation powder is indicated for the long-term, once-daily, maintenance treatment of bronchospasm associated with chronic obstructive pulmonary disease (COPD), including chronic bronchitis and emphysema. It is also indicated to reduce exacerbations in COPD patients.	To improve pulmonary function in conjunction with standard therapy in the management of patients with cystic fibrosis.
Toremifene	Treatment of metastatic breast cancer in postmenopausal women with estrogen positive or receptor unknown tumors.	Treatment of desmoid tumors.
Ursodiol	Ursodiol is indicated for patients with radiolucent, noncalcified gallbladder stones greater than 20 mm in greatest diameter in whom elective cholecystectomy would be undertaken except for the presence of increased surgical risk due to systemic disease, advanced age, idiosyncratic reaction to general anesthesia, or for those patients who refuse surgery. Ursodiol is indicated for the prevention of gallstone formation in obese patients experiencing rapid weight loss.	Treatment of cystic fibrosis liver disease.
Valproic Acid, Sodium	Divalproex sodium extended-release is indicated for the treatment of acute manic or mixed episodes associated with bipolar disorder.	Treatment of familial adenomatous polyposis.

1.3. Repurposing Sulfamethoxazole with a Different Spectrum of Activities

Sulfonamide is a sulpha group of drugs that has been widely used for its antibacterial, anti-carbonic anhydrase, diuretic, hypo glycaemic and antithyroid activities (Strydom et al., 2013). Many sulfonamide groups of drugs are now used as anticancer agents because of their antitumor activities in vivo. Sulfonamide group of drugs share a common chemical structure / motif with some chemical modifications. They exhibit their anticancer mechanism in different mechanistic pathways. Many sulfonamide groups of drugs show their anticancer potential, by supressing carbonic anhydrase activity, introducing cell cycle arrest in G1, G2/M phase by disruption of microtubule network, by inhibiting the functional activities of many transcriptional activators like NF-Y and by inhibiting angiogenesis via inactivating different matrix metalloproteinases (Scozzafava et al., 2003).

Cancer chemotherapy is still a challenge in cancer treatment because most of the anticancer agents are nonspecific in their anti-cancer activities. Moreover, emergence of drug resistance and multidrug resistant p-glycoprotein in various tumours introduce a serious complication in cancer chemotherapy. Thus, the hunt for novel anticancer agent with a cancer cell specific target is never over.

1.4. Sulfonamides as Carbonic-Anhydrase Inhibitors in Cancer

Carbonic anhydrase (CA) is an enzyme which catalyses the hydration of CO_2 that produces bicarbonate (Claudiu et al., 2002). This bicarbonate is very important for many biochemical processes like gluconeogenesis, amino acid synthesis, urea synthesis, membrane lipid production, nucleotide synthesis (Berg et al., 2002). These carbonic anhydrases are also involved in respiration and transport of CO_2 in lungs. Among different carbonic anhydrases isoenzymes, two isoenzymes are mostly involved in many cancer cells because in a cancer cell higher rate of respiration occurs rather than in a normal cell (Claudiu et al., 2002). In this condition high amount of bicarbonate is needed to provide for the process gluconeogenesis, nucleotide biosynthesis which are important metabolic pathways for the survival of cancer cells in hypoxic microenvironment. Carbonic anhydrase is also responsible for the H^+ ion production which has been produced by metabolism and pumped into the cytosol and released by the cell (Seok et al., 2008). Some previous work has shown that hypoxia and expression of carbonic anhydrases are strongly corelated. Hypoxia induced factors are the biomarkers of many cancer types. Hypoxia induced factors elevate carbonic anhydrase IX level among all isoenzymes (Innocenti et al., 2007). CA-IX is expressed in low lwels in normal cells but malignant pancreatic, colon, lungs, kidney, ovary, brain, skin, breast, oesophagus tissues shows higher amounts of CA-IX activity (Benej et al., 2014). Although inhibition of CAs by aromatic and heterocyclic sulfonamides have long been used to treat a variety of diseases such as glaucoma, epilepsy, congestive heart failure, mountain sickness, gastric and duodenal ulcers or as diuretic agents, very little information has been reported about their anticancer effects (Benej et al.,2014). Several derivatives of this class include acetazolamide, methazolamide or ethoxzolamide (Teicher et al., 1993). There are reports which indicate that, acetazolamide, a member of this group of drugs and a strong inhibitor of several CA isozymes is a potential modulator of anticancer therapies in combination with different cytotoxic agents (alkylating agents; nucleoside analogues; platinum derivatives, etc.). It is probably due to the CA inhibition in tumor microenvironment, although other mechanisms of action of this drug could not be excluded.

1.5. Anticancer Activities of Chloroquinoxaline Sulfonamide (CQS)

Chloroquinoxaline Sulfonamide (CQS) contains a secondary sulfonamide moiety which has been used as antibacterial infection purposes. From some research work it had been observed that CQS exhibits its anticancer effects in various cancer cell lines and in solid tumors in breast, ovary, melanoma. In murine melanoma cell line CQS shows its anticancer effects by arresting cell at G0/G1 phase (Branda et al., 1988).

1.6. Antimitotic Sulfonamide Agents in Clinical Trial

Yoshino et al. suggested that specific sulfonamide group of drugs have a potency to inhibit cancer cell growth. Further derivatives of these sulfonamides show higher potency against many cancers cell lines both in vitro and in vivo (Yoshino et al., 1992). E7010 is a specific sulfonamide agent which interacts with β tubulin in the colchicine binding site and inhibits microtubule polymerization (Yoshimatsu et al., 1997). E7010 binds to tubulin in a reversible manner. E7010 shows its anticancer effects in a panel of 26 human cancer cell lines with a lower IC_{50} value (Koyanagi et al., 1994). A second-generation antimitotic sulfonamide drug had been developed which was more efficient and potent than E7010. Owa et al., showed another class of sulfonamide agent which induces cell death in murine leukaemia cells by arresting cells in specifically G1 phase (Yokoi et al., 2002). E7070 which is known as indisulam performs significant anti tumor activity both in vitro and in vivo in a variety of cancer cell lines (Ozawa et al., 1997). It also reduces tumor size in significant amount in HCT -116 xenografts (Ozawa et al., 1997).

1.7. Anticancer Activities of Sulfonylurea

Sulfonylurea is a structural derivative of sulfonamide group of drugs. It has been reported that sulfonylurea shows anti tumor activities in many human cancers cell lines and in vivo system which selects sulfonylurea as a potent anticancer agent (Howbert et al., 1990).

1.8. Microtubule Targeting Sulfonamide Agents

Some sulfonamide group of drugs exhibit their anticancer potential by disrupting microtubule network in cell. Microtubule is a polymer composed of tubulin heterodimer (α and β). Microtubule is highly involved in many important cellular events like cell division, cell motility, maintaining cell shape, vesicular trafficking and many others (Fletcher et al., 2010). During cell division it forms mitotic spindle which is composed of many microtubular proteins. Moreover, the dynamics of microtubule is very important for maintaining cellular homeostasis. Any alternations in this dynamic nature leads to cell death by apoptosis (Estève et al., 2007). There are many antimitotic agents which exhibit their anti-mitotic effects by targeting microtubule dynamics in cells like colchicine, vinblastine, paclitaxel etc. Colchicine and vinblastine are the microtubule destabilising agents whereas taxol derivatives are the microtubule stabilising agents. These three drugs have three separate binding sites on a tubulin dimer (Dumontet et al., 2010). Medina et al. showed that a group of perfluorophenylsulfonamide derivatives inhibit the growth of various cancer cells with their IC_{50} values in the nanomolar range (Medina et al.,1999). Some derivatives of these compounds show anticancer properties by interacting with tubulin. This group of drugs bind with cys-239 residue of β tubulin by nucleophilic aromatic substitution reaction (Medina et al., 1999).

1.9. Sulfonamides Inhibiting Matrix Metalloproteinase (MMPS)

Extracellular matrix (ECM) provides integrity to the various tissues in higher vertebrates. Expression of extracellular matrix proteins is tightly regulated. ECM is involved in many physiological processes like ovulation, morphogenesis, development, wound healing, angiogenesis, metastasis and in many others (Nagase et al., 1999). Matrix metalloproteinases (MMPs) are basically a class of enzymes which exhibit endonuclease activity and contains zinc ion in their structure. These MMPs are involved in the above-mentioned processes and are critically involved in metastasis. During metastasis, MMP helps to loosen attachments of the cancer cells with the ECM and helps them to migrate (Supuran et al., 2003). During epithelial to mesenchymal transition MMPs play an important role. There are about 20 isoenzymes of MMPs present in cells which generally share a wide sequence homology among each other and performs various kinds of actions. They are classified into different classes like collagenase (MMP-1, -8, -13, -18); gelatinase (MMP-2, -9); stromelysins (MMP-3, -10, -11); membrane type of MMP (MMP -14, 15, 16, 17) (Nagase et al., 1999). Inhibition of MMP by specific inhibitors can resist the epithelial mesenchymal transition in a cancer cell which in turn resist cancer metastasis (Supuran et al., 2003).

Recent studies have shown that sulfonylated amino acids have potential to inhibit MMP activity (MacPherson et al., 1997). Some reports suggest that various derivatives of aryl sulfonyl hydroxamates derived from glycine, L alanine, L valine, L-leucine show anticancer effects by binding with MMPs. Some MMP inhibitors are used in combination with other cytotoxic agents in cancer therapy (Clare et al., 2001).

1.10. Sulfonamide Involved in Epigenetics

Eukaryotic gene transcription is a tightly regulated event. DNA is condensed in the form of chromatin by histone protein (Zhou et al., 2019). Two enzymes, histone deacetylase and histone acetyl transferase play key roles in chromatin modification and chromatin remodelling complex (Meinke et al., 2001). Histone deacetylase (HDAC) enzyme has many isoenzyme forms in cell which are evolved in the regulation of cell cycle and tumor formation. Thus, inhibitors of HDAC are effective in cancer therapy (Gray et al., 2001). Many inhibitors including sulfonamide hydroxamic acid group of drugs have been reported as HDAC inhibitors. These compounds show nanomolar affinity against HDAC isoenzymes (Gray SG et al., 2001) and thus are effective potent anticancer agents against human colon cancer HCT -116 cells (Lavoie et al., 2001).

1.11. Sulfonamides against Steroidogenesis

Breast cancer is one of the most familiar cancers among women. Most of the breast cancers are classified as estrogen dependent cancers. Estradiol is the prime factor for development of such types of cancers (Meikle et al., 2001). Estrogen level is very high in breast cancer patients rather than normal woman due to *de novo* cellular biosynthesis of this estrogen hormone (Pasqualini et al., 1996). Production of this hormone in the cell is mainly due to two metabolic pathways. In the first case aromatase converts androstenedione to estrone and in the second pathway estrone sulfatase converts estrone sulphate to estrone which finally gets converted to Estradiol by 1-β-hydroxysteroid dehydrogenase (Pasqualini et al., 1996). Many steroidal and non-steroidal sulfamates were designed for estrone sulfatase inhibitors with lower IC_{50} value (Li et al., 1998). Various non-steroidal derivatives like alkylamoidophenyl sulfamate, coumarin based sulfamates are potential inhibitors of estrone sulfatase (Woo et al., 1998).

Some reports predict that derivatives of 2-mercaptobenzene sulfonamides and benzodithiazines show anticancer properties by some unknown mechanisms. Oxindole based sulfonamides show their anticancer properties by inhibiting cyclin dependent kinase 2 (CDK-2) which is a key regulator of cell cycle (Pogorzelska et al., 2015). These group of drugs show their anticancer efficacy by arresting cell at a particular phase of the cell cycle.

1.12. Repurposing Sulfamethoxazole with a Different Spectrum of Activities

SMX has largely been utilized to prevent varieties of bacterial infections although one of the current challenges often encountered with SMX administration is the resistance against this drug by bacterial species (Majewsky et al., 2014). To overcome this issue attempts have been made to develop potent derivatives of SMX with modified antibacterial activity. Sulfamethoxazolyl-azo-acetylacetone and its Ni complex draw attention for their antibacterial property (Beheshti et al., 2017). However, the effect of SMX or its derivatives on eukaryotic cells has not been deciphered precisely. A group of sulfonamides have been reported with inhibitory activity against a panel of human cancer cell lines. Among them some orally active sulfonamides that bind to the colchicine binding site of tubulin are in clinical trial (Yoshimatsu et al., 1997). They inhibit in vitro tubulin polymerisation (Dumontet et al.,2010). Very few of them have been marketed as anticancer drugs. SMX bears a structural scaffold common to those active compounds. This widely used cheap, antibacterial drug is already in market to treat common bacterial infections. So, it can be explored further to dig out any latent potency related to its anti-mitotic action. Investigation of the mechanistic pathway of SMX interaction with tubulin/MT might shed light on its mode of action and identification of its specific target in the cellular level. SMX itself or its various derivatives could serve as a future lead compound for the development of anti-cancer compounds of future use.

2. Materials and Methods

2.1. Cell Line and Culture Condition

Human cervical cancer cell line (HeLa) was cultured in Dulbecco's modified Eagle medium (DMEM) supplemented with 10% fetal bovine serum (FBS), 100 U/ml penicillin and 100 mg/ml streptomycin following standard protocol. The effects of sulphur drugs on cell proliferations were determined using established assay methods. HeLa cells were grown in the absence or presence of different concentrations of drugs (dissolved in DMSO) for 24 hours, the final concentration of DMSO not exceeding 0.1% of the total volume. Cells were detached from each well by trypsinization (0.025% trypsin) and were counted manually using a hemocytometer.

2.2. Estimation of Cytotoxicity of SMX by MTT Assay

The cytotoxic action of the compound was assayed by MTT. In brief, cells (70% confluent) in 12 well plates were treated with SMX and its derivatives in varying concentrations for 48 hours. At the end of the incubation, 10 µl MTT (3-(4,5-dimethylthiazol-2-yl)-2,5-diphenyl tetrazolium bromide) (5 mg mL^{-1}) was added and the plates were further incubated for 4 hours. The formazan crystals formed within the well were dissolved by adding 100 µL of DMSO and absorbance was monitored at 570 nm.

2.3. Immunofluorescence Microscopy

The effect of SMX on microtubules and chromosomes was tested using fluorescence microscopy. Briefly, HeLa cells were grown on poly lysine coated glass coverslips in the absence and presence of different concentrations of drugs for 24 hours. Subsequently, followed by formaldehyde fixing, permeabilization, blocking with 2% BSA in PBS, cells were incubated with mouse monoclonal anti-α-tubulin antibody (1:300 dilution) and with a 1:350 dilution of Alexa-568-labeled anti-mouse IgG antibody for 1 hour. Nuclear staining was carried out with Hoechst 33258 (1 μg/mL) for 10 min in the dark. The cover slips were observed under microscope after mounting.

2.4. Lactate Dehydrogenase Activity (LDH) Assay

0.3 x 10^6 cells were plated in 6 well plates. After reaching 75% confluency, cells were treated with two different SMX concentrations (IC_{50} and half IC_{50} concentrations). After 24-hour incubation with SMX, cells were washed with 1X PBS buffer. Samples were sonicated and centrifuged at 8000 rpm for 15 minutes. Supernatant was collected and protein concentration was measured using Bradford's Reagent. In a 3 ml cuvette, 1.5 ml 50 mM Tris buffer (pH 7.6), 1 ml 1.8 mM sodium pyruvate, 100 μl 5mM NADH and 100 μL 1:10 diluted (equal protein content) were added and change in OD was measured during 3 minutes reaction. LDH activity was calculated using formula (ΔOD/ 2.0733) X 1000. Where ΔOD = change in OD over 3 minutes (Kim EY et al., 2019).

2.5. Monitoring ROS Production in Presence of Sulfamethoxazole (SMX)

0.3 x 10^6 cells were plated in 6 well plates. In brief, after reaching 75% confluency, treatment with SMX (IC_{50} concentration) was done on Hela cells at three different time points. After washing the cells with 1X PBS, 20 uM 2',7'-Dichlorodihydrofluorescein diacetate (DCFDA) was added to each well and incubated for 30 minutes in the dark (Basu et al., 2018). Cells were collected and centrifuged at 3000 rpm for 5 minutes. After discarding the supernatant, pellets were dissolved in 1XPBS. Fluorescence was measured (E_x/E_m = 485/535 nm) using flow cytometer. Percentage of ROS change over control was determined after background subtraction.

2.6. Cell Cycle Analysis Using PI Staining

0.3 x 10^6 Hela cells were plated in 6 well plates. After reaching 75% confluency, cells were treated with two different SMX concentrations (IC_{50} and half IC_{50} concentrations). Following 24 hours incubation with the drug, cells were collected in microcentrifuge tubes. Cells were centrifuged at 3000 rpm for 5 min. After discarding the media, pellets were resuspended in 1X PBS. 40 μl ice cold methanol was added for fixation. Samples were incubated at -20°C for 3-5 min. 300 μl ice cold PBS was added and incubated further at 4°C for 1 hour. RNase A was mixed (final conc:100μg/ul) and the samples were incubated at 37°C water bath for 1.5 hours. Propidium Iodide (PI) was added (final concentration 120 μg/ul) and flow cytometry was performed (Basu et al., 2018).

2.7. Estimation of Lipid Peroxidation

The extent of lipid peroxidation, HeLa cells were seeded in 6-well plates at a density of 4×10^5 and incubated for 24 hours. Then cells were treated with different concentrations of SMX keeping DMSO as vehicle control. After treatment, cells were grown and lysed by sonicating for 10 sec by ultrasound pulse. Lipid peroxidation was estimated by thiobarbituric acid-reactive substances (TBARS) method by measuring the levels of malondialdehyde (MDA) produced during cellular lipid peroxidation. In short, the cell lysates were then centrifuged at 10,000 g for 10 min at 4°C.

Then equal volume of TBA solution (0.375% TBA, 15% trichloroacetic acid, and 0.25 N HCl) was added to the supernatants and heated for 15 min in a boiling water bath followed by centrifugation at 10,000 g for 5 min. Finally, absorbance of the supernatant was taken at 535nm. The values are represented as fold change over control (Basu et al., 2018).

2.8. Western Blot Analysis

The total protein was collected from Hela cells cultured with IC_{50} concentration (350 μM) of SMX for 24 hours. Protein concentrations were analysed by the Bio-Rad Protein Assay Kit (Merck). Then, the proteins were separated by 8% SDS-PAGE and transferred onto PVDF membranes (Merck Millipore, Billerica, MA, USA). The membranes were blocked with 5% non-fat milk for 2 hours at room temperature followed by incubation overnight at 4°C with a primary antibody (Beclin-1 and alpha Tubulin) at a dilution of 1:1000. Subsequently, the membranes were washed three times with TBST and incubated with the appropriate HRP-conjugated secondary antibody (1:5,000) for 2 hours at room temperature. Protein bands were visualised using the chemiluminescence by adding Luminol (Sigma), P-cumaric acid (Sigma). Alpha tubulin was used as an internal control (Basu et al., 2018).

2.9. Flow Cytometry Analysis for Apoptosis

Flow cytometry assay was performed to measure cell apoptosis rates. Briefly, after treatment with various concentrations (175 μM, 350 μM) of SMX for 24 hours, Hela cells were collected and washed twice in PBS at room temperature. For apoptosis assays, cells (1×10^6) were counted and resuspended in 100 μL annexin-V binding buffer solution (Thermo-sceintific). Subsequently, 5 μL annexin V-FITC (Thermo Fisher sceintific) and 5 μL propidium iodide (HiMedia) were added, and incubated at room temperature for 15 minutes in the dark (Basu et al.,2018). The percentage of apoptotic cells was analysed by flow cytometry using (BD FACS verse, Bose Institute).

2.10. Molecular Modelling

The X ray crystal structure of α and β tubulin complexed with N-deacetyl –N-(2-marcaptoacetyl)- colchicine (DAMA colchicine) was obtained from protein data bank (PDB) (PDB id :1SA0) and M-chain of Lactate dehydrogenase-A (PDB id:1i10) as the target structures in the molecular docking. SMX was docked with the target molecule using Leadit software. 100 possible binding conformations were obtained and the conformation with the lowest binding free energy was selected as the possible binding conformation.

3. Results

3.1. Sulfamethoxazole (SMX) Induces Cytotoxicity in Hela Cells

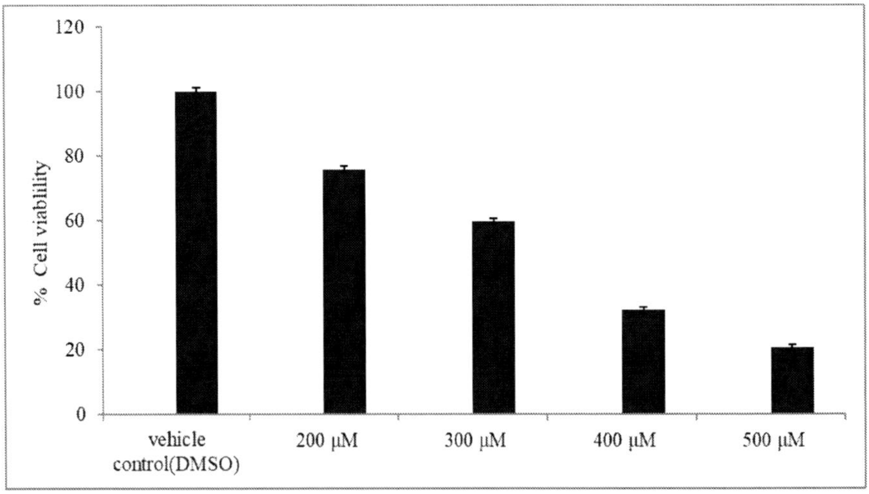

Figure 2A. Gradual inhibition of HeLa cell proliferation upon SMX treatment.

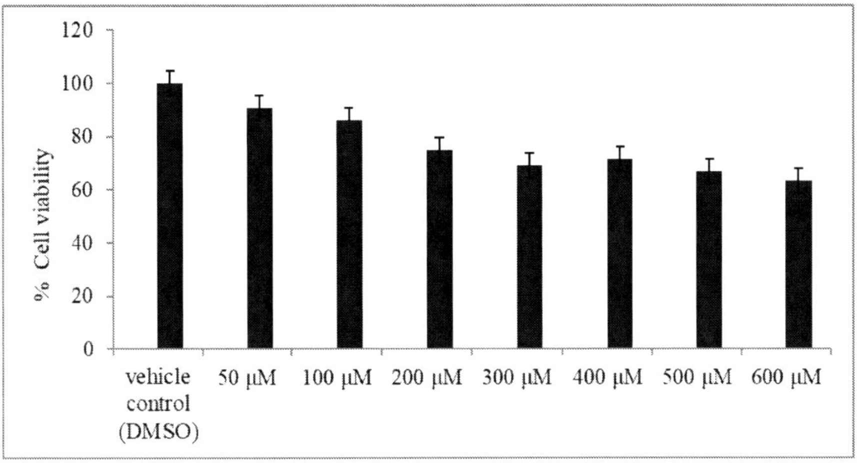

Figure 2B. Effect of Sulfadiazine treatment on HeLa cell proliferation.

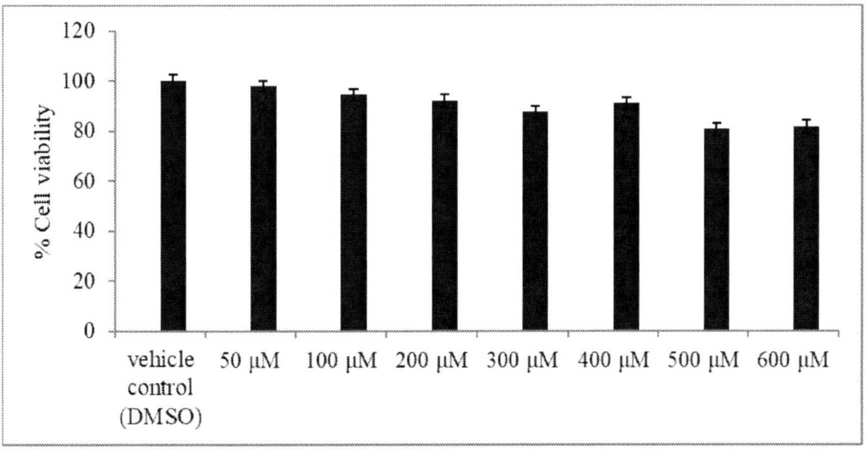

Figure 2C. Effect of Sulfapyridine treatment on HeLa cell proliferation.

SMX induces cytotoxicity in HeLa cell lines in a concentration dependant manner with IC_{50} values 350 μM (Figure 2A). However, sulfadiazine (Figure 2B) and sulfapyridine (Figure 2C) do not show any effective inhibition of HeLa cell which had been confirmed by the MTT assay. This indicates that minute differences in the drug structure might play prominent role for effective antimitotic potential.

3.2. Sulfamethoxazole (SMX) Alters Interphase Microtubules of Hela Cells

To study the alteration in interphase microtubule network and nuclear morphology of HeLa cells upon treatment with SMX, confocal microscopy was performed.

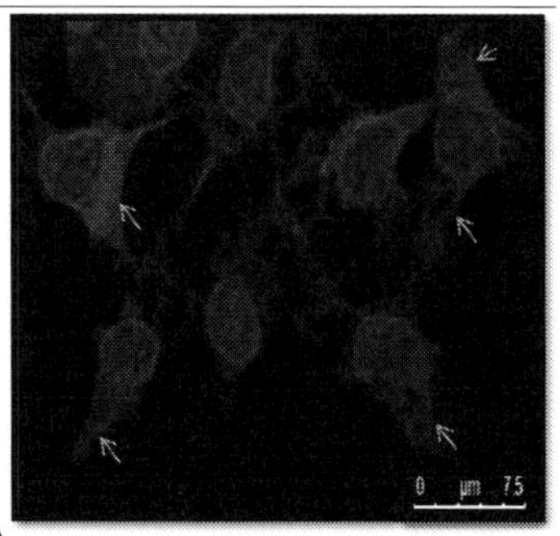

A

Control (HeLa cell line) with intact MT (marked by yellow arrow)

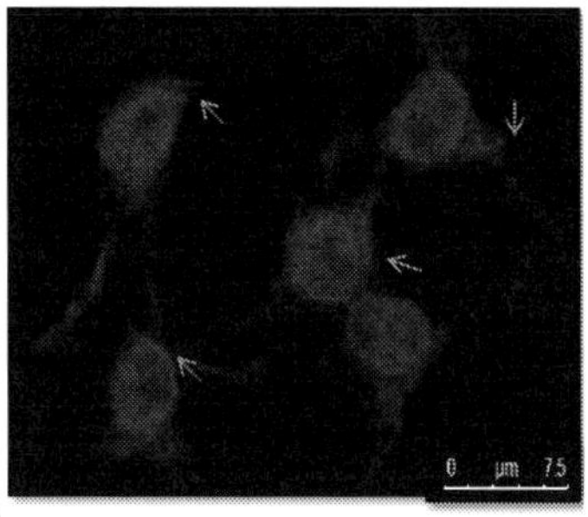

B

Microtube structure of HeLa cells at 175 μM SMX (½ IC_{50} concentration)

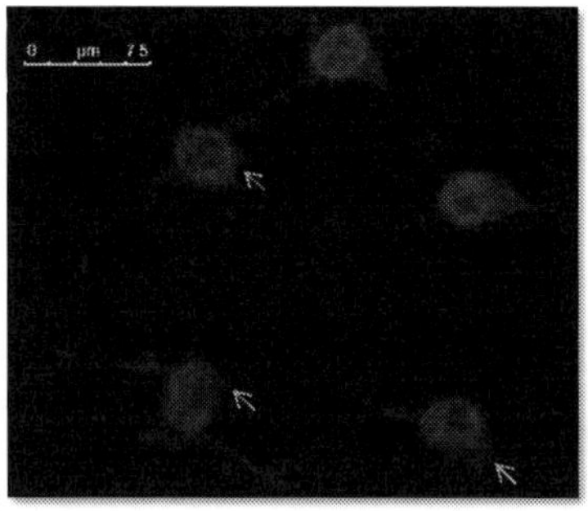

C

Microtube structure of HeLa cells at 350 μM SMX (IC_{50} concentration)

Figure 3. Effect on SMX on microtubule structure in HeLa cells.

Upon treatment with 175 µM SMX (Figure 3B), the interphase microtubule network showed disruption compared to the control treated with vehicle (0.5% DMSO) that displayed normal organization (Figure 3A). The effect was more drastic with 350 µM SMX that revealed further depolymerization of interphase microtubule, leaving behind microtubule in shrinkage form (Figure 3C). Many antimitotic drugs target microtubules and disrupt cytoskeleton as reviewed in many reports.

3.3. Sulfamethoxazole (SMX) Elevates Intracellular ROS Production

Estimation of ROS has been conducted to decipher the cause behind cytotoxicity in case of SMX administration to the Hela cell lines. Elevated levels of reactive oxygen species (ROS) are common in almost all cancer cells (Liou et al., 2010). Optimal levels of ROS promote tumorigenesis, however excessive ROS promotes cell death. ROS might act as mediators of apoptosis involving different caspases or up-regulating death receptor 5 (Redza-Dutordoir et al., 2016). A number of signalling pathways, namely mitogen-activated protein kinase (MAPK) pathway, extracellular signal-regulated kinase (ERK) pathway, phosphoinositide 3-kinase (PI3K) are associated with ROS mediated apoptosis (Son et al.,2013). In reality, the challenge for novel therapeutic strategies will be to steer the cells from ROS-induced tumorigenesis into ROS-induced apoptotic signalling by disruption of the delicate redox balance. ROS level in the resistant cancer cells are usually lower compared to their parental sensitive cells which is consistent with the higher level of antioxidants than the sensitive parental cell lines (Liou et al., 2010). To ascertain whether SMX induces ROS production for its cytotoxic effects on HeLa cells, cells were treated with SMX and ROS production monitored by DCFDA fluorescence method. It has been observed that percentage of ROS production increases with time (Figure 4) upon treatment of 350 □M SMX (IC_{50} concentration) up to 32%over control at 2 hr.

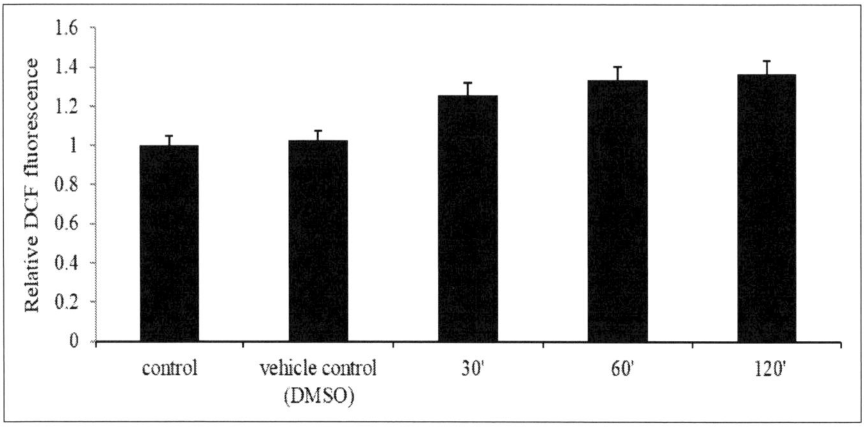

Figure 4. Estimation of ROS production in Hela cells on treatment of 350 M SMX (IC50) at various time points.

3.4. Sulfamethoxazole (SMX) Reduces Intracellular Lactate Dehydrogenase -A Activity

Lactate dehydrogenase (LDH) has been considered as a pivotal player of energy generation in cancer cells. It produces instant, quick energy by "Warburg effect" concentrating on "aerobic glycolysis" compared to the slow route of oxidative phosphorylation. In normal cells, this pathway is active only in specific cases like embryonic development or in the hyper-working skeletal muscle albeit in cancer cells it plays a major role (Liberti et al.,2016). LDH-A level is augmented in certain cancers and promotes tumor growth and invasion as evident from research studies through knocking down LDH-A expression using RNA interference (Yu et al.,2014). This effect is pronounced in hematopoietic malignancies, such as Hodgkin's lymphoma (HL), non-Hodgkin's lymphoma (NHL) or multiple myelomas. From the estimate of LDH activity, prediction of the survival in patients has been carried out as per the International Prognostic Index (IPI) (Feng et al.,2018). Recently, some drug-like inhibitors of LDHA (analogues of gossypol, such as FX11; quinoline 3-sulfonamides; galloflavin, oxamate, AZ-33) have been reported with promising anticancer activity both in vitro and in vivo (Kim et al., 2019). In the present context, role of SMX on LDH-

A activity has been estimated. Compared to control, a steady decrease in LDH-A activity has been observed in the presence of SMX (Figure 5).

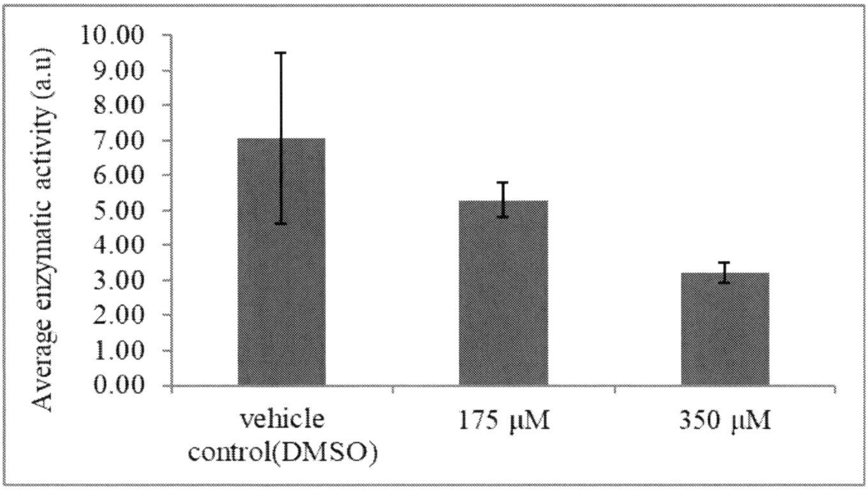

Figure 5. Effect of SMX on Lactate Dehydrogenase (LDH) activity in Hela cells.

3.5. Sulfamethoxazole (SMX) Elevates SUB G1 Cell Population

Propidium Iodide (PI) binds specifically with DNA which reflects different phases of the cell cycle. Amount of DNA is doubled from G1 to G2/M phase. During S phase its amount is intermediate compared to G1 and G2/M phase. From cell cycle analysis using SMX treatment we have found that SMX does not induce any cell cycle arrest but it executes its cytotoxic effects using DNA fragmentation/damage which increased by 1.6-fold compared to its control level (Figure 6). This might have some correlation with the ROS yield as observed during SMX treatment. This might be justified taking into account the role of ROS in the induction of genomic instability of the nuclear as well as mitochondrial DNA caused by several oxidative mutations.

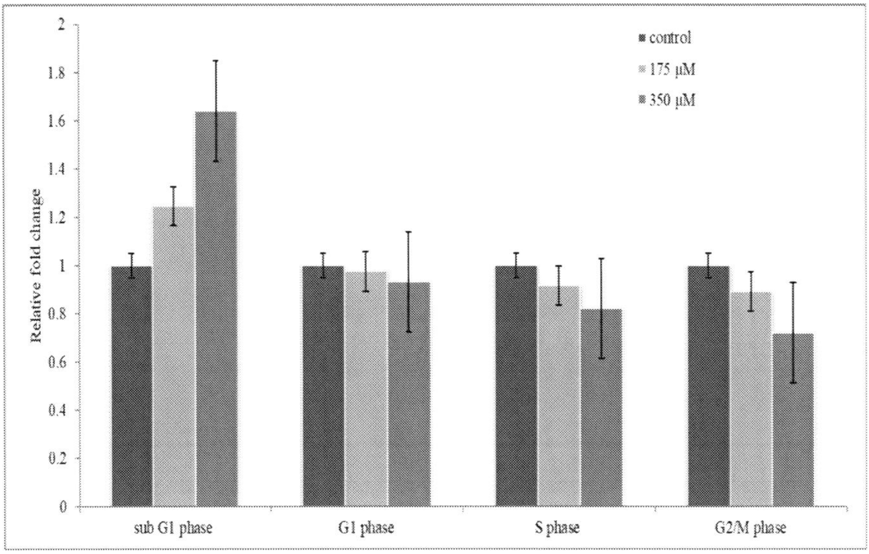

Figure 6. Effect of SMX on cell cycle phases.

3.6. Sulfamethoxazole (SMX) Peroxidises Poly Unsaturated Fatty Acids (PUFAS) in Plasma Membrane

ROS has significantly short half-life, albeit their oxidation products are relatively stable. So, they are good indicators of oxidative stress (Turrens et al., 2003). When ROS attack polyunsaturated fatty acids (PUFAs) of the membranes, they give rise to highly reactive aldehydes namely, malondialdehyde (MDA), 4-hydroxynonenal (HNE), and acrolein (Ayala et al., 2014). These lipid peroxidation products covalently bind to histidine, cysteine, or lysine residues of proteins through Michael addition resulting in structural alteration and impaired functions of these protein residues (Grimsrud et al., 2008). The role of lipid peroxidation is implicated in the pathophysiology or might be associated with many chronic diseases such as Alzheimer's disease, diabetes mellitus, hypertension, and cancers in both animals and humans (Montine et al.,2002). Reports are there where PUFAs in combination with anticancer agents such as doxorubicin and arsenic trioxide have elicited synergistic cytotoxic effect in various cancer cells such as breast, colon, cervical, pancreatic, and renal cancer cells. Increased cytotoxicity in cancer cells is an outcome of augmented lipid peroxidation products that act as an adjunct in radiotherapy (Wang et al., 2001). So, considering its effect in cancer cell lines, effect of SMX (at its IC_{50} value) on lipid peroxidation has been tested (Figure 7). SMX promotes enhanced lipid peroxidation compared to control. Although evidence suggests that little bit ROS is supportive for proliferation and survival of cancer cells however its overproduction induced by the presence of certain drugs like SMX might be detrimental for cells. It might be responsible for SMX mediated cytotoxicity of the cancer cells. Lipid peroxidation biomarkers could also serve as a diagnostic tool to predict the chances of cancer recurrence and is of immense importance.

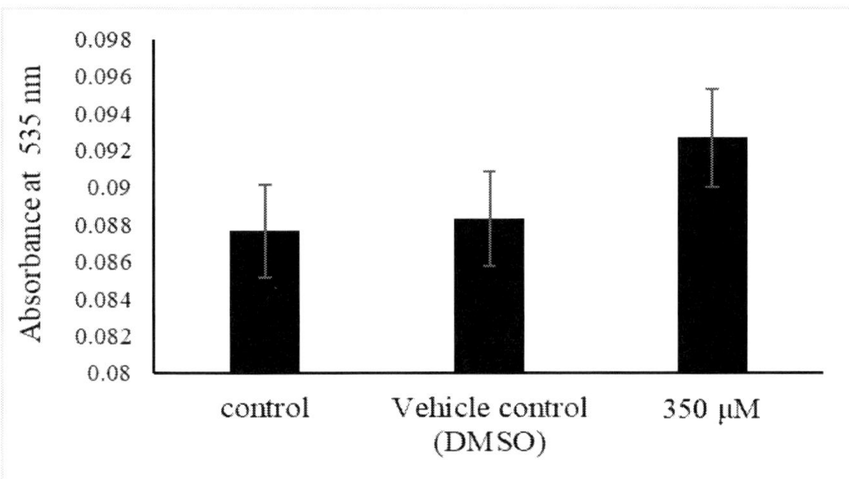

Figure 7. Effect of SMX on lipid peroxidation after treating Hela cells for 24 hours.

3.7. SMX Induces Cell Death in HeLa Cells by Mechanism Other Than Apoptosis

To depict whether SMX introduces cell death in HeLa cell by apoptosis or some other pathway, apoptosis detection assay was performed using FACS analysis by annexin -FITC / PI dual staining method.

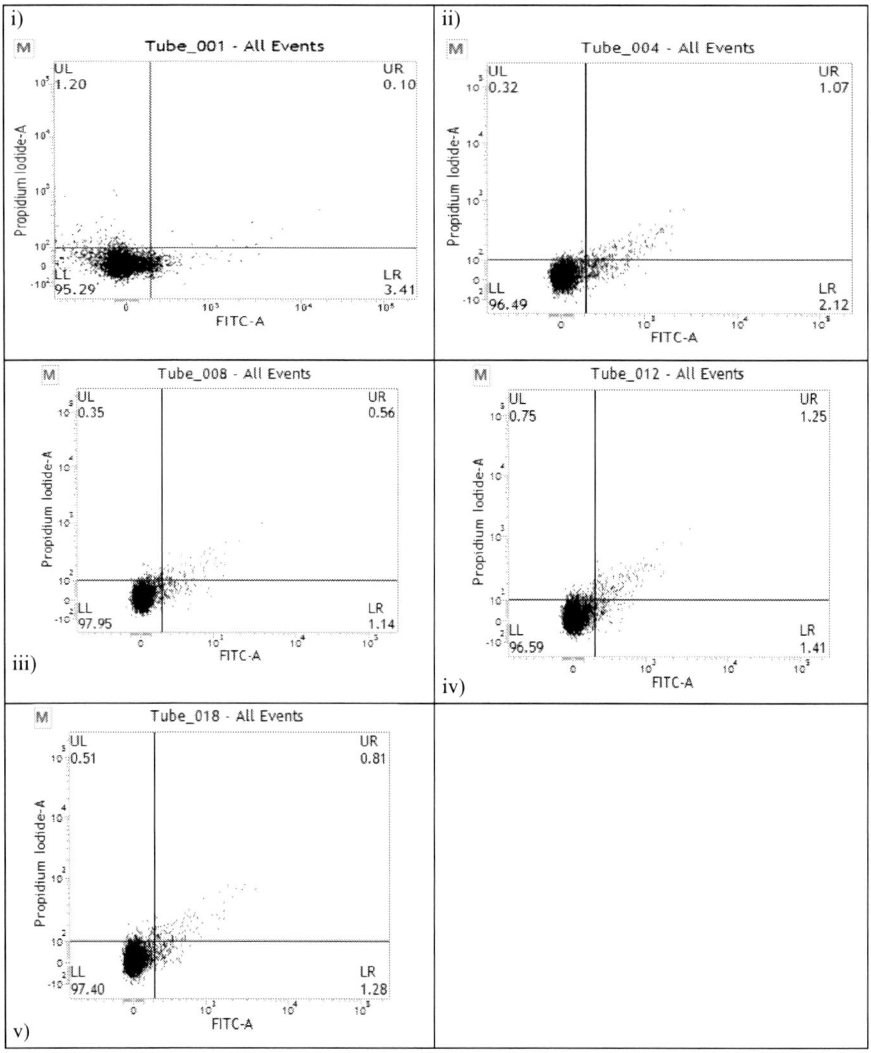

Figure 8A. Effects of SMX on apoptosis in Hela cells during 24 hour treatment i) unstained control; ii) stained control; iii) DMSO control; iv) SMX 175 □M; v) SMX 350 □M.

AnnexinV$^-$/PI$^-$ population indicates healthy cell, Annexin V$^+$/PI$^-$ population indicates early apoptotic cell, Annexin V$^+$/PI$^+$ indicates late apoptotic cells and Annexin V$^-$/PI$^+$ population indicates necrotic population. It was observed that SMX does not induce apoptosis / necrosis significantly (Figure 8).

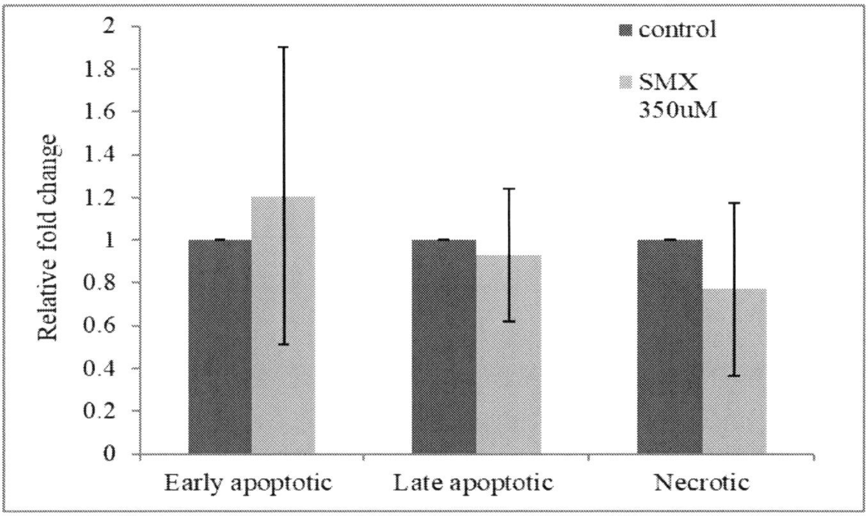

Figure 8B. Fold change of early apoptotic, late apoptotic and necrotic cells compared to control.

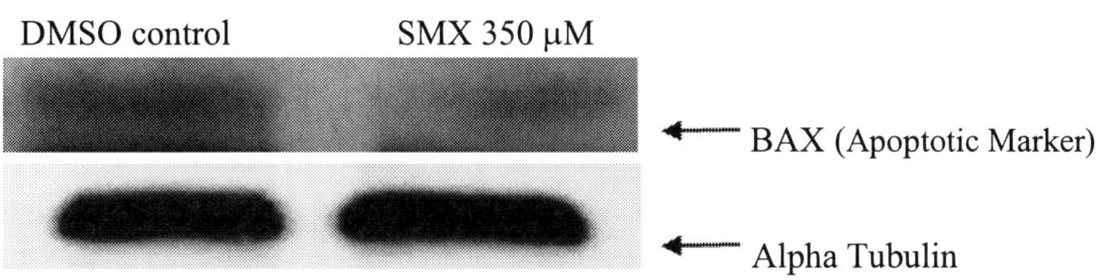

Figure 9. Western blot analysis on proapoptotic Bax expression after SMX treatment for 24 hours compared to control Hela cells.

Insertion of Bax family members into the mitochondrial membrane induces the release of cytochrome C and the induction of apoptotic cell death. The Bax molecule seems to reside in the cytoplasm and responds to various stimuli by migration to the mitochondria where it causes cytochrome

C release, leading to APAF-1 dimerization and the apoptotic cascade. As observed by researchers it was observed that growth-factor starvation can cause translocation of Bax from the cytoplasm to the mitochondria. Withdrawal of growth factor causes an increase in the intracellular pH that allows the unfolding of Bax and the insertion of its C-terminal hydrophobic domain into the mitochondrial membrane, causing apoptosis. However, in spite of several propositions suggested, there is no significant expression of Bax on western blot analysis of SMX treated Hela cells lysate. This is in accordance with the flowcytometry analysis (Figure 9).

3.8. Sulfamethoxazole (SMX) Interacts with LDH-A and Tubulin with H- Bond Interaction

Molecular docking using SMX with Lactate Dehydrogenase-A (LDH-A) and Tubulin has been performed by the LeadIT 2.3.2 software. The 3D structure of Tubulin (PDB id: 1SA0), Lactate Dehydrogenase-A (PDB id:1i10) (LDH-A) was collected from RCSB PDB. As well as, the 3D structure of Sulfamethoxazole was collected from the PubChem (PubChem CID: 5329). During docking all the parameters were kept as default.

3.9. SMX LDH-A Interaction at Residue Level

Sulfamethoxazole (SMX) shows a low binding score with the LDH-A. The binding score is -24.1151 units. SMX interacts with LDH-A mainly via H-bond and Van der Waals interaction. The green line indicates the Van der Waals interaction and red dotted line indicates the H-bond. SMX interacts with the LDH-A at the Trp 249, Lys 244, Ala 250, Arg 168 residues. The overall result shows that SMX has a strong binding affinity with LDH-A (Figure 10).

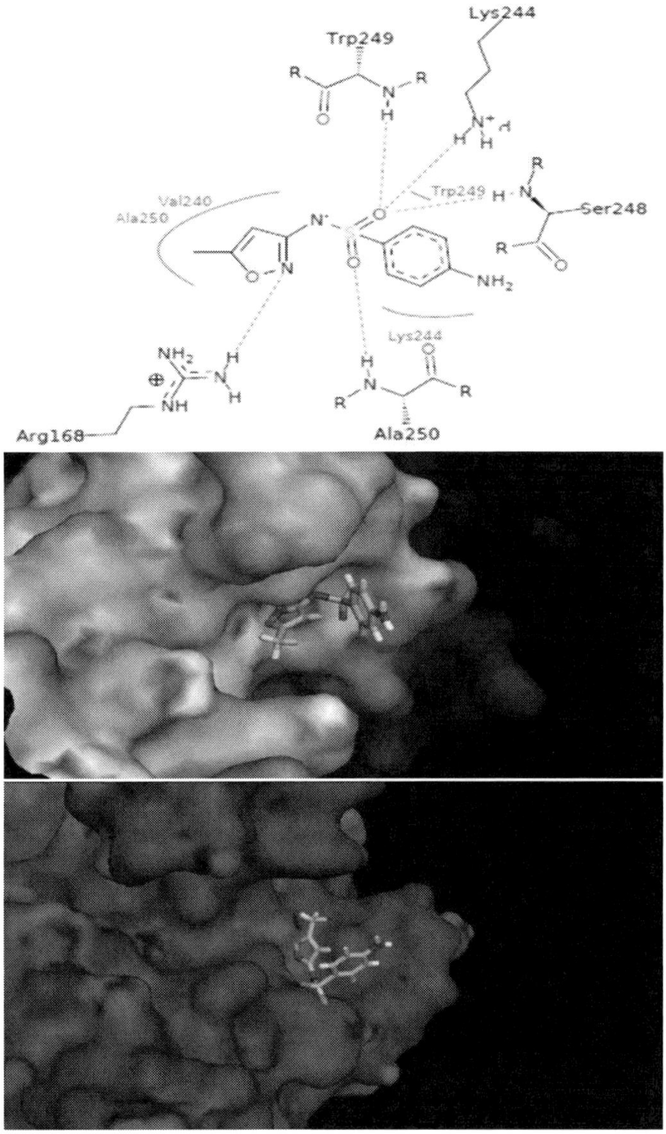

Figure 10. Docking three-dimensional view of SMX – LDH-A complex (Δ G = -24.1151 unit).

3.10. SMX Tubulin Interaction at Residue Level

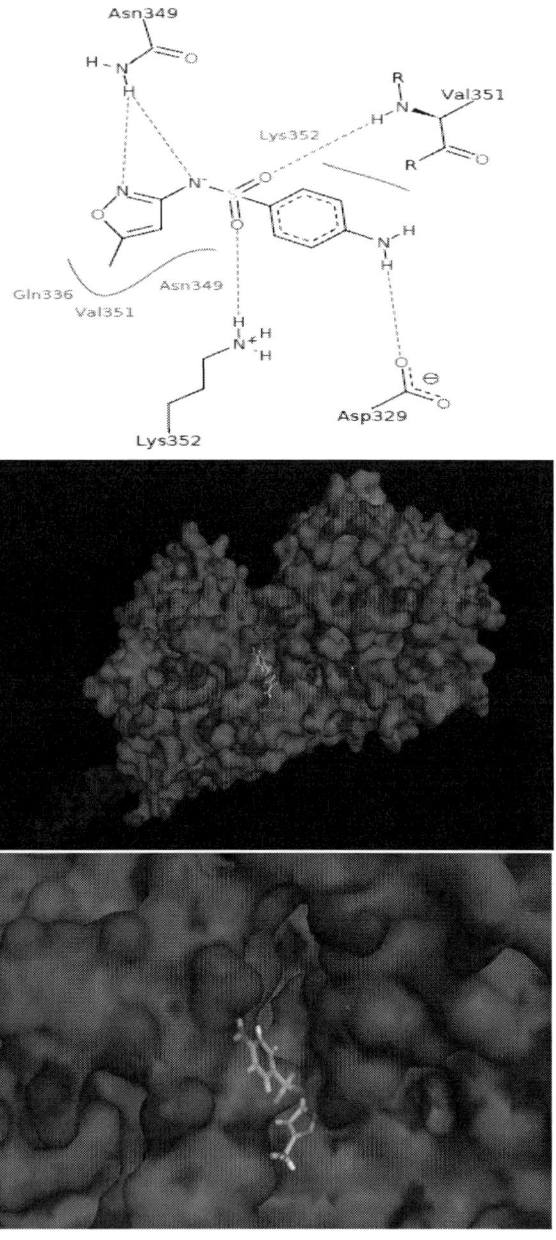

Figure 11. Docking three-dimensional view of SMX – Tubulin complex (Δ G = -20.36 unit).

Sulfamethoxazole (SMX) has a low binding energy with Tubulin. The binding score is -20.36 unit. SMX interacts with Tubulin mainly by the H-bond and Van der Waals interaction. The green line indicates the Van der Waals interaction and red dotted line indicates the H-bond. SMX interacts with Tubulin at the Asn 349, Val 351, Asp 329, Lys 352 residues (Figure 11). The overall result shows that SMX has a strong binding affinity with Tubulin.

4. DISCUSSION

We had shown that SMX shows its anticancer effects in human cervical cancer cell lines in a dose dependent manner. It exhibits its IC50 concentration at 350 μM in HeLa cells. Non-cancerous cells are unaffected by SMX. SMX treatment induces sub G1 population that indicates DNA fragmentation which leads to cell death. SMX also disrupts regular microtubule network in cells confirmed via confocal microscopy that indicates that SMX could be a probable binding partner of tubulin at cellular level. It also inhibits intracellular LDH-A activity dose dependently which in parallel ensures LDH-A as a molecular level binding partner of SMX. Lactate dehydrogenase A (LDH-A) is a crucial enzyme responsible for instant energy production in many types of cancer cells. Due to hypoxic microenvironment and instant energy production cancer cells preferentially choose glycolytic fermentative pathway rather than normal oxidative phosphorylation as reviewed earlier (Zheng et al., 2012). It also elevates intracellular reactive oxygen species level which damages membrane lipids and induces cell death (Lesiów et al., 2019). SMX shows no visible cell death in HeLa cells via apoptosis that in turn suggests alternate modes of cell death mechanism induced by SMX. Western blot analysis also shows that SMX has no effect on the expression of the proapoptotic protein Bax in SMX treated Hela cells. That is also in support of the proposition that SMX induced cell death is operated via some yet unknown mechanism. This could be substantiated by previously published reports suggesting that Sulfathiazole, a sulfonamide group of drugs too executes its cytotoxic effects by cytoprotective autophagy and not through apoptosis (Mohammadpour et al., 2013). The main aim of this chapter is to discuss the probable cell death mechanisms induced by SMX since this area is yet to be explored. Here we have, summarised action of SMX against other eukaryotic targets like tubulin and LDH A (Figure 10 and 11).

CONCLUSION

SMX, an antibacterial agent that interferes in bacterial folic acid biosynthesis pathway also targets tubulin and LDH-A as evident from the previous discussion. We are trying to figure out anti-mitotic potential of SMX keeping in mind the concept of Repurposing of Drugs as many Sulfonamides are potent antimitotic agents (Gwaltney et al., 2001). The quest for the molecular targets of SMX in the mammalian system has identified tubulin as well as LDH-A as potential binding partners of SMX. Many cancer cells show overexpressed LDH-A levels which selects LDH-A as a potent target for many anticancer agents like oxamate, gossypol, 1-(Phenylseleno)-4-(Trifluoromethyl) Benzene (Kim et al., 2019). On the other hand, some sulphonamides like E-7010 and many more are antimitotic agents binding tubulin-MT system. Our preliminary work as well as docking studies reveal that SMX could be studied further to design derivatives that would work as future lead molecules with anti-mitotic potential. It is also noticed that SMX has high IC_{50} value (350 μM) compared to other potent anticancer agents which is an impasse for its direct use as an anticancer drug. Some well-known anti-inflammatory and anti-diabetic medicines like Diclofenac, Metformin used in bulk among a vast pool of diabetic patients/common mass are having their IC_{50} values also in quite high range (Gottfried et al., 2013, Heckman et al., 2017). Very recently Panda's group has shown that Crocin which is a common drug in our medicine cabinet exhibits anti-cancer activity by inhibiting microtubule dynamics (Hire et al., 2017). It opens a new possibility to produce effective derivatives of commonly used drugs as lead compounds with lower IC_{50} value in nanomolar ranges.

Any information delineating anti-cancer property of sulfonamides like SMX would shed new light to propagate research in this direction offering eventual cure and recovery of the vast cancer population. Great socio-economic relief compared to the existing conventional cancer research that involves huge cost, time, manpower and risk has been achieved with drug repurposing. The outcome might have great socio-economic impact with new hope for us minimizing cost, time and labour to bring drugs from bench to bed side.

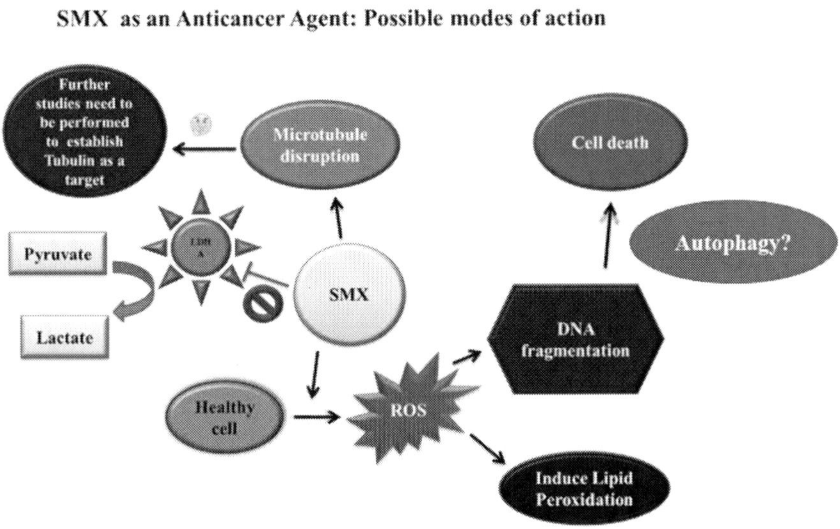

Figure 12. Probable mechanistic action of SMX in Hela cells.

ACKNOWLEDGMENTS

This study was supported by a grant from the Science and Engineering Research Board (SERB).

REFERENCES

Ayala, A., Muñoz, M. F., & Argüelles, S. (2014). Lipid peroxidation: production, metabolism, and signaling mechanisms of malondialdehyde and 4-hydroxy-2-nonenal. *Oxidative medicine and cellular longevity*, 2014, 360438. https://doi.org/10.1155/2014/360438.

Basu, C., & Sur, R. (2018). S-Allyl Cysteine Alleviates Hydrogen Peroxide Induced Oxidative Injury and Apoptosis through Upregulation of Akt/Nrf-2/HO-1 Signaling Pathway in HepG2 Cells. *BioMed research international,* 2018, 3169431. https://doi.org/10.1155/2018/3169431.

Beheshti, A., Hashemi, F., Behavndi, F., Zahedi, M., Kolahi, M., Motamedi, H., & Mayer, P. (2017). Synthesis, structural characterization, QSAR and docking studies of a new binuclear nickel (II) complex based on the flexible tetradentate N-donor ligand as a potent antibacterial and anticancer agent. *International journal of biological macromolecules*, 104(Pt A), 1107–1123. https://doi.org/10. 1016/j.ijbiomac.2017.06.098

Benej, M., Pastorekova, S., & Pastorek, J. (2014). Carbonic anhydrase IX: regulation and role in cancer. *Sub-cellular biochemistry*, 75, 199–219. https://doi.org/10.1007/978-94-007-7359-2_11.

Berg JM, Tymoczko JL, Stryer L. *Biochemistry. 5th edition*. New York: W H Freeman; 2002. Section 16.3, Glucose Can Be Synthesized from Noncarbohydrate Precursors. Available from: https://www.ncbi.nlm. nih.gov/books/NBK22591/.

Branda RF, McCormack JJ, Perlmutter CA. Cellular pharmacology of chloroquinoxaline sulfonamide and a related compound in murine B16 melanoma cells. *Biochemical Pharmacology*. 1988 Dec;37(23):4557-4564. doi: 10.1016/0006-2952(88)90672-7.

Bray, F., Jemal, A., Grey, N., Ferlay, J., & Forman, D. (2012). Global cancer transitions according to the Human Development Index (2008-2030): a population-based study. *The Lancet. Oncology*, 13(8), 790–801. https://doi.org/10.1016/S1470-2045(12)70211-5.

Clare, B. W., Scozzafava, A., & Supuran, C. T. (2001). Protease inhibitors: synthesis of a series of bacterial collagenase inhibitors of the sulfonyl amino acyl hydroxamate type. *Journal of medicinal chemistry*, 44(13), 2253–2258. https://doi.org/10.1021/jm010087e.

Claudiu T Supuran, Andrea Scozzafava (2002) 'Carbonic anhydrase inhibitors and their therapeutic potential,' *Expert Opinion on Therapeutic Patents,* Volume 12(2).

Dumontet, C., & Jordan, M. A. (2010). Microtubule-binding agents: a dynamic field of cancer therapeutics. *Nature reviews. Drug discovery*, 9(10), 790–803. https://doi.org/10.1038/nrd3253.

Estève, M. A., Carré, M., & Braguer, D. (2007). Microtubules in apoptosis induction: are they necessary?. *Current cancer drug targets*, 7(8), 713–729. https://doi.org/10.2174/156800907783220480.

Feng, Y., Xiong, Y., Qiao, T., Li, X., Jia, L., & Han, Y. (2018). Lactate dehydrogenase A: A key player in carcinogenesis and potential target in cancer therapy. *Cancer medicine*, 7(12), 6124–6136. https://doi.org/10.1002/cam4.1820.

Fletcher, D. A., & Mullins, R. D. (2010). Cell mechanics and the cytoskeleton. *Nature*, 463(7280), 485–492. https://doi.org/10.1038/nature08908.

Gottfried, E., Lang, S. A., Renner, K., Bosserhoff, A., Gronwald, W., Rehli, M., Einhell, S., Gedig, I., Singer, K., Seilbeck, A., Mackensen, A., Grauer, O., Hau, P., Dettmer, K., Andreesen, R., Oefner, P. J., & Kreutz, M. (2013). New aspects of an old drug--diclofenac targets MYC and glucose metabolism in tumor cells. *PloS one*, 8(7), e66987. https://doi.org/10.1371/journal.pone.0066987.

Gray, S. G., & Ekström, T. J. (2001). The human histone deacetylase family. *Experimental cell research*, 262(2), 75–83. https://doi.org/10.1006/excr.2000.5080.

Grimsrud, P. A., Xie, H., Griffin, T. J., & Bernlohr, D. A. (2008). Oxidative stress and covalent modification of protein with bioactive aldehydes. *The Journal of biological chemistry*, 283(32), 21837–21841. https://doi.org/10.1074/jbc.R700019200.

Gwaltney, S. L., 2nd, Imade, H. M., Li, Q., Gehrke, L., Credo, R. B., Warner, R. B., Lee, J. Y., Kovar, P., Frost, D., Ng, S. C., & Sham, H. L. (2001). Novel sulfonate derivatives: potent antimitotic agents. *Bioorganic &*

medicinal chemistry letters, 11(13), 1671–1673. https://doi.org/10.1016/s0960-894x(01)00279-7.

H John Smith, Paul J Nicholls, Claire Simons &Regis Le Lain (2001) 'Inhibitors of steroidogenesis as agents for the treatment of hormone-dependent cancers,' *Expert Opinion on Therapeutic Patents*, 11(5), pp. 789-824.

Hay, M., Thomas, D. W., Craighead, J. L., Economides, C., & Rosenthal, J. (2014). Clinical development success rates for investigational drugs. *Nature biotechnology*, 32(1), 40–51. https://doi.org/10.1038/nbt.2786.

Heckman-Stoddard, B. M., DeCensi, A., Sahasrabuddhe, V. V., & Ford, L. G. (2017). Repurposing metformin for the prevention of cancer and cancer recurrence. *Diabetologia*, 60(9), 1639–1647. https://doi.org/10.1007/s00125-017-4372-6.

Hire, R. R., Srivastava, S., Davis, M. B., Kumar Konreddy, A., & Panda, D. (2017). Antiproliferative Activity of Crocin Involves Targeting of Microtubules in Breast Cancer Cells. *Scientific reports*, 7, 44984. https://doi.org/10.1038/srep44984.

Howbert, J. J., Grossman, C. S., Crowell, T. A., Rieder, B. J., Harper, R.W., Kramer, K. E., Tao, E. V., Aikins, J., Poore, G. A., Rinzel, S. M., Grindey, G. B., Shaw, W. N., Todd, G. *J. Med. Chem.* 1990, 33, 2393-2407.

Innocenti, A., Vullo, D., Pastorek, J., Scozzafava, A., Pastorekova, S., Nishimori, I., & Supuran, C. T. (2007). Carbonic anhydrase inhibitors. Inhibition of transmembrane isozymes XII (cancer-associated) and XIV with anions. *Bioorganic & medicinal chemistry letters*, 17(6), 1532–1537. https://doi.org/10.1016/j.bmcl.2006.12.113.

Kim, E. Y., Chung, T. W., Han, C. W., Park, S. Y., Park, K. H., Jang, S. B., & Ha, K. T. (2019). A Novel Lactate Dehydrogenase Inhibitor, 1-(Phenylseleno)-4-(Trifluoromethyl) Benzene, Suppresses Tumor Growth through Apoptotic Cell Death. *Scientific reports*, 9(1), 3969. https://doi.org/10.1038/s41598-019-40617-3.

Kim, E. Y., Chung, T. W., Han, C. W., Park, S. Y., Park, K. H., Jang, S. B., & Ha, K. T. (2019). A Novel Lactate Dehydrogenase Inhibitor, 1-(Phenylseleno)-4-(Trifluoromethyl) Benzene, Suppresses Tumor

Growth through Apoptotic Cell Death. *Scientific reports*, 9(1), 3969. https://doi.org/10.1038/s41598-019-40617-3.

Koyanagi, N., Nagasu, T., Fujita, F., Watanabe, T., Tsukahara, K., Funahashi, Y., Fujita, M., Taguchi, T., Yoshino, H., & Kitoh, K. (1994). In vivo tumor growth inhibition produced by a novel sulfonamide, E7010, against rodent and human tumors. *Cancer research*, 54(7), 1702–1706.

Lavoie, R.; Bouchain, G., Frechette, S.; Woo, S. H., Khalil, E. A., Leit, S.; Fournel, M., Yan, P. T.;Trachy-Bourget, M. C., Beaulieu, C.; Li, Z.; Besterman, J., Delorme, D. *Bioorg. Med. Chem. Lett.* 2001, 11, 2847-2850.

Lesiów, M. K., Komarnicka, U. K., Kyzioł, A., Bieńko, A., & Pietrzyk, P. (2019). ROS-mediated lipid peroxidation as a result of Cu(ii) interaction with FomA protein fragments of F. nucleatum: relevance to colorectal carcinogenesis. *Metallomics: integrated biometal science*, 11(12), 2066–2077. https://doi.org/10.1039/c9mt00179d.

Li, P. K., Chu, G. H., Guo, J. P., Peters, A., & Selcer, K. W. (1998). Development of potent non-estrogenic estrone sulfatase inhibitors. *Steroids*, 63(7-8), 425–432. https://doi.org/10.1016/s0039-128x(98)00044-0.

Liberti, M. V., & Locasale, J. W. (2016). The Warburg Effect: How Does it Benefit Cancer Cells?. *Trends in biochemical sciences*, 41(3), 211–218. https://doi.org/10.1016/j.tibs.2015.12.001.

Liou, G. Y., & Storz, P. (2010). Reactive oxygen species in cancer. *Free radical research*, 44(5), 479–496. https://doi.org/10.3109/ 107157 61003667554.

MacPherson, L. J., Bayburt, E. K., Capparelli, M. P., Carroll, B. J., Goldstein, R., Justice, M. R., Zhu, L., Hu, S., Melton, R. A., Fryer, L., Goldberg, R. L., Doughty, J. R., Spirito, S., Blancuzzi, V., Wilson, D., O'Byrne, E. M., Ganu, V., & Parker, D. T. (1997). Discovery of CGS 27023A, a non-peptidic, potent, and orally active stromelysin inhibitor that blocks cartilage degradation in rabbits. *Journal of medicinal chemistry*, 40(16), 2525–2532. https://doi.org/10.1021/jm960871c.

Majewsky, M., Wagner, D., Delay, M., Bräse, S., Yargeau, V., & Horn, H. (2014). Antibacterial activity of sulfamethoxazole transformation products (TPs): general relevance for sulfonamide TPs modified at the para position. *Chemical research in toxicology*, 27(10), 1821–1828. https://doi.org/10.1021/tx500267x.

Medina, J. C., Roche, D., Shan, B., Learned, R. M., Frankmoelle, W. P., Clark, D. L., Rosen, T., & Jaen, J. C. (1999). Novel halogenated sulfonamides inhibit the growth of multidrug resistant MCF-7/ADR cancer cells. *Bioorganic & medicinal chemistry letters*, 9(13), 1843–1846. https://doi.org/10.1016/s0960-894x(99)00276-0.

Meinke, P. T., & Liberator, P. (2001). Histone deacetylase: a target for antiproliferative and antiprotozoal agents. *Current medicinal chemistry*, 8(2), 211–235. https://doi.org/10.2174/0929867013373787.

Mohammadpour, R., Safarian, S., Sheibani, N., Norouzi, S., & Razazan, A. (2013). Death inducing and cytoprotective autophagy in T-47D cells by two common antibacterial drugs: sulphathiazole and sulphacetamide. *Cell biology international*, 37(4), 348–358. https://doi.org/10.1002/cbin.10047.

Montine, T. J., Neely, M. D., Quinn, J. F., Beal, M. F., Markesbery, W. R., Roberts, L. J., & Morrow, J. D. (2002). Lipid peroxidation in aging brain and Alzheimer's disease. *Free radical biology & medicine*, 33(5), 620–626. https://doi.org/10.1016/s0891-5849(02)00807-9.

Nagase, H., & Woessner, J. F., Jr (1999). Matrix metalloproteinases. *The Journal of biological chemistry*, 274(31), 21491–21494. https://doi.org/10.1074/jbc.274.31.21491.

Ozawa, Y., Sugi, N. H., Nagasu, T., Owa, T., Watanabe, T., Koyanagi, N., Yoshino, H., Kitoh, K., & Yoshimatsu, K. (2001). E7070, a novel sulphonamide agent with potent antitumour activity in vitro and in vivo. *European journal of cancer* (Oxford, England: 1990), 37(17), 2275–2282. https://doi.org/10.1016/s0959-8049(01)00275-1.

Ozawa, Y.; Funahashi, Y.; Senba, T.; Sonoda, J.; Yoshimatsu, K. Proc. Am. Assoc. Cancer Res. San Diego, USA 1997, 38, Abstract 3163.

Pantziarka, P., Bouche, G., Meheus, L., Sukhatme, V., Sukhatme, V. P., & Vikas, P. (2014). The Repurposing Drugs in Oncology (ReDO) Project.

Ecancermedicalscience, 8, 442. https://doi.org/10.3332/ ecancer. 2014.442.

Pasqualini, J. R., Chetrite, G., & Nestour, E. L. (1996). Control and expression of oestrone sulphatase activities in human breast cancer. *The Journal of endocrinology*, 150 Suppl, S99–S105.

Pogorzelska, A., Sławiński, J., Brożewicz, K., Ulenberg, S., & Bączek, T. (2015). Novel 3-Amino-6-chloro-7-(azol-2 or 5-yl)-1,1-dioxo-1,4,2-benzodithiazine Derivatives with Anticancer Activity: Synthesis and QSAR Study. *Molecules* (Basel, Switzerland), 20(12), 21960–21970. https://doi.org/10.3390/molecules201219821.

Pushpakom, S., Iorio, F., Eyers, P. A., Escott, K. J., Hopper, S., Wells, A., Doig, A., Guilliams, T., Latimer, J., McNamee, C., Norris, A., Sanseau, P., Cavalla, D., & Pirmohamed, M. (2019). Drug repurposing: progress, challenges and recommendations. Nature reviews. *Drug discovery*, 18(1), 41–58. https://doi.org/10.1038/ nrd.2018.168.

Redza-Dutordoir, M., & Averill-Bates, D. A. (2016). Activation of apoptosis signalling pathways by reactive oxygen species. *Biochimica et biophysica acta,* 1863(12), 2977–2992. https://doi.org/10.1016/j. bbamcr.2016.09.012.

Scozzafava, A., Owa, T., Mastrolorenzo, A., & Supuran, C. T. (2003). Anticancer and antiviral sulfonamides. *Current medicinal chemistry*, 10(11), 925–953. https://doi.org/10.2174/0929867033457647.

Seung-Hyeok Seok, Min-Won Baek, Hui-Young Lee, Dong-Jae Kim, Kiho Cho, Jae-Hak Park (March 2008) 'Carbonic anhydrase II gene upregulation and tumorigenesis in Lewis lung carcinoma-bearing mice,' *Basic and Applied Pathology,* 1(1), pp. 9-11 [Online]. Available at: https://onlinelibrary.wiley.com/doi/abs/10.1111/j.1755-9294.2008. 00002.x (Accessed:).

Son, Y., Kim, S., Chung, H. T., & Pae, H. O. (2013). Reactive oxygen species in the activation of MAP kinases. *Methods in enzymology*, 528, 27–48. https://doi.org/10.1016/B978-0-12-405881-1.00002-1.

Strydom, S. J., Rose, W. E., Otto, D. P., Liebenberg, W., & de Villiers, M. M. (2013). Poly(amidoamine) dendrimer-mediated synthesis and stabilization of silver sulfonamide nanoparticles with increased antibacterial activity. *Nanomedicine: nanotechnology, biology, and medicine*, 9(1), 85–93. https://doi.org/10.1016/j.nano.2012.03.006.

Supuran C. T. (2018). Carbonic anhydrase inhibitors and their potential in a range of therapeutic areas. *Expert opinion on therapeutic patents*, 28(10), 709–712. https://doi.org/10.1080/13543776.2018.1523897.

Supuran, C. T., Casini, A., & Scozzafava, A. (2003). Protease inhibitors of the sulfonamide type: anticancer, antiinflammatory, and antiviral agents. *Medicinal research reviews*, 23(5), 535–558. https://doi.org/10.1002/med.10047.

Teicher, B. A., Liu, S. D., Liu, J. T., Holden, S. A., Herman, T. S. *Anticancer Res.* 1993, 13, 1549-1556.

Turrens J. F. (2003). Mitochondrial formation of reactive oxygen species. *The Journal of physiology*, 552(Pt 2), 335–344. https://doi.org/10.1113/jphysiol.2003.049478.

Wang, W., Qin, S. K., Chen, B. A., & Chen, H. Y. (2001). Experimental study on antitumor effect of arsenic trioxide in combination with cisplatin or doxorubicin on hepatocellular carcinoma. *World journal of gastroenterology*, 7(5), 702–705. https://doi.org/10.3748/wjg.v7.i5.702.

Woo, L. W., Howarth, N. M., Purohit, A., Hejaz, H. A., Reed, M. J., & Potter, B. V. (1998). Steroidal and nonsteroidal sulfamates as potent inhibitors of steroid sulfatase. *Journal of medicinal chemistry*, 41(7), 1068–1083. https://doi.org/10.1021/jm970527v.

Yokoi, A., Kuromitsu, J., Kawai, T., Nagasu, T., Sugi, N. H., Yoshimatsu, K., Yoshino, H., & Owa, T. (2002). Profiling novel sulfonamide antitumor agents with cell-based phenotypic screens and array-based gene expression analysis. *Molecular cancer therapeutics*, 1(4), 275–286.

Yoshimatsu, K., Yamaguchi, A., Yoshino, H., Koyanagi, N., & Kitoh, K. (1997). Mechanism of action of E7010, an orally active sulfonamide antitumor agent: inhibition of mitosis by binding to the colchicine site of tubulin. *Cancer research*, 57(15), 3208–3213.

Yoshimatsu, K., Yamaguchi, A., Yoshino, H., Koyanagi, N., & Kitoh, K. (1997). Mechanism of action of E7010, an orally active sulfonamide antitumor agent: inhibition of mitosis by binding to the colchicine site of tubulin. *Cancer research*, 57(15), 3208–3213.

Yoshino, H., Ueda, N., Niijima, J., Sugumi, H., Kotake, Y., Koyanagi, N., Yoshimatsu, K., Asada, M., Watanabe, T., & Nagasu, T. (1992). Novel sulfonamides as potential, systemically active antitumor agents. *Journal of medicinal chemistry*, 35(13), 2496–2497. https://doi.org/10.1021/jm00091a018.

Yu, Y., Liao, M., Liu, R., Chen, J., Feng, H., & Fu, Z. (2014). Overexpression of lactate dehydrogenase-A in human intrahepatic cholangiocarcinoma: its implication for treatment. *World journal of surgical oncology*, 12, 78. https://doi.org/10.1186/1477-7819-12-78.

Zheng J. (2012). Energy metabolism of cancer: Glycolysis versus oxidative phosphorylation (Review). *Oncology letters*, 4(6), 1151–1157. https://doi.org/10.3892/ol.2012.928.

Zhou, B. R., & Bai, Y. (2019). Chromatin structures condensed by linker histones. *Essays in biochemistry*, 63(1), 75–87. https://doi.org/10.1042/EBC20180056.

INDEX

B

C

D

E

H

I

J

K

L

N

O

P

R

S

T

U

V

X